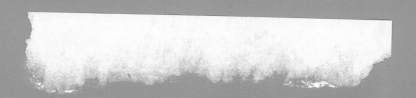

WUIS DAS £65

Glossary of Orthodontic Terms

by

John Daskalogiannakis, DDS, MSc

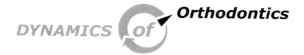

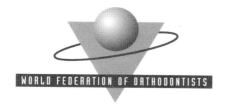

WORLD FEDERATION OF ORTHODONTISTS

Glossary of Orthodontic Terms

by

John Daskalogiannakis

Editorial Board

Frans P.G.M. van der Linden
Rainer R. Miethke
James A. McNamara, Jr.

National Collaborators

J. A. McNamara, Jr. (USA)
R. R. Miethke (Germany)
H. G. Sergl (Germany)
Ch. Bolender (France)
J. Duran von Arx (Spain)
F. A. Miotti (Italy)
K. Faltin (Brazil)

Advisory Board

William R. Proffit
Dieter Drescher
Ralf J. Radlanski
Friedrich Sernetz

Project Director

A. Ammann

Illustration Support

Rainer Landsee

Quintessence Publishing Co, Inc

Chicago, Berlin, London, Tokyo, Paris, Barcelona,
São Paulo, Moscow, Prague, and Warsaw

Sources of Illustrations

The majority of the illustrations in this book were computer-generated by Dr. R. Landsee. These illustrations are not labeled with a number. The remaining illustrations were reproduced from previous publications with permission from the respective authors or publishers. These illustrations are labeled by a number identifying the source, as follows:

1 Dentaurum product catalog, 2 F.P.G.M. van der Linden, 3 L.M. Carter and P. Yaman, 4 L.J. Peterson, 5 J.A. McNamara, Jr., 6 W.R. Proffit, 7 H.G. Sergl, 8 D.E. Enlow, 9 P.R. Begg, 10 H. Boersma, 11 American Orthodontics product catalog, 12 C.H. Tweed, 13 T.M. Graber, 14 E. Krüger, 15 E.W. Renfroe, 16 A. Dürer

World Federation of Orthodontists

401 N. Lindbergh Blvd.
St. Louis, MO 63141-7816
(314)993-1700
Fax (314)993-5208
e-mail: wfo@wfo.org
Web site: www.wfo.org

John Daskalogiannakis

Department of Orthodontics and Oral Biology
University of Nymegen
P.O. Box 9101
6500 HB Nymegen
The Netherlands

German Library—Cataloging-in-Publication Data

Daskalogiannakis, John
Glossary of Orthodontic Terms / by John Daskalogiannakis.—Berlin : Quintessence Publ., 2000
    (Quintessence books)
    ISBN 3-87652-760-0

© 2000 Quintessence Publishing Co, Inc
All rights reserved.

Lithography: Fotolito Veneta, Verona
Printing and Binding: Jütte, Leipzig

Printed in Germany

ISBN 3-87652-760-0

Foreword

Glossary of Orthodontic Terms is another step forward toward the globalization of orthodontics and orthodontic treatment. As the world of orthodontics becomes more interdependent, the glossary will provide a commonality of scientific language that enhances our communication.

The World Federation of Orthodontists (WFO) is pleased to endorse the work and to compliment its author, Dr. John Daskalogiannakis, his editors, and his advisors for providing well thought-out and easily understood definitions. This terminology will provide a core basis for orthodontic communication.

The purpose of the WFO is to advance the art and science of orthodontics throughout the world. To accomplish that purpose, a universal scientific language is nesessary. *Glossary of Orthodontic Terms* will be helpful to every orthodontist and any other professional interested in the communication of the vast array of terms used to describe the intricacies of orthodontics and dentofacial orthopedics.

The reader will find this volume comprehensive, but not all-inclusive. The beauty and excitement of orthodontics is that new concepts, new terms, and new solutions discovered each day will make the next edition of *Glossary of Orthodontic Terms* a requirement before the pages of this magnificent volume are dry.

The WFO has attached its logo and endorsement to this work with care and pride. We believe the glossary will help both the WFO and the orthodontic scientific community achieve a mutual goal of effective communication in orthodontics worldwide.

Congratulations to all involved!

EXECUTIVE COMMITTEE, WORLD FEDERATION OF ORTHODONTISTS

William H. DeKock, President, Iowa, USA
Lee W. Graber, Vice-President, Illinois, USA
Ronald S. Moen, Sec.-Gen., Missouri, USA
A.E. Athanasiou, Thessaloniki, Greece

Jae Chan Kim, Seoul, Korea
Takayuki Kuroda, Tokyo, Japan
Robert P. Max, Auckland, New Zealand
Per Rygh, Bergen, Norway

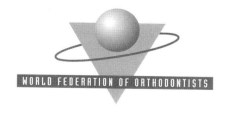

Preface

This *Glossary of Orthodontic Terms* is written so as to cover, in a comprehensive, albeit succinct manner, much of the material that orthodontic residents are likely to encounter during their postgraduate education and/or preparation for Board examinations. It also is meant to contribute to the education of undergraduate dental students getting acquainted with orthodontics, and to serve as a practical aid to orthodontists and general dentists with an interest in orthodontics, when keeping up with scientific literature or during their clinical practice. Finally, it is my hope that this work will prove valuable to specialists in related fields who work in collaboration with orthodontists.

To meet its obligation to record accurate usage of terminology in the current interdisciplinary practice of orthodontics, the *Glossary* draws subject matter from a multitude of topics including biomechanics, cephalometrics, clinical orthodontics, embryology, growth and development, history of orthodontics, implantology, materials science, occlusion, oral biology, oral and maxillofacial surgery, pediatric dentistry, periodontology, syndromology, and temporomandibular disorders. All in all, more than 2,800 terms are defined. The definitions were written by referral to the original publications in peer-reviewed journals and to leading textbooks in their respective fields. Where deemed necessary, they are supplemented by carefully selected illustrations.

Glossaries, perhaps more than any other form of scientific publication, represent not so much the research of their authors or editors but mainly that of others, who are conventionally mentioned in a list of references. One of the most difficult decisions of editorial policy concerned the inclusion of such a list. A compromise between the space requirements and the desirability and significance of authentication was reached by including selected references. Nevertheless, I would like to acknowledge from this position all those whose scientific publications of any type contributed to the writing of this volume.

A large amount of effort by many people has been placed into this first edition. Special mention is due to Dr. F. van der Linden, whose experience and wisdom were critical in bringing this project to completion, and to Dr. R. Miethke, who most generously offered his hard work, advice and friendship. I am grateful to Dr. J. McNamara, Jr. for his thorough editorial review, as well as to Drs. D. Drescher, W. Proffit, W. DeKock, F. Sernetz and L. Graber for kindly contributing their knowledge, ideas and criticism upon request. Thanks also to Dr. R. Landsee for lending his skills with the computer-generated illustrations, and to the staff at Quintessence Publishing Co. for their dedicated work and excellent cooperation throughout the project. Finally, my appreciation to the World Federation of Orthodontists for honoring this volume with its endorsement.

It is my hope that *Glossary of Orthodontic Terms* will contribute to the promotion of this wonderful discipline, dentistry's first specialty, which we are fortunate enough to practice and serve. However, this is only a first effort and as such, it is perhaps flawed with omissions or imperfections. I would like to assure anyone willing to send their suggestions or criticism to me at the Department of Orthodontics and Oral Biology, University of Nymegen, P.O. Box 9101, 6500 HB Nymegen, The Netherlands, that they will be received with gratitude and appreciation.

John Daskalogiannakis

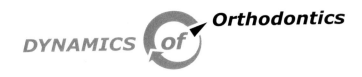

DYNAMICS of Orthodontics

An interactive multimedia learning series

Dynamics of Orthodontics

"Dynamics of Orthodontics" is an interactive multimedia learning series offering flexible, individualized instruction in the study of orthodontics. The series consists of several discrete multimedia components that together form a comprehensive learning network. (A complete list of the various components appears on the previous page.) Designed for students and experts alike, as well as for dentists and other specialists engaged in multidisciplinary care, the "Dynamics of Orthodontics" series makes innovative use of multimedia technology for educational purposes. Available in six languages, it is expected to increase knowledge in orthodontics and to lead to better patient care worldwide.

Glossary of Orthodontic Terms, the first component of this series to be released, represents a major step forward in the effort to reach international agreement on the meaning and usage of orthodontic terminology. In preparing the *Glossary*, which is available in book and CD-ROM format, every effort was made to ensure the accuracy, completeness, and currency of the information provided. A CD-ROM of the *Glossary* in six languages, designed to facilitate translations and the use of uniform definitions, is now under development.

Both the International Quintessence Publishing Group and Dentaurum are to be complimented for taking the initiative to develop the "Dynamics of Orthodontics" series and for their leadership role in using multimedia techniques to improve the distribution of information and knowledge in this field.

Frans P.G.M. van der Linden
William R. Proffit
James A. McNamara, Jr.
Rainer R. Miethke

Editors of the "Dynamics of Orthodontics" series

A

A-point See Cephalometric landmarks (Hard tissue), A-point.

A-B plane See Cephalometric lines, A-B plane.

ABO See Board, American Board of Orthodontics.

ABO diplomate (ABO-certified) The status of an orthodontist who has completed the Certification Examination of the American Board of Orthodontics. [Modified from the AAO Glossary of Dentofacial Orthopedic Terms, 1993.]

ABO-eligible The status of an orthodontist who has completed Parts I and II, but not Part III of the Certification Examination of the American Board of Orthodontics. [Modified from the AAO Glossary of Dentofacial Orthopedic Terms, 1993.]

Abrasion Exaggerated mechanical wear of tooth structure caused by a foreign abrasive material (e.g. improper toothbrushing technique or deleterious habits such as pipe smoking, tobacco chewing and chewing on pens or pencils). Toothbrush abrasion is the most common example, which may sometimes present as a sharp V-shaped notch in the gingival portion of the labial surface of the teeth. [Compare with Attrition.]

Abrasive strips (Finishing strips, Lightening strips, Coated abrasive strips) Strips containing abrasive particles on a flexible backing material (heavyweight paper, metal or plastic). Used mainly for interproximal enamel reduction. [Also see Interproximal stripping.]

Acceleration, Law of See Newton's laws.

ACCO appliance See Appliance, ACCO.

Achondroplasia An autosomal dominant condition characterized by failure of the primary growth cartilages of the limbs and cranial base to grow properly. Early fusion of the sphenoethmoidal, intersphenoidal and sphenooccipital synchondroses and early closure of the epiphyseal plates of the long bones result in very short arms and legs and a characteristic midface deficiency that is most accentuated at the bridge of the nose. The anterior cranial base appears to be of approximately normal length, whereas the posterior cranial base is extremely short (i.e. the sphenooccipital synchondrosis seems to be affected more than the sphenoethmoidal).

Affected patients also exhibit short bodies with thick extremities and stubby fingers, often associated with limited motion of the joints, lumbar lordosis, protruding abdomen, and inability to straighten the elbows.

Correction of the midface deficiency and the resulting Class III malocclusion in achondroplasia may require a Le Fort III, or modified Le Fort II osteotomy to advance the entire midface.

Acid etching An enamel bonding technique invented by M. G. Buonocore in 1955. During this process a selected area of tooth substance is prepared for bonding via the application of a corrosive agent (most commonly a solution or gel of 37% orthophosphoric acid). The effect is a removal of a small amount of less mineralized, interprismatic enamel and opening of pores between the enamel prisms, substantially enlarging the surface area of the bonded part so the adhesive can penetrate into the enamel, providing micromechanical retention.

Acromegaly Chronic metabolic disorder caused by hyperfunction of the anterior pituitary gland after maturity, usually due to an adenoma. The resulting overproduction of growth hormone induces an overgrowth of the bones, connective tissue and viscera. Skeletal changes principally involve the skull, with frontal bossing, prominent cheek bones, grossly overdeveloped mandible with a protrusive chin and consequent mandibular prognathism. The small bones of the hands and feet are also affected, and there is associated broadening of the hands, fingers and feet.
Enlargement of the soft tissue usually is manifested by large ears and nose, thick lips and macroglossia. The tongue, which exhibits a lobulated margin and papillary hypertrophy, fills the oral cavity and results in associated labial and buccal tipping of the teeth. There is generalized splanchnomegaly and hypertrophy of the target organs for anterior pituitary hormones, including the adrenal cortex, thyroid gland, parathyroid glands and gonads. [Also see Gigantism.]

Acrylic (Methyl methacrylate) An organic resin commonly used for the construction of dental removable appliances, including appliances used during orthodontic treatment and retention. [Modified from the AAO Glossary of Dentofacial Orthopedic Terms, 1993.]

Action and reaction, Law of See Newton's laws.

Activation The process of storing mechanical energy into an active member of an orthodontic appliance (e.g. stretching an elastic, or compressing an open coil spring) in order for it to produce the desired force system, which will be delivered to the dentition. The force system that must be applied for activation of a spring is the opposite to the force system desired (during deactivation).

Activation angle See Angle of activation.

Activator See Appliance, Activator.

Active member The part of an orthodontic appliance that is involved directly in tooth movement. [Compare with Reactive member.]

Active myofascial trigger point See Myofascial trigger point, Active.

Active segment See Segment, Active.

Active torque See Torque, Active.

Active vertical corrector See Appliance, Active vertical corrector.

Adams clasp See Clasp, Adams.

Adams pliers See Orthodontic instruments, Adams pliers.

Adaptability (Adaptive capacity, Adaptive potential) Relative ability to adjust to the demands of the environment.

Adaptation 1. The progressive adjustive changes in sensitivity that regularly accompany continuous sensory stimulation or lack of stimulation. The process by which an organism responds to the functional demands of its environment.
2. The process by which a dental device is fitted to another structure (e.g. adaptation of a band to a tooth).

"Adenoid facies" A long-standing descriptive term implying a relationship between mouth breathing (due to enlarged adenoids) and the development of malocclusion through altered function. The classic description of "adenoid facies" consists of narrow nasal and alar width, hypotonic musculature, "dull" or "vacant" facial expression and lips separated at rest. It is important to stress that the presence of "adenoid facies" does not necessarily mean that the patient is an obligatory mouth breather, or in other words, mouth breathing is habitual in certain patients.

Adenoidectomy Surgical removal of the adenoids.

Adenoids Masses of lymphoid tissue in the nasopharynx which classically have been associated with airway obstruction and mouth breathing, with all the suggested consequences—hence the term "adenoid facies."

Adhesion 1. Attractive force between atoms or molecules of dissimilar materials, when they are in close approximation. [Compare with Cohesion.] The attachment of one substance to another. [See Bonding.]
2. The abnormal fibrous joining of adjacent structures following an inflammatory process or as a result of injury repair.

Capsular adhesion Fibrosis of the capsular tissues of a joint.

Extracapsular adhesion Fibrosis of pericapsular tissues such as muscles or ligaments.

Intracapsular adhesion (Fibrous ankylosis, Pseudoankylosis) Fibrosis between intra-articular surfaces within a joint capsule, resulting in reduced mobility of the affected joint.

Adhesive system See Bonding agent.

Adjustment, Occlusal See Occlusal equilibration.

Adolescent growth spurt See Pubertal growth spurt.

Adult occlusal equilibrium See Occlusal equilibrium, Adult.

Advanced arch See Arch, Stopped.

Advancement (of the mandible) An orthognathic surgical procedure aiming at sagittal (anterior) augmentation of the mandible, most often performed through a standard, or modified bilateral sagittal split ramus osteotomy (BSSO). [Compare with Setback of the mandible; also see Osteotomy, Bilateral sagittal split.]

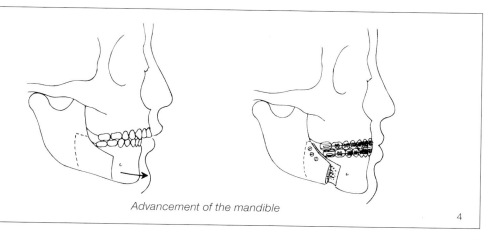

Advancement of the mandible

4

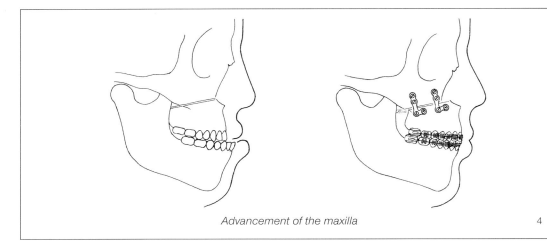

Advancement of the maxilla 4

Advancement (of the maxilla) Anterior repositioning of the maxilla by orthognathic surgery. It most often involves a Le Fort I osteotomy. [Also see Osteotomy, Le Fort I.]

Aesthetic See Esthetic.

Agenesis Congenital absence of a tooth.

Ala The lateral rim of the nostril.

Alar cinch A procedure performed during any orthognathic surgery that includes mobilization of the entire maxilla, in order to prevent excessive widening of the alar bases. It involves passing a permanent suture in a figure-eight fashion through the alar base tissues and through a bur hole placed in the region of the anterior nasal spine. This is repeated on the opposite side. Each suture is tightened independently, taking care to maintain symmetry, until the desired alar base width is attained (as determined from measurements before surgery). A situation in which an alar cinch may not be performed during maxillary orthognathic surgery is when very narrow alar bases exist preoperatively.

Alginate An irreversible hydrocolloid consisting of salts of alginic acid (an extract of marine kelp). The most widely used impression material in orthodontics.

Aligner, Spring See Spring aligner.

Allogenic graft See Graft, Allogenic.

Allograft See Graft, Allogenic.

Alloplast See Graft, Alloplastic.

Alloplastic graft See Graft, Alloplastic.

Alloy A material that exhibits metallic properties (high electrical and thermal conductivity) and is composed of two or more elements, at least one of which is a metal (e.g, steel is an alloy of iron and carbon, brass is an alloy of copper and zinc).

Alpha position The anterior component of an orthodontic spring or the anterior point of attachment of a spring. [Compare with Beta position.]

Alveolar arch See Arch, Alveolar.

Alveolar bone See Bone, Alveolar.

Alveolar bone graft See Graft, Alveolar bone.

Alveolar crest The most coronal portion of the alveolar process.

Alveolar mucosa See Mucosa, Alveolar.

Alveolar process The U-shaped ridge of maxillary or mandibular alveolar bone that surrounds and supports the roots of the erupted teeth, as well as the unerupted tooth buds.

Alveolar ridge See Ridge, Alveolar.

Alveolo-gingival fibers See Gingival fibers.

Alveolus The socket in the bone into which a tooth is attached by means of the periodontal ligament.

Amalgam-plugger See Orthodontic instruments, Serrated amalgam-plugger.

American Board of Orthodontics See Board, Orthodontic, American Board of Orthodontics.

ANB angle See Cephalometric measurements (Hard tissue), ANB angle.

Anchorage The sites that provide resistance to the reactive forces generated as a (most commonly, undesirable) consequence of the activation of an orthodontic or orthopedic appliance. [Short definition: resistance to unwanted tooth movement].

Cervical anchorage Anchorage provided by the back of the neck when extraoral appliances such as a cervical pull headgear are used.

Extraoral anchorage Anchorage provided by sites located outside the oral cavity.

Infinite anchorage The term is commonly used when referring to implants used as anchorage in orthodontics, to indicate that they show no movement (zero anchor-

age loss) as a consequence of reaction forces. [Also see Implant, Orthodontic.]

Intermaxillary anchorage Anchorage for tooth movement provided by the teeth of the opposing arch.

Intramaxillary anchorage Anchorage provided by teeth within the same arch as the ones that are to be moved.

Maximum anchorage (Type A anchorage) A situation in which the treatment objectives require that no or very little anchorage can be lost.

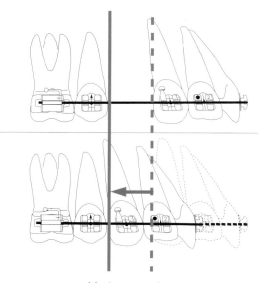

Maximum anchorage

Minimum anchorage (Type C anchorage) A situation in which, for an optimal result, a considerable movement of the anchorage segment (anchorage "loss") is desirable, during closure of space. *See illustration next page.*

Moderate anchorage (Type B anchorage) A situation in which anchorage is not critical and space closure should be performed by reciprocal movement of both the active and the anchorage segment. *See illustration next page.*

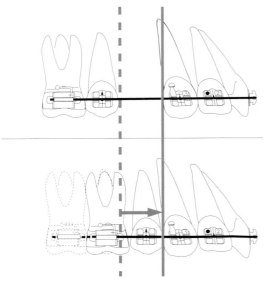

Minimum anchorage

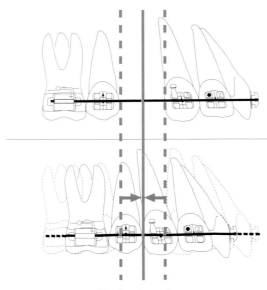

Moderate anchorage

Occipital anchorage Anchorage provided by the superior and posterior portions of the head, when extraoral appliances such as a high-pull headgear are used.

Reciprocal anchorage A situation in which the movement of one or more dental units is balanced against the movement of another, or more dental units, on which the reaction forces are placed. [The term generally means that the movement of both the active and the reactive component is desirable.]

Anchorage loss The undesirable movement of the reactive anchorage segment, which happens as a side effect of the movement of the active segment (e.g. mesial movement of the maxillary molars during retraction of maxillary incisors with intramaxillary mechanics).

Anchorage preparation A procedure commonly used in the Tweed technique, during which the molars and premolars are tipped distally prior to retraction of the anterior teeth. The theory behind it is that it increases the anchorage value of the posterior segments, allowing further retraction of the canines and incisors with less anchorage loss.

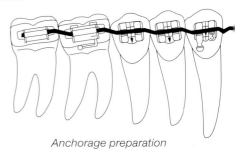

Anchorage preparation

Anchorage reinforcement The process of increasing the anchorage value of the reactive segment to resist anchorage loss. This can be done in a number of ways, e.g. by incorporating more teeth into the reactive segment; by using additional stabilizing arches such as a lingual arch, a Nance holding arch or a transpalatal arch; or by using extraoral or intermaxillary traction.

Anchorage segment See Segment, Anchorage.

Anchorage value   Relative resistance of a tooth (or a segment of teeth) in comparison to another, which usually is estimated on the basis of comparison of root surface areas and density of the supporting bone.

Andresen appliance   See Appliance, Activator.

Andrews' six keys of the optimal occlusion   See Six keys of occlusion.

Angle classification   A classification of malocclusion introduced by E.H. Angle, based on the anteroposterior relationship of the maxillary and mandibular first permanent molars. Angle's assumption when formulating this classification was that the maxillary first permanent molar always is in the physiologically correct position and the variability comes from the mandible.
Angle's classification, which is still popular, only can serve as a framework, as it does not take into account many other important relationships in the anteroposterior (e.g. overjet, canine relationship), transverse (e.g. buccolingual crossbites), or vertical (e.g. overbite) planes of space. It also does not identify intra-arch problems, such as crowding, spacing, rotations, missing or impacted teeth.

Class I malocclusion (Neutroclusion)
A malocclusion in which the buccal groove of the mandibular first permanent molar occludes with the mesiobuccal cusp of the maxillary first permanent molar.

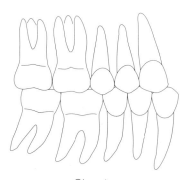

Class I

The term *Class I* is sometimes used incorrectly as a synonym for normal occlusion, although in reality, it only signifies a normal relationship of maxillary and mandibular first molars in the sagittal plane.

Class II malocclusion (Distoclusion, Postnormal occlusion)   A malocclusion in which the buccal groove of the mandibular first permanent molar occludes posterior (distal) to the mesiobuccal cusp of the maxillary first permanent molar. The severity of the deviation from the Class I molar relationship usually is indicated in fractions (or multiples) of the mesiodistal width of a premolar crown ("cusp" or "unit").

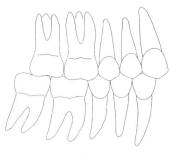

Class II

"Divisions" are used in Class II malocclusion, based on the inclination of the maxillary incisors:

Division 1   A Class II malocclusion with proclined maxillary incisors, resulting in an increased overjet.

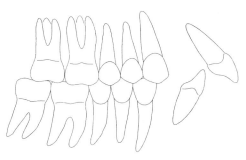

Class II Division 1

Division 2 A Class II malocclusion typically with the maxillary central incisors tipped palatally, a short anterior lower face height and an excessive overbite.

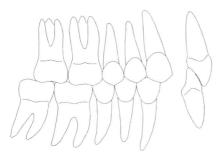

Class II Division 2

Three types of Class II Division 2 malocclusion can be distinguished, based on differences in the spatial conditions in the maxillary dental arch:

Type A: The four maxillary permanent incisors are tipped palatally, without the occurrence of crowding.

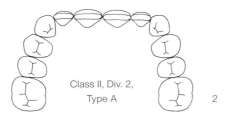

Class II, Div. 2,
Type A   2

Type B: The maxillary central incisors are tipped palatally and the maxillary laterals are tipped labially.

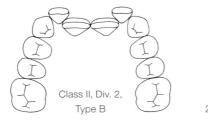

Class II, Div. 2,
Type B   2

Type C: The four maxillary permanen incisors are tipped palatally, with the canines labially positioned.

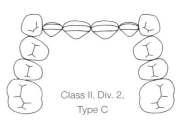

Class II, Div. 2,
Type C   2

Class III malocclusion (Mesioclusion Prenormal occlusion) A malocclusion in which the buccal groove of the mandibular first permanent molar occludes anterio (mesial) to the mesiobuccal cusp of the maxillary first permanent molar. The same conventions as described above are used to indicate the severity of deviation from a Class I molar relationship.

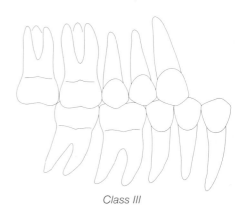

Class III

"Subdivisions" (left or right) are used in asymmetrical situations to indicate the side that deviates from a Class I molar relationship.

Angle of activation A measure (in degrees of the activation placed into an orthodontic wire by bending or torsion, with regard to its initial passive state. When the wire characteristics and the interbracket distance are known, the clinician can estimate the magnitude of the force produced.

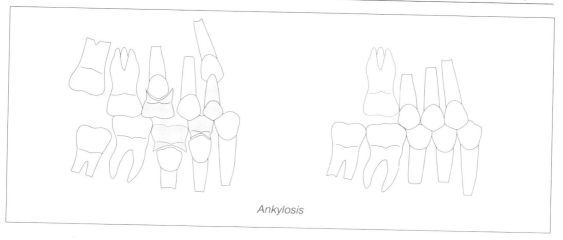

Ankylosis

Angle of convexity See Cephalometric measurements (Hard tissue), Angle of convexity.

Angle of facial convexity See Cephalometric measurements (Soft tissue), Angle of facial convexity.

Angle of flexure See Cephalometric measurements (Hard tissue), Cranial base angle.

Angle of the mandible See Cephalometric measurements (Hard tissue), Gonial angle.

Angle's normal occlusion theory See Extraction vs. non-extraction debate.

Angulation (Second order, "Tip") Angular deviation of the long axis of a tooth from a

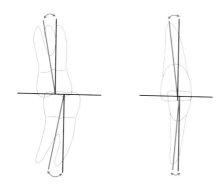

Angulation

line perpendicular to the occlusal plane, in the mesiodistal direction. [Compare with Inclination.]

Ankyloglossia (Tongue-tie) Restriction of tongue movements, possibly accompanied by speech difficulties, resulting from a short lingual frenum, or one that is attached too close to the tip of the tongue.

Ankylosis Abnormal immobility, union or fusion that may occur between two bones at their articulation (e.g. ankylosis of the TMJ) or between teeth and alveolar bone.
In the instance of the TMJ, bony or fibrous ankylosis can be caused by conditions such as congenital defects, trauma, inflammation, infections, arthritis or neoplasms.
In the case of an ankylosed tooth, the periodontal ligament is obliterated in one or more localized areas, and a "bony bridge" is formed by penetration of alveolar bone into the cementum. Dental ankylosis eliminates the potential for both eruption and orthodontic movement. In a growing individual, an ankylosed tooth is accompanied by a localized vertical deficiency of the alveolar ridge, and consequently appears to "submerge" as adjacent, unaffected teeth continue to erupt. Ankylosis of deciduous teeth (usually molars) is a more common phenomenon than ankylosis of permanent teeth. [Also see Tooth mobility, Reduced.]

Annealing A heat treatment and cooling schedule used to reduce the hardness and increase the ductility of a metal by removing residual stress.

Anodontia A rare condition characterized by congenital absence of all teeth (both deciduous and permanent). Most commonly related to ectodermal dysplasia. [Compare with Oligodontia.]

Anomalad A malformation, together with its subsequently derived structural changes (e.g. the Robin anomalad).

ANS See Anterior nasal spine.

ANS-PNS See Cephalometric lines, Palatal plane.

Antagonist(s) The tooth (teeth) of the opposing arch, with which a tooth is supposed to have occlusal contact in centric occlusion.

Antegonial notch A depression or concavity usually present in the inferior border of the mandible, immediately anterior to the angle, near the insertion of the masseter muscle.

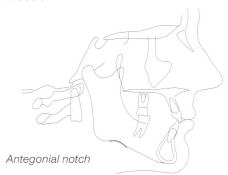

Antegonial notch

A deeper than normal antegonial notch may be indicative of a dolichofacial pattern or of mandibular underdevelopment. Pronounced antegonial notching also is a common characteristic of some syndromes with micrognathia of the lower jaw, such as Treacher Collins syndrome.

Anterior band-removing pliers See Orthodontic instruments, Band-removing pliers.

Anterior component of occlusal force A theory attempting to explain the tendency of posterior teeth to drift mesially with time. Factors that are considered related to this phenomenon are: morphology and angulation of teeth, occlusal and muscular forces and transseptal fibers.

Anterior cranial base The anterior aspect of the floor of the cranial vault, commonly delimited cephalometrically by sella turcica and nasion.

Anterior crossbite See Crossbite, Anterior.

Anterior debanding pliers See Orthodontic instruments, Band-removing pliers.

Anterior diagonal elastics See Orthodontic elastics, Anterior diagonal.

Anterior facial height See Cephalometric measurements (Hard tissue), Facial height.

Anterior forced bite See Forced bite, Anterior.

Anterior guidance Term used to describe a particular scheme of disclusion of the dental arches during a protrusive mandibular excursion. Contacts between the maxillary incisors and the mandibular anterior teeth guide the mandible downward, to create disarticulation (separation) of all other teeth.

Anterior lower face height See Cephalometric measurements (Hard tissue), Facial height.

Anterior maxillary segmental osteotomy See Osteotomy, Anterior maxillary segmental.

Anterior nasal spine (ANS) See Cephalometric landmarks (Hard tissue), Anterior nasal spine.

Anterior non-occlusion See Non-occlusion, Anterior.

Anterior oblique elastics See Orthodontic elastics, Anterior diagonal.

Anterior open bite See Open bite.

Anterior repositioning appliance See Splint, Anterior repositioning.

Anterior repositioning splint See Splint, Anterior repositioning.

Anterior rotation (of the mandible) See Mandibular rotation, Counter-clockwise.

Anterior teeth The maxillary and mandibular incisors and canines.

Anteroposteriorly In a direction parallel to the sagittal plane; in radiology it denotes beam direction from front to back.

Anthropometry Measurement of dimensions of the human body and its parts.

Antrum A cavity or chamber. The term usually refers to the maxillary sinus.

Apertognathia See Open bite.

Apical area (of the bone) The apical area in the newborn child and during the first year of life is the region in which the developing deciduous and permanent teeth are found. In the deciduous dentition it comprises the area occupied by the apices of the deciduous teeth and the developing permanent teeth. In the mixed dentition, the apical area is the region in which lie the apices of the deciduous and erupted permanent teeth, as well as the developing unemerged permanent teeth.
In the adult, the apical area consists of the region in which normally the apices of the permanent teeth can be located. The concept of the apical area was introduced by F.P.G.M. van der Linden in 1979.

Apical base Maxillary and mandibular bone that supports and is continuous with the alveolar processes, as well as with the maxillary and mandibular bodies. Although the

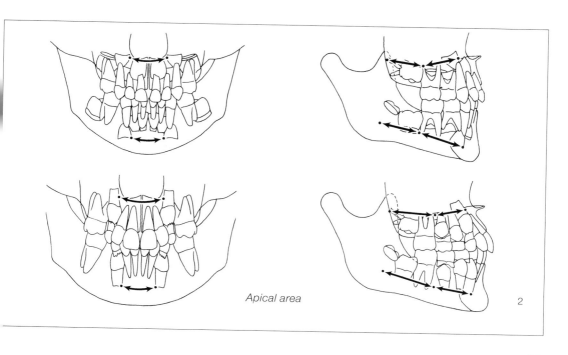

Apical area

2

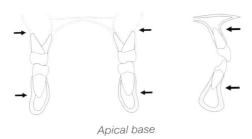

Apical base

demarcation between alveolar and basal bone is not specific, it generally is thought to lie at or slightly above the level of the apices of the roots. The concept of the apical base was introduced by A.F. Lundström in 1923. [Also see Bone, Basal.]

Apparent rotation (of the mandible) See Mandibular rotation, Matrix.

Appliance Any device used for a particular functional, diagnostic and/or therapeutic effect.

ACCO appliance A combination of a modified maxillary removable appliance with a straight-pull J-hook headgear. The acronym "ACCO" was suggested by H.I. Margolis (1976) and stands for ACrylic-Cervical-Occipital.
The maxillary removable appliance includes an anterior bite plane, a labial bow, clasps for retention and finger springs for distalization of the maxillary molars.
The J-hook headgear is attached to loops on the labial bow that are bent between the maxillary central and lateral incisors. Its purpose is to counteract the reaction force on the maxillary anterior teeth caused by the distalizing force of the finger springs on the maxillary molars. A cervical headgear also may be attached on the maxillary molars to complement the action of the ACCO.
In the original design of the appliance by Margolis, molar distalization took place one side at a time. During distalization on one side, ball clasps or passive finger springs on the other side enhanced retention of the appliance. Once a Class I molar relationship

was achieved on the active side, a new ACCO was made. The new acrylic configuration and clasps on the completed side would retain the correction achieved, at the same time providing anchorage to correct the residual Class II relationship on the contralateral side of the arch.

Activator (Monobloc) The first removable functional appliance, developed by V. Andresen. Historically, the term "activator" was introduced to describe the "activation of mandibular growth," to which the achieved correction of a Class II malocclusion was attributed. The term currently is used in a generic sense, referring to a family of functional appliances used to treat Class II malocclusions characterized, at least in part, by mandibular deficiency. [For activators designed for patients with Class III malocclusions, see Appliance, Class III functional.] These appliances position the mandible forward, promoting a new mandibular postural position. The reactive forces from the stretch of the muscles and soft tissues are transmitted to the maxillary dentition and through that, to the maxilla.

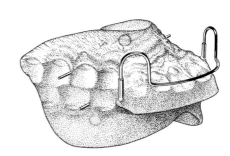

Activator 2

The acrylic body of the Andresen activator covers part of the palate and the lingual aspect of the mandibular alveolar ridge. (Note: In its original design the appliance contacted the mandibular anterior teeth only on the lingual side and did not extend over the incisal edges.) A labial bow fits anterior to the maxillary incisors and carries U-loops for adjustment. On the palatal aspects of the maxillary incisors, the acrylic is relieved to allow their retraction.

A main feature of the appliance is the faceting of the acrylic on palatal and lingual aspects of the maxillary and mandibular posterior teeth, respectively, designed to direct their eruption. On the palatal aspect of the maxillary posterior teeth the facets are cut so as to allow occlusal, distal and buccal movement of these teeth. This movement is achieved by keeping the acrylic in contact with only the mesiopalatal surfaces of the premolars and molars. On the lingual aspect of the mandibular posterior teeth the facets only permit occlusal and mesial movement, with the acrylic contacting the distolingual surface of these teeth. [Also see Appliance, Functional.]

Active vertical corrector An appliance introduced by E.L. Dellinger, attempting to correct anterior open bites by intrusion of posterior teeth. The appliance consists of maxillary and mandibular posterior bite blocks with incorporated repelling samarium-cobalt magnets. A commonly reported side effect of treatment with the appliance is the creation of a posterior crossbite owing to the lateral force components of the repelling magnets. [Also see Orthodontic magnets.]

Bass appliance A removable functional appliance designed by N.M. Bass, consisting of a basic maxillary expansion plate on which various other parts can be mounted. The expansion plate covers the occlusal surfaces of all maxillary teeth and has torquing

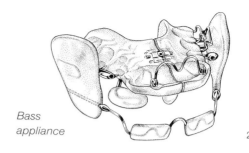

Bass appliance 2

springs for the maxillary central incisors. The appliance also carries tubes in which buccal shields can be attached, and has mandibular lip pads extending in the vestibule in a fashion similar to the Fränkel appliance. On the lingual side there are specially designed flanges that can be gradually advanced. The Bass appliance also can be combined with a high-pull headgear.

Begg appliance (Light-wire appliance)
Fixed multi-banded orthodontic appliance developed by P.R. Begg for his light-wire technique. The appliance consists of narrow (single-wing), ribbon-arch brackets (originally developed by E.H. Angle as the "pin and tube" appliance) and light, round stainless steel archwires. It allows a series of tipping movements of teeth in conjunction with intermaxillary elastics.

Treatment with the Begg technique is classically divided into three stages:
The first stage includes initial alignment by simple tipping, with the exception of the anchor teeth. Any spaces present between the anterior teeth are closed and any rotations or crossbites are corrected. Deep ante-

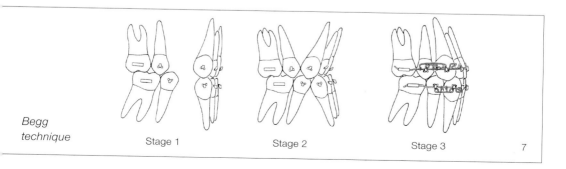

Begg technique   Stage 1   Stage 2   Stage 3   7

rior overbites or open bites are eliminated, and the anteroposterior occlusal relationship between the maxillary and mandibular teeth is overcorrected. Arch forms are coordinated and extraction spaces are reduced, to some degree, during the first stage.

During the second stage all extraction spaces are closed completely, by allowing significant lingual tipping of the anterior teeth (incisors and canines), brought upon by a combination of intramaxillary and intermaxillary elastic traction.

The third and final stage basically includes uprighting of the teeth by movement of the roots. This root movement is performed by round archwires with bent-in torquing loops, in combination with root-torquing auxiliaries of various designs. Individual tooth positioning is performed with bends and root-tipping springs. [Also see Differential force theory; Orthodontic wire, Australian; Appliance, Tip-Edge.]

Bidimensional appliance See Bidimensional technique.

Bimler appliance (Bite former, Bimler stimulator) A modification of the activator by H.P. Bimler. There are three main kinds of Bimler appliance: type A for patients with Class II Division 1 malocclusions, type B for those with Class II Division 2 and type C for patients with a Class III malocclusion.

All of the above appliances are flexible and carry springs and bows on the labial and lingual side in both arches. The springs and bows are connected together by two acrylic wings which extend toward the palatal and lingual mucosa. Each appliance type is subdivided further into two main categories, space creation or space closure; the space creation variety carries additional active springs.

In the type A appliance the mandible is held in its advanced position by engagement of the mandibular incisors in a splint. The splint contacts the labial aspect of the mandibular incisors while special springs engage on their lingual aspect. A mandibular labial wire holds the splint in place, extending distally

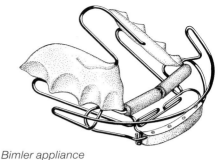

Bimler appliance

to connect with the maxillary part of the appliance. The maxillary part of the appliance carries a labial arch and palatal springs for the maxillary incisors.

In the type B appliance the palate is covered by acrylic, with an incorporated midline screw. No labial arch exists for the maxillary incisors.

In the type C appliance occlusal wires covered with plastic tubing are used to achieve bite opening. There is no labial splint, but the mandibular incisors are retracted by a labial bow originating from the maxillary part of the appliance.

Bionator A modification of the activator developed by W. Balters in the 1950s. Its design is significantly less bulky compared to the activator, thus reducing interference with speech. The bionator consists of a lingual horseshoe of acrylic, with a palatal spring shaped like a (reversed) Coffin spring. Facets are created in the acrylic to guide the maxillary and mandibular posterior teeth and hold them in the postured relationship. A labial bow exists anterior to the

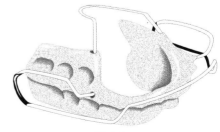

Bionator

maxillary incisors that extends distally to keep the buccal musculature away from the teeth. In the original design of the appliance, the mandibular incisors were not capped with acrylic.

Bruxism appliance See Nightguard.

Chin cap (Chin cup) Extraoral orthopedic appliance that consists of a cap that fits on the patient's chin and a headstrap similar to that of a high-pull headgear. It is designed to deliver a superiorly and posteriorly directed force to the mandibular condyles, via the chin. The appliance has been used for decades in an attempt to correct mandibular prognathism in young patients by restraining or redirecting mandibular condylar growth.

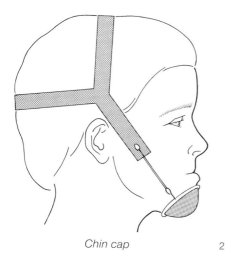

Chin cap   2

Class Class III functional appliances (Reverse functional appliances) Various types of functional appliances that position the mandible posteriorly and rotate it open. Such appliances are advocated for the correction of maxillary deficiency and/or mild mandibular prognathism in a growing child.

The mode of action of Class III functional appliances includes correction of any anterior crossbite by labial tipping of the maxillary incisors and retroclination of mandibu-

lar incisors (introducing an element of dental compensation for the existing skeletal discrepancy). The prominence of the chin is decreased by causing the mandible to rotate down and back and by increasing the lower face height. Treatment with such appliances generally is not indicated for patients with excessive lower face height, as is often the case with Class III problems.

Combined functional/extraoral traction appliance A functional appliance on which a facebow can be attached for extraoral traction (e.g. the Bass and the Teuscher appliances), or on which a facebow is rigidly fixed (e.g. the Van Beek appliance).

Crefcoeur appliance A removable appliance designed by J. Crefcoeur, most often used to increase space at a specific location in the dental arch. The appliance is in essence a Hawley-type acrylic plate, sectioned (split) at the point where space creation is necessary. A heavy-gauge stainless steel wire (Crefcoeur spring) is embedded in the acrylic at the posterior aspects of the appliance bilaterally. This wire runs parallel

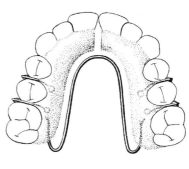

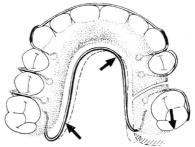

Crefcoeur appliance   10

to the edges of the acrylic on the lingual aspect and can be activated appropriately to increase the separation between the two sectioned parts of the appliance. After sufficient space has been created, the two parts of the appliance can be reconnected with rapid-curing acrylic. The appliance also can be used to reduce a localized space in the dental arch and to expand or constrict the dental arches. Good retention and adequate clasps are very important for the Crefcoeur appliance, particularly in the area of the separation. The retention of the appliance can be enhanced by creating artificial undercuts with composite on certain teeth.

Crib 1. An interceptive appliance used for correction of deleterious habits such as a deviating tongue position and/or digit-sucking. A crib typically consists of a fixed transpalatal [0.036-inch (0.90-mm) or heavier gauge] wire, soldered on two maxillary first permanent molar bands. The wire extends toward the anterior palate where it forms a crib-shaped "fence" meant to interfere with the habit. A crib also can be incorporated in a removable appliance. Posterior (lateral) tongue cribs can be used as part of removable appliances in patients with unilateral or bilateral posterior open bite. [See also Appliance, Habit-breaking.]
2. The basic retention clasp of a Crozat appliance. [See also Appliance, Crozat.]

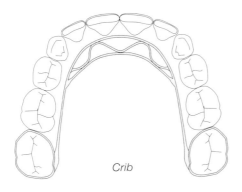

Crib

Crozat appliance Removable orthodontic appliance which was developed by G. Crozat in the early 1900s. In its original design the appliance was fabricated entirely of precious metal. Heavy gold wires constituted the framework and lighter gold fingersprings produced the desired tooth movement.

The Crozat appliance can be used in the maxilla and/or mandible. Tight circumferential clasps (*cribs*) on the molars provide adequate retention to permit the use of light intermaxillary elastics with the appliance.

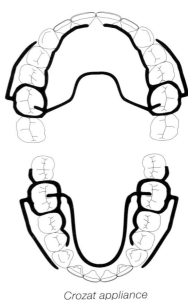

Crozat appliance

Delaire appliance See Appliance, Face mask.

Edgewise appliance (Standard edgewise) Fixed multi-banded orthodontic appliance, introduced by E.H. Angle in 1928. It involves a rectangular labial archwire ligated into attachments (brackets) that are fixed on bands which are cemented to individual teeth, or that are directly bonded to individual teeth. The term *edgewise* refers to the fact that the bracket slot is fabricated in a way that permits insertion of the archwire with its long dimension perpendicular to the long axis of the tooth, instead of parallel to it, as in the (earlier) *ribbon arch* bracket. *See illustration next page.*

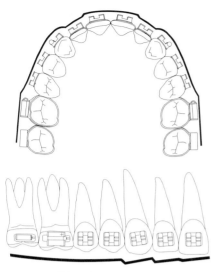

Edgewise appliance

Elastic open activator A modification of the activator developed by G. Klammt. The appliance has reduced acrylic bulk, facilitating increased appliance wear. The acrylic is replaced by wires which increase the flexibility of the appliance. The flexible design allows isotonic muscular contractions (in contrast to rigid appliances, which only allow isometric contractions).

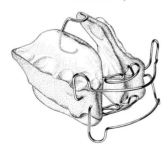

Elastic open activator 2

Expansion appliance An orthodontic appliance used to expand the maxillary or, less frequently, the mandibular dental arch. An expansion appliance can be removable (e.g. split-plate appliance with a jackscrew) or fixed on the teeth (e.g. the Hyrax appliance or the Quad-helix). [See also

Expansion, Rapid maxillary; Expansion, Slow maxillary.]

Extraoral traction appliance An orthodontic appliance that makes use of extraoral anchorage (e.g. headgear, face mask).

Face mask (Reverse-pull headgear, Protraction headgear, Face frame) Extraoral appliance that utilizes rests on the chin and forehead (and occasionally the cheek bones) as anchorage for elastic traction, with the purpose of orthopedically protracting the maxilla. This maxillary protraction is performed as an early treatment modality in Class III malocclusions associated with maxillary hypoplasia.

The face mask also can be used as an orthodontic appliance, to provide extraoral anchorage for protraction of posterior teeth. Usual side effects of face mask treatment include elongation of the face (caused by extrusion of the teeth to which the elastic traction is applied) and proclination of the maxillary incisors, when the traction is applied to the maxilla. The appliance was designed by J. Delaire and subsequently modified by H. Petit and others.

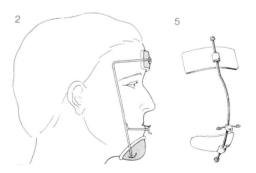

Face mask

Fixed appliance An appliance that is cemented or bonded to the teeth and thus cannot be removed by the patient. The term commonly refers to fixed attachments (brackets, tubes, bands) placed on the teeth in conjunction with archwires to move them to a new position.

Fixed/removable appliance Orthodontic appliance that is fixed to the teeth but can be removed by the clinician for adjustment and subsequently re-inserted, without taking off any brackets or bands. Fixed/removable appliances make use of special sheaths welded on the palatal or lingual aspect of molar bands (e.g. the fixed/removable lingual arch or transpalatal arch). [Also see Sheath.]

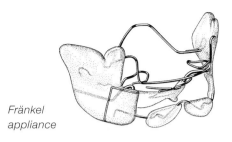

Fränkel appliance

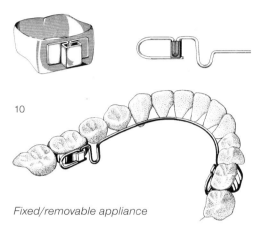

Fixed/removable appliance

Fränkel appliance (Function Regulator) Group of functional appliances developed by R. Fränkel to treat malocclusions, while aiding in the maturation, training and reprogramming of the orofacial neuromuscular system. Four main types of appliances have been described by Fränkel: Function Regulator (FR)-I was designed for treatment of Class I and Class II Division 1 malocclusions. The FR-II appliance is meant for patients with Class II Division 1 and 2 malocclusions, the FR-III was designed for patients with Class III malocclusions and the FR-IV for patients with hyperdivergent facial patterns and anterior open bite. The appliances consist of acrylic buccal (vestibular) shields and lip pads, connected by wires, to restrain and retrain aberrant musculature and to prevent the effects of restricting muscle forces on the dentition. The extension of the buccal shields into the full depth of the vestibule is supposed to stimulate the periosteum in order to achieve

a skeletal expansion of the apical bases. Lingual shields also are included to accomplish a gradual, stepwise advancement of the mandible.

Functional appliance A removable or fixed appliance that alters the posture of the mandible and transmits the forces created by the resulting stretch of the muscles and soft tissues and by the change of the neuromuscular environment to the dental and skeletal tissues to produce movement of teeth and modification of growth.

Haas appliance (Haas rapid maxillary expansion appliance, Haas palatal separator) A fixed expansion appliance that was popularized by A.J. Haas. The appliance consists of bands cemented on the maxillary first premolars and first molars that are rigidly connected to each other with heavy-gauge wires on the buccal and palatal aspect of the teeth. Two acrylic pads encase the palatal connecting wires and are joined with a midline jackscrew. The acrylic pads

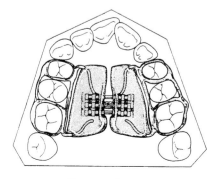

Haas appliance

are in close contact with the palatal mucosa. The Haas appliance was designed to expand the maxillary arch by opening the mid-palatal suture, thereby causing a skeletal expansion of the maxilla. According to Haas, the contact of the pads with the palate allows the forces from the appliance to be dissipated against the underlying hard and soft tissues of the palate, thus minimizing the amount of dental tipping and maximizing the skeletal effect. Others consider this a disadvantage of the appliance with regard to hygiene, resulting in inflammation of the palatal tissues. [Also see Expansion, Rapid maxillary.]

Habit-breaking appliance (Habit reminder)

Any removable or fixed appliance designed to correct undesirable habits such as digit-sucking, tongue interposition, tongue-thrusting, or infantile swallow. [Also see Appliance, Vestibular shield; Appliance, Crib.]

Harvold-Woodside activator

A modification of the activator developed by E.P. Harvold and D.G. Woodside. Its distinguishing feature is the overextended vertical opening to which the appliance is constructed. The bite is opened by 5 mm to 6 mm beyond the freeway space. The rationale is that maximum stretching of the muscles will produce a force that will be transmitted to the bones and teeth, inducing a compensatory anatomic correction. It is claimed that the Harvold-Woodside activator requires minimal mandibular advancement to produce the desired sagittal correction, as the extreme muscle stretch can cause intrusion (or inhibition of eruption) of the maxillary posterior teeth, resulting in "closure" or counterclockwise rotation of the mandible with a relative Class II correction (bite-block effect). Relieving the acrylic occlusally to the mandibular posterior teeth allows them to erupt in a mesial direction, which also facilitates Class II correction.

Hawley appliance

See Retainer, Hawley.

Headgear appliance

See Headgear.

Herbst appliance

Tooth-borne, fixed type of functional appliance originally developed by E. Herbst in the early 1900s, which was re-introduced by H. Pancherz in the 1970s. This appliance was one of the first attempts to produce a "jumping of the bite" effect. Its components originally were produced by Dentaurum in Germany and now are available from several suppliers internationally.

The Herbst appliance consists of frameworks cemented or bonded to the maxillary and mandibular dental arches (but occasionally can be removable). These frameworks are connected to each other bilaterally with a piston-and-tube device, whose telescopic action encourages forward repositioning of the mandible as the patient closes into occlusion. Alternatively, the Herbst appliance can be used in combination with fixed orthodontic appliances.

Since the force is delivered directly to the teeth, there is an increased tendency for mandibular incisor proclination during treatment with the Herbst appliance. On the other hand, because of the enforced full-time wear, the occlusal changes can be brought about quite rapidly. [Also see "Jumping of the bite."]

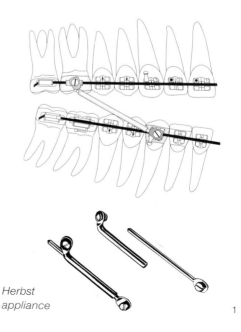

Herbst appliance

1

Herren activator (L.S.U. activator) A modification of the activator developed by P. Herren (also known as the Louisiana State University modification of the same appliance). It is essentially an activator made to a construction bite that positions the mandible forward and downward to a significant degree. According to P. Herren, the wearing of this appliance is not supposed to increase the activity of the lateral pterygoid muscle.

Hickham protraction appliance A modification of the face mask developed by J.H. Hickham. It consists of a chin cup with hooks extending upwards and forwards, for application of anterior elastic traction to the maxilla and/or the maxillary (or mandibular) dentition.

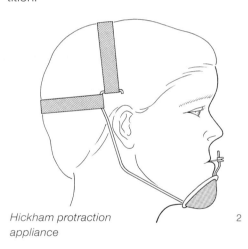

Hickham protraction appliance   2

"Hybrid" functional appliance A non-specific functional appliance (usually asymmetrical) combining various features of other functional appliances. Such appliances sometimes are used to aid in leveling a transversely canted occlusal plane and to improve symmetry in patients with hemifacial microsomia, or with growth disturbances after trauma to the mandibular condyle.

Hyrax appliance (Hygienic rapid pa latal expander) A commonly used type o banded rapid maxillary expansion app ance developed by W. Biederman and orig inally licensed to Dentaurum. The compo nents now are available from several supp ers internationally. The framework of th appliance is made entirely of stainless ste or cobalt-chromium alloy, with no acryl contacting the palatal mucosa. Bands a cemented (usually) on the maxillary first pr molars and first molars. The bands are co nected by means of rigid wires to a speci expansion screw which is located in th midline of the palate, in close proximity the palatal contour. Hyrax-type expansio screws are available in various sizes (mo commonly 7 mm, 11 mm and 13 mm) d pending on the application. Buccal an palatal support wires also may be added f rigidity. [Also see Expansion, Rapid max lary.]

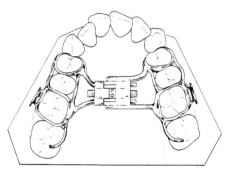

Hyrax appliance

Jasper jumper appliance A type of fixe functional appliance developed by J. Jasper. In essence it is a flexible versio of the Herbst appliance. The Jasper jumpe is used in combination with fixed appliance for correction of Class II malocclusions. It consists of two polyurethane-coated stai less steel coil springs (force modules attached at both ends to stainless steel en caps. The force modules are available seven lengths (from 26 to 38 mm, 2-mm increments). The end-caps carr holes so they can be attached to the ancho

ing unit. One end-cap is attached to the distal aspect of the headgear tube of the maxillary molar by means of a special ball pin attachment. The other end-cap is attached to the mandibular arch, between the canine and the first premolar, either directly onto the main archwire, or on a segment utilizing the auxiliary slot of the mandibular molar. Upon insertion, the appliance bows out towards the cheek, promoting an anterior mandibular position.

The Jasper jumper may be used as an alternative to intermaxillary elastics and requires minimal patient cooperation, as it is fixed on the archwires.

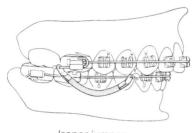

Jasper jumper 5

Jones jig A fixed orthodontic appliance designed by R.D. Jones for unilateral or bilateral maxillary molar distalization without patient cooperation. The appliance consists of a heavy-gauge wire and an open-coil nickel-titanium spring delivering a force of approximately 0.7 to 0.8 N (70 to 80 g) over a compression range of 1 to 5 mm. The distal end of the jig assembly carries a sol-

dered additional wire that is inserted into the main tube of the maxillary first molar band, whereas the heavy-gauge wire is placed in the headgear tube. The sliding part of the jig is attached on the anchor teeth by a stainless steel ligature so that the coil spring is compressed. The bands on the anchor teeth (which can be either the first premolars, second premolars, or deciduous second molars) are soldered to a large, modified Nance button to make maximal use of palatal anchorage.

Kinetor A removable functional appliance developed by H. Stockfisch. The appliance consists of two acrylic plates joined by vestibular steel loops and supported by occlusal rubber tubes. This design gives the appliance a certain degree of flexibility, which is supposed to reinforce muscular impulses and stimulate function.

Kingsley appliance (Bite-jumping appliance) Probably the first removable functional appliance (developed by N.W. Kingsley in 1877). The appliance consisted of a vulcanite palatal plate with an anterior inclined plane, which forced the mandible in an anterior direction ("jumping of the bite"). It also contained a mechanism for retraction of maxillary incisors and was retained by silk threads to the maxillary molars. [Also see "Jumping of the bite."]

Labiolingual appliance Early orthodontic fixed appliance system introduced by

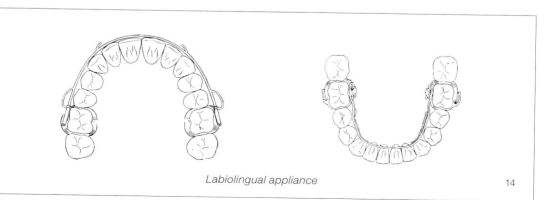

Labiolingual appliance 14

O.A. Oliver. The appliance consisted of bands on the molar teeth in conjunction with heavy mandibular lingual and maxillary labial base arches. Movement of individual teeth with this system was achieved by activating fingersprings and other accessory springs soldered on the base archwires.

Lehman appliance (Lehman activator)

A combination activator-headgear appliance developed by R. Lehman. It consists of a maxillary acrylic plate that carries two rigidly fixed outer bows and a mandibular lingual shield. The acrylic plate covers the palate and it extends over the occlusal and incisal surfaces of the maxillary teeth, up to the occlusal third of their buccal and labial surfaces.

Selective expansion of the maxillary arch is possible by appropriately activating the two transverse expansion screws (one anterior and one posterior) that are embedded in the plate.

Occipital traction is applied through a headstrap attached on the outer bows, which are fixed at the anterior aspect of the appliance. The mandibular lingual shield is connected to the maxillary plate by means of two heavy S-shaped wires. Unlike many activator-type appliances which are constructed with the mandible in a protruded position, this appliance is made from a bite registration taken in centric occlusion. According to R. Lehman, the S-shaped wires are activated by approximately 2 mm every 4 to 6 weeks, to achieve a gradual advancement of the mandible.

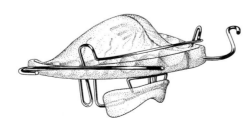

Lehman appliance 2

Light-wire appliance See Appliance Begg.

Lingual appliance 1. Any removable c fixed orthodontic appliance, placed on th lingual (palatal) side of the dental arches.
2. An esthetic, "invisible" fixed orthodonti appliance consisting of special orthodonti attachments bonded on the lingual surface of the teeth. The principle of a rectangula wire in a rectangular pre-adjusted (straigh wire) slot is the same, but the design of th attachments is modified.

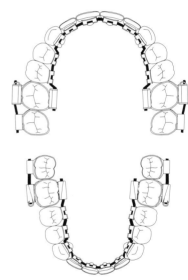

Lingual appliance

The maxillary anterior brackets have a fla surface that occludes with the mandibula incisors in patients with deep bite and act as an anterior bite plane. The archwire shap also is modified to fit the configuration of th lingual surface of the dental arch ("mush room" configuration). Accuracy of bracke placement is critical, so indirect bonding i advocated.

Disadvantages of the lingual applianc include smaller interbracket distance, mor difficult access, arguably reduced comfor for the patient due to tongue impingemen and usually higher treatment fee.

Lip bumper Intraoral removable orthodontic appliance consisting of a U-shaped 0.036-inch (0.90-mm) stainless steel wire, which in its anterior portion may carry a plastic or acrylic pad. The ends of the lip bumper are inserted into tubes on the mandibular first or second permanent molars. Its anterior portion is adjusted to lie in the vestibular area, 2 to 3 mm away from the alveolar process and the mandibular incisors (the vertical height varies).

Lip bumpers commonly are worn on a full-time basis and occasionally may be ligated in place (in case of reduced patient compliance). They are used to control or increase the mandibular dental arch length, to upright mesially or lingually tipped mandibular molars and to prevent the interposition of the lower lip between the maxillary and mandibular incisors.

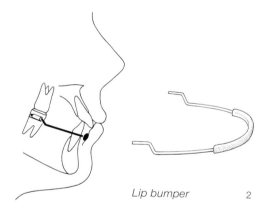

Lip bumper   2

Depending on the anterior configuration (with or without lip pads) the appliance has two effects: First, by removing the soft tissue forces from the labial aspect of the mandibular incisors it can cause labial tipping of these teeth. Second, by transmitting the force from the lip to the mandibular first molars, the lip bumper causes distal movement (mainly tipping) of these teeth. This distal movement is accomplished more easily when the second molars are still unerupted or have been extracted as part of the treatment plan.

Monobloc See Appliance, Activator.

Mouthguard A removable appliance, usually made from flexible or rigid thermoplastic material, used to cover and protect the teeth while engaging in contact sports.

Mühlemann appliance See Appliance, Propulsor.

Muscle relaxation appliance See Splint, Relaxation.

Nance appliance See Arch, Nance holding.

Nightguard See Nightguard.

Obturator See Obturator.

Open activator An activator with reduced acrylic coverage of the anterior palate in comparison to the classic activator. It is meant to facilitate speech by allowing contact between the tongue and palate.

Oral screen A removable appliance placed in the anterior vestibular region to improve lip position and reduce the overjet. In patients with a persistent tongue thrust or tongue interposition habit, it can be used in conjunction with a tongue crib. [Also see Appliance, Vestibular shield.]

Orthodontic appliance Any appliance used to prevent, intercept and/or correct different forms of malocclusion, malrelationship and malfunction of the teeth and associated surrounding structures.

Orthopedic appliance Any appliance used to prevent, intercept and/or correct improper relationships between the maxilla and mandible, as well as various functional deviations, by influencing growth, development and function.

Pendulum appliance A fixed orthodontic appliance introduced by J.J. Hilgers as a means for molar distalization without patient compliance.

The appliance makes use of palatal anchorage through a large Nance button, which is retained with bands on the maxillary first premolars and occlusal rests on the distal aspect of the maxillary second premolars.

Two "pendulum" springs fabricated out of 0.032-inch (0.81-mm) TMA wire extend from the posterior edge of the Nance button. Each spring contains a closed helix (close to the midline), a small horizontal adjustment loop and a recurved portion that inserts into palatal sheaths soldered on the bands of the maxillary first molars. The thickness of the palatal sheaths on the molar bands is 0.036 inch (0.90 mm), so that the 0.032-inch (0.81-mm) diameter wire fits loosely in them. If expansion of the maxillary arch is necessary, the appliance can be fabricated in a split-plate design (*Pend-X* or *Pendex* appliance) by incorporating a midpalatal screw in the center of the Nance button. Prior to cementation the springs are bent (preactivated) so that they lie parallel to the midsagittal plane, and they subsequently are inserted into the sheaths.

As the molar is driven distally, it also moves palatally (on an arc). This palatal movement can be counteracted by slightly opening the adjustment loop. Distal root movement of the molars also can be produced by adjusting the recurved portion of the "pendulum" springs in order to avoid distalization by mere tipping.

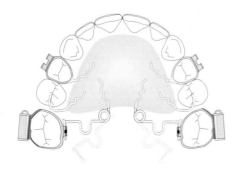

Pendulum appliance

Pin-and-tube appliance Early fixed orthdontic appliance (now archaic) consistin of vertical tubes soldered onto bands place on the permanent teeth. Movement of th teeth was achieved by use of an archwi with soldered vertical pins that were force into the tubes. The system, originally deve oped by E.H. Angle, was later replaced by the ribbon-arch appliance.

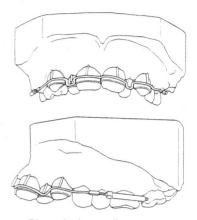

Pin-and-tube appliance

Positioner (Tooth positioner) A remo able orthodontic appliance originally deve oped for closing band spaces after deban ing. It currently is used mainly to achieve fir adjustments and retain corrected positior following fixed appliance treatment.

The positioner is fabricated of rubber or ela tomeric plastic material covering the max lary and mandibular dental arches, as we as part of the alveolar process. For it construction, individual teeth are cut from plaster model and are reset subsequent in an ideal relationship.

The patient is instructed to wear the pos tioner immediately following fixed applianc removal and to clench the teeth into it. Th appliance functions by molding of the inc vidual teeth into the correct position withi the arch through the forces generated by th elastic material in contact with the teeth When used in patients who exhibited a Clas II malocclusion prior to treatment, the pos tioner can be constructed in a slightly ove corrected Class I relationship, providing a "functional appliance" component.

Advantages of the positioner include its resistance to fracture, stimulation of tissue tone and continuous improvement of tooth position if it is worn properly. Disadvantages are its bulkiness (making it less comfortable for the patients), and the possibility that it may keep teeth loose by producing intermittent forces on them.

Positioners are contraindicated in patients with airway obstruction and in patients with a history of temporomandibular disorders. Their use often is preferred in patients with minimal overbite or open bite tendency, as they tend to deepen the bite.

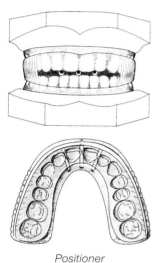

Positioner 5

Preadjusted appliance See Appliance, Straight-wire.

Propulsor (Mühlemann appliance) A removable functional appliance similar to the activator. The appliance carries a vestibular acrylic extension over the maxillary alveolar process. The intention is to distribute the posteriorly directed force over the basal bone to maximize the skeletal and to minimize the dentoalveolar effect.

Quad-helix appliance An all-wire fixed orthodontic expansion appliance originally developed by E. Herbst and popularized by R.W. Ricketts, among others. It typically consists of a 0.036-inch (0.90-mm) stainless steel wire, containing four helices (two anteriorly and two posteriorly) to increase its range and flexibility. The wire is soldered (or attached in a fixed/removable design) onto bands on the maxillary first molars (and occasionally also on the maxillary first premolars). Various other designs, such as a tri- or a bi-helix, also are described.

The appliance is used for symmetrical or asymmetrical expansion of the maxillary dental arch, as well as for derotation of the molars. It has a tendency to produce buccal tipping of the teeth, and is not advocated in patients who require a significant amount of expansion. It is considered advantageous for patients with cleft lip and palate, in whom a localized expansion of the anterior aspect of the collapsed lesser maxillary alveolar segment often is necessary.

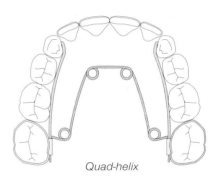

Quad-helix

Rapid maxillary expansion appliance See Expansion, Rapid maxillary.

Removable appliance An appliance that is not fixed to teeth, but can be removed by the patient.

Ribbon-arch appliance A fixed multi-banded orthodontic appliance developed by E.H. Angle, which marked another stage towards the development of the edgewise appliance. Each band carried a vertical slot capable of receiving a rectangular wire in a vertical orientation (with the longer dimension of the cross-section parallel to the long axis of the tooth), hence the term *ribbonwise*. The archwire was retained in place by pins. Control of buccolingual (third-order) root position was difficult with the appliance. This problem was overcome later with the development of the edgewise appliance. [Also see "Ribbonwise."]

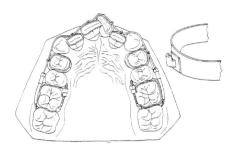

Ribbon-arch appliance   13

RPE appliance See Expansion, Rapid maxillary.

Sagittal appliance An active removable appliance with expansion screws in the anteroposterior direction bilaterally (*two-way sagittal*) or additionally in the transverse direction (*three-way sagittal*), when expansion is also necessary. Retention is achieved by a combination of Adams clasps and arrowhead clasps. Sagittal appliances are used mainly in patients with labially displaced canines to increase the arch length by advancing the incisors and to apply a distalizing force on the posterior teeth.

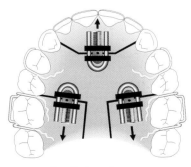

Sagittal appliance

Schwarz appliance A removable orthodontic appliance introduced by A.M. Schwarz for expansion of the maxillary and/or the mandibular dental arch. The appliance consists of a horseshoe-shaped acrylic plate fitting along the lingual surface of the teeth and covering a large portion of the lingual aspect of the alveolar process or palate. A midline expansion screw is incorporated in the acrylic, and ball or arrowhead clasps on the deciduous and permanent molars provide the necessary retention.
Although Schwarz developed a variety of "split-plate" appliances, the mandibular appliance is widely considered as the one that bears his name.

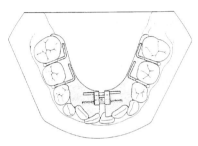

Schwarz appliance   5

Segmental appliance (Sectional appliance) See Mechanics, Segmental arch.

Space-regaining appliance See Space regainer.

Space-retaining appliance See Space maintainer.

SPEED appliance (Strite Industries, Ltd. Fixed, self-ligating orthodontic appliance system developed by H.G. Hanson. The appliance consists of miniaturized self-ligating brackets with built-in flexible, escape proof spring-clips that obviate the need for conventional elastomeric or stainless steel ligatures and permit light force delivery. The spatial relationship between the spring loaded clip and the archwire allows a continuous dynamic interaction between them while maintaining three-dimensional contro

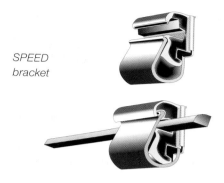

SPEED bracket

of tooth position. [SPEED is an acronym of the words Spring-loaded, Precision, Edgewise, Energy and Delivery.]

Split-plate appliance See Appliance, Expansion.

Stabilization appliance See Splint, Relaxation.

Stöckli-Teuscher activator See Teuscher-Stöckli activator/headgear combination appliance.

Straight-wire appliance (Preadjusted appliance, SWA) A modification of the edgewise appliance, introduced by L.F. Andrews in 1972.

In the standard edgewise appliance the orientation of the bracket slot was at right angles to the long axis of the tooth and the thickness of the bracket base was the same for all types of teeth. During treatment, bends were placed in the archwire to individually position each tooth in the buccolingual direction (in-out or first-order bends), as well as to idealize the angulation of the long axis of the tooth in the mesiodistal direction (tip or second-order bends) and in the buccolingual direction (torque or third-order bends).

In the straight-wire appliance this information is incorporated in the brackets and tubes for each individual tooth, by varying the thickness of the base and the angulation of the slot relative to the long axis of the tooth, in both the mesiodistal and buccolingual

directions. As a result, a "straight" archwire can be used to ideally position the teeth, avoiding—though not completely eliminating—the need for placing such bends in the archwire. Accurate placement of the brackets on the teeth is of paramount importance with this appliance.

Straight-wire appliances of various prescriptions (sets of characteristic values for each individual tooth) are available on the market. [Also see Appliance prescription; Appliance, Edgewise.]

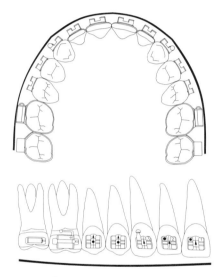

Straight-wire appliance

Teuscher-Stöckli activator/headgear combination appliance A modified activator used in combination with a high-pull headgear. The appliance was introduced by U.M. Teuscher and P.W. Stöckli as a means to avoid the detrimental profile effects of cervical traction when treating Class II malocclusions in growing individuals.

Buccal headgear tubes are incorporated in the interocclusal acrylic at the level of the maxillary second premolar or first molar. The vector of the high-pull headgear force is directed through a point midway between the estimated center of resistance of the maxilla and that of the maxillary dentition. In this way it is claimed that the best compromise is reached between a resulting counterclockwise rotation of the maxillary occlusal plane and a clockwise rotation of the maxilla itself, possibly maintaining the inclination of the maxillary occlusal plane.

The design includes reduced palatal acrylic coverage to provide more space for the tongue. The acrylic covers the occlusal and incisal surfaces of the maxillary teeth to distribute the headgear force over the entire dentition. The labial bow can be substituted by torquing springs to counteract palatal tipping of the maxillary incisors.

Long lingual flanges extend from the lower portion of the appliance to enhance forward positioning of the mandible. In addition, Fränkel-type lower lip pads may be added to enhance normal perioral muscle function. Finally, a jackscrew is added occasionally for controlled expansion.

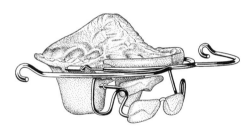

Teuscher-Stöckli appliance   2

Tip-Edge appliance Fixed orthodontic appliance developed by P.C. Kesling as a combination of the Begg and the straight-wire appliance (marketed by TP Orthodontics). The appliance consists of specially designed brackets with modified slots that have the shape of an asymmetric bowtie. The brackets are equipped with auxiliary vertical slots that can receive a variety of auxiliaries, including rotation springs, uprighting springs, power pins and position indicators to facilitate bonding.

The shape of the main slots allows tipping of the teeth during space closure (a basic principle of the Begg technique). After space closure the angulation of the teeth is idealized by uprighting springs (side-winders). When a rectangular archwire is

used during this uprighting process, the beveling and the dimensions of the modified, fully programmed slot permit gradual expression of the torque to simultaneously control tooth inclination. [Also see Appliance, Begg.]

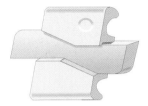

Tip-Edge bracket

Tongue crib See Appliance, Crib.

Tri-helix appliance A modification of the quad-helix, used in situations in which the constriction of the anterior maxilla is too severe to accommodate two helices in the anterior aspect of the appliance (e.g. in patients with a history of cleft lip and palate).

Twin arch appliance (Twin wire appliance) An early orthodontic fixed appliance introduced by J. Johnson in 1931. The appliance made use of the resilience of two thin gauge stainless steel wires ranging in size from 0.09 inch (0.23 mm) to 0.014 inch (0.35 mm) in diameter. Two end-tubes were soldered onto the first molar bands, capable of receiving the twin wire strands. The bands on the remaining teeth carried special locks forming channels with a rectangular cross-section. The twin wires were

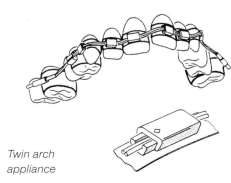

Twin arch appliance

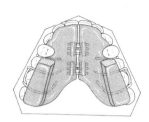
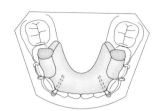
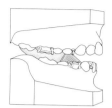

Twin block appliance

5

held in the locks by special sliding caps. Differential crown or root movement was achieved by using two archwires of different sizes (one longer than the other) and by appropriately squeezing both into the lock so that they lie on top of each other (in a coronal-apical direction). Occasionally, a lingual arch also was used in conjunction with the appliance.

Twin block appliance   Tooth-borne removable functional appliance that was developed by W.J. Clark. It consists of a maxillary and mandibular portion, which carry inclined planes constructed in such a way that an anterior displacement of the mandible and a certain amount of vertical separation of the arches are effected upon closure of the mouth. Due to the two-part design, the appliance is tolerated easily by the patient and thus increased wear is facilitated. The maxillary portion of the appliance includes capping of the molars, with an inclined plane at its mesial end. This plane engages a similar incline on the mandibular portion of the appliance, thus causing the mandible to assume the desired protruded position. Retention of the maxillary portion is achieved by modified Adams clasps [see Clasp, Delta] that span the second premolars and first molars. A labial bow with U-loops also is included in the maxillary portion. A headgear can be attached to the maxillary portion of the appliance by inserting a facebow into special coils incorporated in the delta clasps. The occasional addition of a midline expansion screw can pro-

vide compensatory maxillary arch expansion as the anteroposterior relationship improves.

The mandibular portion of the appliance carries capping in the premolar region only and is retained by delta clasps on the first premolars and C-clasps on the canines.

Two-by-four appliance (2x4)   A term denoting partial use of fixed orthodontic appliances, only including the 2 first permanent molars and the 4 permanent incisors. A 2x4 is most often used for treatment in the mixed dentition, e.g. for alignment, intrusion, or proclination of the incisors.

U-bow activator   A removable functional appliance developed by R. Karwetzky consisting of a maxillary and a mandibular part, which are connected by a U-shaped bow on either side. These U-bows allow gradual displacement of the mandible from its original position in small increments. The appliance

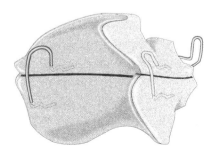

U-bow activator

exists in three variations, proposed for the treatment of Class II, Class III, or asymmetric malocclusions.

Universal appliance   An early fixed orthodontic appliance developed by S.R. Atkinson, combining some of the principles of edgewise and ribbon-arch appliances to achieve precise control of individual teeth in all planes of space. The appliance consisted of bands for all the teeth in both arches. Each band carried a bracket with two horizontal slots, of which the larger, occlusal slot opened occlusally and the smaller, gingival slot opened buccally. The occlusal slot could accommodate a ribbon arch of up to 0.015 x 0.028 inch (0.38 x 0.70 mm) in cross-section, or alternatively up to three 0.010-inch (0.25-mm) archwires. The wires for the gingival slot were 0.008 inch (0.20 mm) to 0.014 inch (0.35 mm) in diameter. Special lock pins held the archwires in place. A lingual arch was used, which was secured in horizontal sheaths soldered on the lingual aspect of the molar bands.

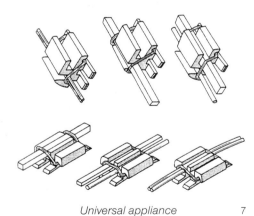

Universal appliance   7

Van Beek appliance   A removable functional appliance/high-pull headgear combination, developed by H. Van Beek. The facebow of the headgear is embedded rigidly in the acrylic at the anterior aspect of the appliance and is its only metal part. The appliance provides labial acrylic coverage of the maxillary incisors.

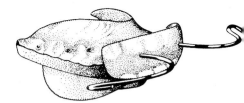

Van Beek appliance

Vestibular shield (Vestibular screen)   A simple removable appliance made of 2- t[o] 3-mm-thick acrylic or thermoplastic mater[i]al, occupying the vestibule and extendin[g] posteriorly to the distal margin of the las[t] erupted molar. The appliance can be co[n]structed with the mandible placed in an ante[-] rior position so that the incisors are in a[n] edge-to-edge relationship.

The appliance is intended to eliminate a[n] abnormal sucking habit or lip dysfunctio[n,] to establish a competent lip seal and t[o] interrupt contact between the tip of th[e] tongue and the lower lip, promoting mat[u]ration of the swallowing pattern. In patient[s] with a persistent tongue thrust, the vestibu[-] lar shield can be combined with a tongu[e] crib. [Also see Appliance, Oral screen.]

Appliance prescription   The set of charac[-] teristic values (in degrees) for mesiodist[al] tip ("angulation"), buccolingual inclinatio[n] ("torque"), and rotational offset, which ar[e] incorporated into each bracket for every ind[i-] vidual tooth; the "specifications" of a fixe[d] orthodontic appliance. The prescription [of] an orthodontic appliance usually is spec[i-] fied by the clinician at the time of placing th[e] order with the manufacturer or distributor.

Appliance setup   See Bracket setup.

Appliance trimming   Selective grinding awa[y] of acrylic from a removable appliance a[t] areas that contact the teeth. The purpose [of] this process is to guide tooth eruption an[d] aid in the development of a proper arch for[m.] Trimming is an important aspect of trea[t-] ment with removable and functional appl[i]ances.

Applied force system See Force system, Applied.

Apposition of bone See Bone apposition.

Approximal drift See Drift (of teeth), Mesial.

Ar See Cephalometric landmarks (Hard tissue), Articulare.

Arch A structure with a curved or bow-like outline. The term sometimes is used in orthodontics as a synonym for archwire.

Alveolar arch The arch formed by the ridge of the U-shaped maxillary and mandibular alveolar processes.

Auxiliary arch An accessory archwire commonly used in addition to the main or base archwire.

Base arch The main archwire occupying the bracket slots of a fixed orthodontic appliance system. Use of the term "base arch" implies the presence of other auxiliary arches or springs active at the same time.

Bypass arch An orthodontic archwire that is stepped around one or more teeth, so that these teeth are not included in it (due to their severe malposition, or other reasons).

Closing-loop arch An archwire in which closing loops are incorporated (unilaterally or bilaterally), commonly used for retraction of the incisors. A closing loop arch usually is made out of full-dimension stainless steel wire in an attempt to maintain the inclination

and angulation of the teeth as they are being retracted.

Dental arch The arch formed by the maxillary or the mandibular teeth, when viewed from the occlusal.

E-arch (High labial arch) Early orthodontic appliance used by E.H. Angle, consisting of bands on the molars and a heavy labial archwire extending around the dental arch. The end of the wire was threaded, and a small nut placed on the distal end of the archwire allowed it to be advanced to increase the arch perimeter. Individual teeth were ligated to this arch by means of stainless steel ligatures. The term still is used occasionally to signify a type of overlay arch made of heavier gauge wire, inserted into the headgear tubes of molar bands in order to aid in posterior expansion (or compression) of the dental arch, or to function as a lip bumper. [See also Arch, Overlay.]

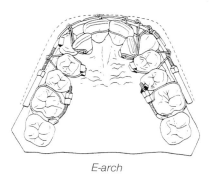

E-arch 13

Horseshoe arch Special type of transpalatal arch with the shape of a horseshoe, oriented in the horizontal plane.

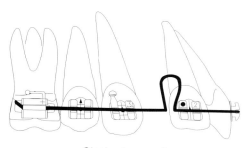

Closing-loop arch

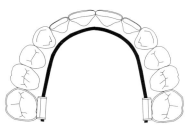

Horseshoe arch

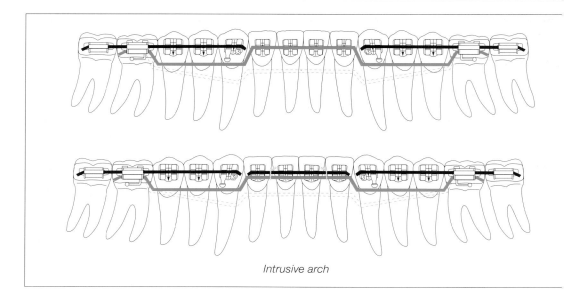

Intrusive arch

Intrusive arch An archwire used as the main wire, or as an auxiliary in the segmented arch technique, to achieve leveling of the dental arch by intrusion of the incisors. An intrusive arch is activated for incisor intrusion by placing tip-back bends mesial to the molar tubes. [Also see Arch, Utility.]

Lingual arch A single, heavy-gauge orthodontic wire, adapted to the lingual aspect of (usually) the mandibular arch, attached to bands on the first permanent molars. Two U-loops, often bent into the wire mesial to the first molars, offer the possibility of adjustment in the sagittal direction.
The lingual arch is generally used for stabilization (anchorage reinforcement), as a holding arch for space maintenance, for expansion, for increase of dental arch length, or for anchorage when intermaxillary traction is used. Lingual arches can be of fixed (soldered) or fixed/removable design.

Nance holding arch Maxillary fixed appliance developed by H.N. Nance, consisting of a heavy palatal wire soldered to the palatal aspect of the first molar bands. The wire is directed from the molars anteriorly and is attached to an acrylic button that rests against the most superior and anterior aspect of the palatal vault. Used as a space maintainer, or as a means to reinforce anchorage.

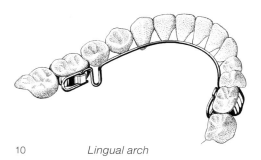

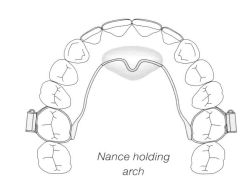

10   *Lingual arch*

Nance holding arch

Overlay arch (Piggyback arch) An auxiliary archwire added to the main (base) archwire, most commonly used to achieve transverse changes in the dental arch or individual tooth movements. An overlay arch can be inserted in the auxiliary slots or the headgear tubes of the molar attachments, or it may be simply tied onto the main archwire.

Porter arch (W-arch) Maxillary fixed/removable appliance consisting of a heavy-gauge (0.036 inch or 0.90 mm) transpalatal wire with a W-shaped configuration, secured to the palatal aspect of the first molar bands. It is used to achieve expansion of the maxillary dental arch and/or derotation of the molars.

Transpalatal arch (TPA, Palatal bar, Goshgarian-type palatal arch) Maxillary fixed or fixed/removable appliance consisting of a 0.036-inch (0.90-mm) or higher gauge wire that extends from one maxillary first molar, along the contour of the palate, to the maxillary first molar on the opposite side. The arch is adapted to the curvature of the palatal vault, so that it lies 2 to 3 mm away from the palatal mucosa. A U-loop, which usually is incorporated midway across its span, can be activated for expansion or constriction of the intermolar width. The TPA also is used commonly for anchorage reinforcement, for derotation of the molars, or for producing root movements of these teeth.

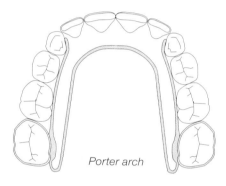

Porter arch

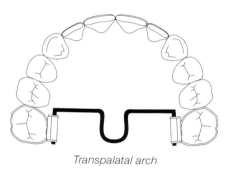

Transpalatal arch

Stopped arch (Proclination arch, Advanced arch) An orthodontic archwire with stops or loops (usually placed mesial to the first molar tubes) to procline the incisors, or to maintain the existing arch length.

Utility arch A maxillary or mandibular continuous archwire bypassing the canines and/or premolars to achieve leveling of the arch and/or uprighting of the molars, or to function as a stopped arch for incisor proclination. The utility arch, which was introduced by R.W. Ricketts, usually is made out of 0.016 x .0016-inch (0.41 x 0.41-mm) or 0.016 x 0.022-inch (0.41 x 0.56-mm) stainless steel or cobalt-chromium wire. The wire is stepped away from the occlusal plane between the first molars and lateral incisors for convenience and comfort. Avoiding engagement of the premolars and canines results in improved load/deflection properties because of the length of wire between the molar and incisor segments. The stepping of the archwire in a gingival direction in

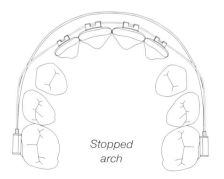

Stopped arch

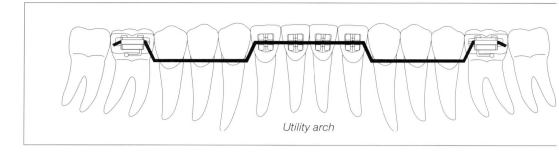

Utility arch

the buccal segments also reduces the risk of deformation during mastication. The utility arch can be used for movement of the incisors in the vertical and/or sagittal plane of space.

Arch bars Half-round, oval, round or flat wire bars, bent to fit the labial surface of the dental arches, in the cervical third of the crowns. Arch bars may carry special bases so they can be bonded to the teeth, or more commonly, they can be attached to them with interdental ligature wires. They may contain supporting elements, such as hooks or eyelets, for attaching elastic bands or tie wires. Arch bars are used to facilitate intermaxillary fixation in orthognathic surgery, or for stabilization of fractures of the maxilla or mandible. Single arch bars also are used sometimes for stabilization of traumatized teeth.

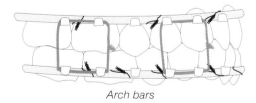

Arch bars

Arch-contouring pliers See Orthodontic instruments, Arch-forming pliers.

Arch coordination One of the aspects of fixed appliance orthodontic treatment by which it is made sure that the maxillary and mandibular dental arches fit harmoniously with each other, with corresponding arch forms and good anterior and buccal overjet. [Also se Archwire coordination.]

Arch depth The perpendicular distance in th midsagittal plane from the most labial mi point between the central incisors to a lir connecting the distal surfaces of two po terior corresponding teeth in a dental arc usually the second premolars (or secon deciduous molars).

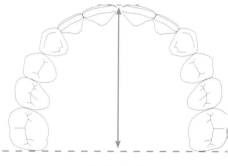

Arch depth

Arch form The shape of an individual denta arch, or of an archwire formed to fit or shap that arch. The arch form can be paraboli hyperbolic, ellipsoidal, square, tapering, \ shaped etc.

Arch-forming pliers See Orthodontic instru ments, Arch-forming pliers.

Arch length (Arch perimeter) A measure ment of space available in the dental arct for alignment of the teeth. *See illustratio next page.*

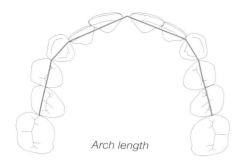

Arch length

Arch length discrepancy A difference between the space available in the dental arch and the space required to align the teeth. An arch length discrepancy can either be in the form of a deficiency or an excess of arch length.

Arch length deficiency (Crowding) A negative difference between the space available in the dental arch and the space required to align the teeth. With regard to the severity of space deficiency, crowding is divided into three categories: first-degree (mild) crowding, second-degree (moderate) crowding and third-degree (severe) crowding.

The classification into primary, secondary and tertiary crowding takes into account the etiology of the space deficiency.

Primary (hereditary) crowding is determined genetically and is caused by disproportionately sized teeth and jaws. *Secondary* crowding is an acquired anomaly caused by mesial drifting of the posterior teeth after premature loss of deciduous teeth in the lateral segments and/or lingual or distal displacement of the anterior teeth.

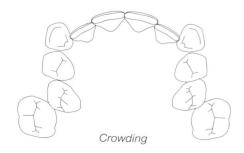

Crowding

The etiopathogenesis of *tertiary* crowding is still under debate. This type of crowding—primarily in the mandibular anterior teeth—occurs during and after adolescence and was previously thought to be associated with third molar eruption. Others attribute the anomaly to differential anteroposterior growth of the maxilla and mandible terminating at different times, in combination with differential rotation of the maxilla and mandible with growth. Malocclusions with crowding are more common in modern populations than those involving interdental spacing and wide arches.

Arch length excess (Spacing) A positive difference between the space available in the dental arch and the space required to align the teeth.

As with crowding, a distinction can be made between primary, secondary and tertiary spacing.

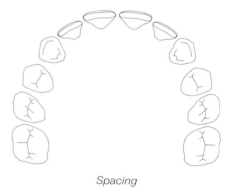

Spacing

Primary (hereditary) spacing is determined genetically and is caused by disproportionately sized teeth and jaws, including tooth agenesis.

Secondary spacing is an acquired anomaly caused by drifting of teeth, subsequent to loss of a permanent tooth.

Tertiary spacing is caused by bone loss due to periodontal disease, resulting in a disturbance of the equilibrium of forces acting on the teeth and associated tooth movement.

Arch marker See Marking pencil.

Arch perimeter See Arch length.

Arch turret See Orthodontic instruments, Turret.

Arch width The breadth of the dental arch, determined by measuring distances between corresponding contralateral teeth (e.g. intercanine width, intermolar width).

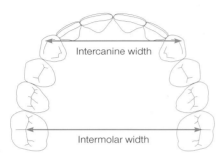

Arch width

Archwire (Arch wire) A wire engaged in orthodontic attachments that are affixed to the crowns of two or more teeth to cause or guide tooth movement.

Continuous archwire An archwire that engages, through crown attachments (brackets and tubes), many or all of the erupted teeth in the maxillary or mandibular dental arch (i.e. from molar to molar).

Finishing archwire The archwire used in the finishing stage of treatment.

"Full dimension" archwire A large re[c]tangular archwire that will practically "fi[ll]" the bracket slot. Usually referring to a[n] 0.017 x 0.025-inch (0.43 x 0.64-mm) [or] 0.018 x 0.025-inch (0.46 x 0.64-mm) arc[h] wire, when a 0.018 x 0.025-inch (0.4[6] x 0.64-mm) slot size is used, or an 0.0[21] x 0.025-inch (0.53 x 0.64-mm) archwi[re] when a 0.022 x 0.028-inch (0.56 x 0.7[1] mm) slot is used.

Main archwire See Arch, Base.

Multiloop archwire A stainless ste[el] archwire with loops of various configur[a]tions bent in the interbracket spaces, [to] increase the flexibility of the wire to facilita[te] bracket engagement. The use of multiloo[p] archwires was very common in earlier day[s] of orthodontics, when the only way to reduc[e] the load/deflection characteristics of th[e] appliance was to increase the length of wir[e] between brackets. It has now been large[ly] replaced by multistrand wires, or wire[s] made of various superelastic material[s]. [Also see Loop; Load/deflection rate.]

Overlay archwire See Arch, Overlay.

Piggyback archwire See Arch, Overlay.

Sectional archwire (Segmental arch wire) An archwire that engages only [a] few teeth within an arch (e.g. only the fo[ur] incisors, or only the teeth in a posterio[r] dental segment.) [Also see Mechanic[s]; Segmental arch.]

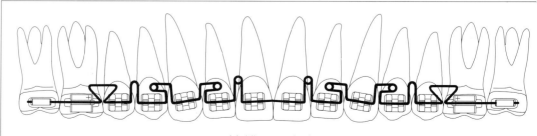

Multiloop archwire

Stabilizing archwire A stiff, full-dimension archwire, used to maintain the actual position of the teeth (e.g. prior to orthognathic surgery), or to consolidate a number of teeth, forming a large anchorage segment.

Stopped archwire See Arch, Stopped.

Surgical archwires The stabilizing archwires that are in place during the orthognathic surgical procedure. They usually are rectangular stainless steel wires to which hooks have been added in the interbracket spaces to facilitate intermaxillary fixation. Surgical archwires must fit passively to be effective. If they create any tooth movement after the impressions are made for the model surgery and for splint construction, the splint will no longer fit.

Archwire bends See Bends, Archwire.

Archwire coordination The process of superimposing the maxillary and mandibular archwires prior to placing them in the patient's mouth, to ensure that their arch form fits with each other, with the objective of achieving coordinated dental arches. [Also see Arch coordination.]

Archwire cross-section Various diameters and cross-sectional shapes of orthodontic archwires exist. The ones most commonly used, specified by the size of the cross-section in inches (mm) are:

Round:
0.012 inch (0.30 mm),
0.014 inch (0.35 mm),
0.016 inch (0.40 mm),
0.017 inch (0.43 mm),
0.018 inch (0.46 mm),
0.019 inch (0.48 mm),
0.020 inch (0.51 mm)
Square:
0.016 x 0.016 inch (0.41 x 0.41 mm),
0.017 x 0.017 inch (0.43 x 0.43 mm),
0.018 x 0.018 inch (0.46 x 0.46 mm),
0.019 x 0.019 inch (0.48 x 0.48 mm)

Rectangular:
0.016 x 0.022 inch (0.41 x 0.56 mm),
0.017 x 0.022 inch (0.43 x 0.56 mm),
0.017 x 0.025 inch (0.43 x 0.64 mm),
0.018 x 0.025 inch (0.46 x 0.64 mm),
0.019 x 0.025 inch (0.48 x 0.64 mm),
0.020 x 0.025 inch (0.51 x 0.64 mm),
0.021 x 0.025 inch (0.53 x 0.64 mm).

Archwire locks See Gurin lock.

Archwire size See Archwire cross-section.

Archwire stop A bend, auxiliary attachment, or occasionally a drop of solder placed on an archwire to prevent it from sliding mesially or distally through the orthodontic attachments.

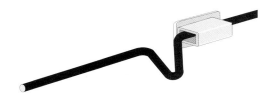

Archwire stop

Arcon articulator See Articulator, Arcon.

Arm, Moment See Moment arm.

Arm, Power See Power arm.

Arrow clasp See Clasp, Arrowhead.

Arrowhead clasp See Clasp, Arrowhead.

Arthritis Inflammation of a joint, usually accompanied by pain.

    Degenerative arthritis See Osteoarthritis.

    Hypertrophic arthritis See Osteoarthritis.

Juvenile rheumatoid arthritis (JRA, Still's disease) Idiopathic arthritis that begins before the age of 16 years, with rheumatoid factor found in 70% of the patients. It is more common in women, with onset most often between 12 and 15 years of age. Resorption of the condylar head is a common finding, creating a severe Class II malocclusion with a progressively worsening anterior open bite. Any orthognathic surgical treatment must be deferred until the active inflammatory process subsides.

Rheumatoid arthritis Chronic polyarticular erosive inflammatory disease, more common in women, characterized by bilateral involvement of joints, with proliferative synovitis, atrophy and rarefaction of bones.

Arthrodial joint See Joint, Arthrodial.

Arthrography of the TMJ Radiographic visualization of the TMJ.

Single-contrast arthrography Arthrography following injection of a radiopaque contrast medium into the joint space(s) to determine the location and integrity of intra-articular soft tissue structures, including disc position, soft tissue contours, presence of perforations, joint motion, intra-articular free bodies and adhesive capsulitis.

Double-contrast arthrography A procedure similar to single-contrast arthrography but with injection of a small amount of radiopaque contrast agent followed by inflation of the joint with air.

Single-space arthrography Contrast arthrography with injection of a radiopaque contrast medium into either the upper or the lower synovial joint compartment of the TMJ.

Double-space arthrography Contrast arthrography with injection of a radiopaque contrast agent into both the upper and lower synovial joint spaces.

Arthrokinetics of the TMJ Temporomandibular joint motion.

Depression of the mandible Movement of the mandibular alveolar process away from that of the maxilla.

Distraction of the mandible Separation of the surfaces of the TMJ by extension, without injury or dislocation of the parts.

Elevation of the mandible Movement of the mandibular alveolar process toward that of the maxilla.

Lateral excursion of the mandible Right or left movement of the mandible away from the median plane. [Compare with Laterotrusion and Mediotrusion.]

Protrusion of the mandible Anterior mandibular movement with bilateral forward condylar translation.

Retrusion of the mandible Posterior mandibular movement with bilateral backward condylar translation.

Arthroscopy Direct visualization of a joint with an endoscope.

Arthrosis Degeneration of a joint, evidenced by bony alterations.

Articular disc (Intra-articular disc, Meniscus) A thin biconcave pad of dense fibrous connective tissue, interposed between the temporal bone and the mandibular condyle, that divides the articular space into an upper and a lower compartment. It is devoid of any blood vessels or nerve fibers and its anterior and posterior borders (bands) are thick, whereas its central part (where the condylar head fits) is thinner. Anteriorly it may be attached to fibers of the superior head of the lateral pterygoid muscle. Posteriorly it attaches to a structure consisting of loose connective tissue, which is richly vascularized and innervated, known as the retrodiscal tissue (retrodiscal lamina). The medial and lateral aspects of the disc are attached to the lateral poles of the condyle by the collateral ligaments, which permit rotational movement of the disc on the condyle during opening and closing of the mouth.

Articular disk See Articular disc.

Articular eminence A convex bony ridge situated immediately anterior to the glenoid fossa of the temporal bone, that also is involved in the temporomandibular joint. The degree of convexity of the articular eminence is highly variable but important because the steepness of this surface dictates the pathway of the condyle when the mandible is positioned anteriorly.

Articular fossa of the temporal bone See Glenoid fossa.

Articulare (Ar) See Cephalometric landmarks (Hard tissue), Articulare.

Articulator A mechanical instrument that represents the temporomandibular joints and the jaws, to which maxillary and mandibular casts may be attached, with the intention of reproducing mandibular movements. Depending on the amount of adjustments that an articulator can accommodate (which increases the accuracy and precision of the simulation of the clinical situation), there are non-adjustable, semi-adjustable (anatomic) and fully adjustable (gnathologic) articulators. Articulators have all the mechanical limitations imposed by their construction. The various types and models show great variation in their function depending on the way they were constructed and the occlusal concepts on which they were based.

Arcon articulator An articulator that imitates the human anatomical relations of the maxilla and mandible, in that the condylar parts (balls) of the instrument are incorporated in the lower member of the articulator. [Compare with Articulator, Non-arcon.]

Non-arcon articulator An articulator built in such a way that the condylar parts of the instrument are incorporated in its upper member and the articular surfaces are part of the lower member (in this respect the instrument does not simulate the anatomical characteristics of the human skull). [Compare with Articulator, Arcon.]

Artificial undercuts See Undercuts, Artificial.

Artistic bends See Bends, Artistic.

Association A recognized pattern of morphological defects or malformations that currently is not considered to constitute a syndrome or an anomalad, but that may be reclassified as a syndrome or as an anomalad as knowledge advances.

Asymmetric elastics See Orthodontic elastics, Asymmetric.

Asymmetric expansion See Expansion, Asymmetric.

Asymmetric headgear See Headgear, Asymmetric.

Atherton's patch The small red triangular patch of thin and non-keratinized gingival epithelium often observed on the side opposite from the direction in which a tooth is moving. The first report of this phenomenon was made by J.D. Atherton and N.W. Kerr in 1968, associated with the mesial aspect of maxillary canines being distalized after extraction of the first premolars.

Attached gingiva See Gingiva, Attached.

Attachment, Gingival The part of the gingiva that is bound down to the underlying cementum and bone.

Attachment, Orthodontic A precision component that can be welded or soldered to a band, or bonded directly to a tooth, to facilitate the application of forces during orthodontic treatment. The general term encom-

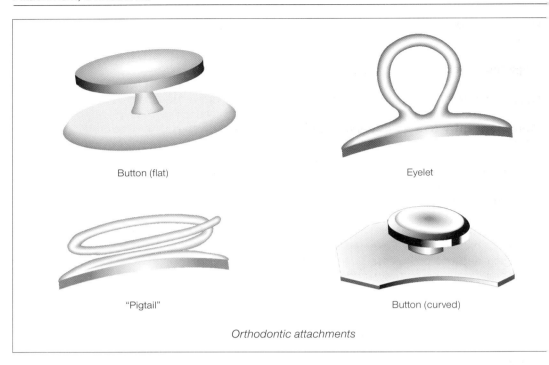

Button (flat)	Eyelet
"Pigtail"	Button (curved)

Orthodontic attachments

passes items such as brackets, tubes, buttons, eyelets, and "pigtail" attachments.

Attrition (Dental wear, Occlusal wear)
Loss of tooth structure due to repetitive physiological or parafunctional occlusal contact between the teeth. Attrition results in the formation of flat areas on the surface of teeth (*wear facets*) that have a polished appearance and readily reflect light. Although a certain degree of attrition is con-

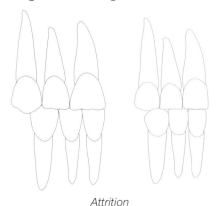

Attrition

sidered physiological with age, the presence of deleterious parafunctional habits such as bruxism may accelerate it. Attrition also affects the interproximal surfaces of the teeth. [Compare with Abrasion.]

Auriculo-orbital plane See Cephalometric lines, Frankfort horizontal plane.

Austenite The face-centered cubic (FCC) crystalline structure of iron and steel, or the body-centered cubic (BCC) structure in nickel-titanium alloys, at higher temperatures. In stainless steels, certain elements such as nickel maintain the austenitic structure at room temperature. Appropriate cooling of nickel-titanium alloys can induce transformation to a close-packed hexagonal martensitic phase (martensitic transformation). The transformation from austenite to martensite and vice versa is what gives alloys such as nickel-titanium the characteristic properties of *shape memory* and *superelasticity* (*pseudoelasticity*). [Also see Martensitic transformation.]

Australian wire   See Orthodontic wire, Australian.

Autogenous graft   See Graft, Autologous.

Autologous graft   See Graft, Autologous.

Autoradiography (Radio-autography)   A histological research technique used to determine the sites of synthesis of a substance within a tissue. A precursor of the substance, labeled by a radioactive material, is administered by either incubation (in the case of a culture) or injection (in the case of an experimental animal) and incorporated into the tissue. Following that, histological sections of the tissue are covered with a photographic emulsion and placed in the dark for some time. The final image on the photographic film is a two-dimensional representation of the pattern of synthesis of the substance within the tissue.

Autorotation (of the mandible)   The rotation of the mandible around the condylar axis (or an axis in the region of the condyles), after repositioning of the osteotomized maxilla. Mandibular autorotation can be simulated approximately during preparation of the surgical prediction tracing by rotating the mandibular template until the mandibular teeth contact the repositioned maxillary teeth. The same can be accomplished during model surgery using an articulator or one of the various operation simulation systems. This significant step in the surgical treatment planning process will determine the feasibility of a single-jaw (maxilla only) procedure, versus the need for bimaxillary surgery.

For example, in a patient with a Class II, Division 1, anterior open bite malocclusion, it may be feasible to achieve an ideal overjet/overbite relationship and to decrease the elongated lower anterior face height just by a maxillary differential impaction and subsequent mandibular autorotation, without the need for a mandibular osteotomy.

Autotransplantation (of a tooth)   The insertion into a prepared alveolar socket of a tooth, or a developing tooth germ from another site in the mouth of the same individual. Replacement of an avulsed tooth, while technically an autograft, is considered a replantation, rather than a transplant. [Also see Replantation.]

The most common potential side effects of the procedure, which is thought to be very technique- and operator-sensitive, are ankylosis, arrested root development and root resorption of the transplant. It is generally agreed that the best time to harvest a tooth for transplantation is when it has completed 1/4 to 3/4 of its root formation and has not yet emerged.

Auxiliary   An accessory device or appliance.

Torquing auxiliary   See Orthodontic springs, Torquing.

Auxiliary arch   See Arch, Auxillary.

Auxiliary tube   See Tube, Auxillary.

Avascular necrosis   Bone infarction not associated with sepsis, but with circulatory impairment (occlusion of blood vessels), leading to bony necrosis.

Avulsion   The complete separation of a tooth from its alveolus as a result of trauma.

Axes, System of   See Global reference frame.

Axis of rotation   The line about which rotation of a three-dimensional object actually occurs.

B

B-point   See Cephalometric landmarks (Hard tissue), B-point.

Ba   See Cephalometric landmarks (Hard tissue), Basion.

Ba-N   See Cephalometric lines, Basion-Nasion.

Ba-Pt-Gn   See Cephalometric measurements (Hard tissue), Facial axis angle of Ricketts.

Backward rotation (of the mandible)   See Mandibular rotation, Clockwise.

Bacterial plaque   See Plaque.

Balancing contact   See Occlusal contact, Non-working side.

Balancing interference   See Occlusal interference, Non-working side.

Balancing side   See Non-working side.

Ball clasp   See Clasp, Ball.

Band   See Orthodontic band.

"Band and bar" space maintainer   See Space maintainer, "Band and bar."

"Band and loop" space maintainer   See Space maintainer, "Band and loop."

Band biter   See Orthodontic instruments, Band seater.

Band burnisher   See Orthodontic instruments, Band burnisher.

Band-contouring pliers   See Orthodontic instruments, Band-contouring pliers.

Band pusher   See Orthodontic instruments, Band pusher.

Band-removing pliers   See Orthodontic instruments, Band-removing pliers.

Band seater   See Orthodontic instruments, Band seater.

Banding   The process of cementing an orthodontic band in place, which involves the selection of the appropriate band for certain tooth, its fitting and adaptation and finally, its fixation on the tooth by means of cement.

Barrer retainer   See Retainer, Spring.

Basal bone   See Bone, Basal.

Base arch   See Arch, Base.

Basilar kyphosis (Kyphosis of the cranial base)   A term indicating a reduce cranial base angle (NSBa). [Compare with Platybasia.]

Basion (Ba)   See Cephalometric landmark (Hard tissue), Basion.

Basion-Nasion line (Ba-N)   See Cephalometric lines, Basion-Nasion.

Bass appliance See Appliance, Bass.

Bayonet bends See Bends, First-order.

Beaver-tail burnisher See Orthodontic instruments, Band burnisher.

Begg appliance See Appliance, Begg.

Begg bracket See Appliance, Begg.

Behavioral therapy An attempt to change the attitude and habits of an individual, without the use of appliances or medications; a means to improve patient cooperation and compliance. Behavioral therapy is performed under the assumption that all elements of behavior can be learned. Essential in this approach is a clear explanation of the rationale of the therapy and the importance of the necessary motivation and persistence.

Bending test Experimental setup to determine the material properties of a specimen in bending. This involves the measurement of angular or linear deflection of an archwire segment, resulting from a bending moment or an applied force. A bending test designed for orthodontic wires is the American National Standards Institute/American Dental Association (ANSI/ADA) Specification No 32.

Bends (Archwire bends) Localized permanent deformations, placed into an archwire, that change its direction and/or orientation from the original. Bends are added to an archwire for various reasons. Some bends are placed without the purpose of generating any forces (e.g. bends placed to account for discrepancies in bracket positioning or tooth anatomy, to bypass teeth that will not be included in the archwire, or to avoid possible deformation of the archwire due to chewing). However, most bends are added with the purpose of generating a force system necessary for a specific tooth movement. Archwire bends were an indispensable part of treatment with the standard edgewise appliance, whereas with the straight-wire appliance they are supposed to be either avoided or greatly reduced. According to the orthodontic coordinate system introduced by C.H. Tweed, bends on an orthodontic wire are roughly categorized as 1st-order, 2nd-order and 3rd-order bends (see below).

Artistic bends (Esthetic bends) Bends to position anterior teeth for optimal esthetic appeal. (Usually referring to second-order bends on anterior teeth).

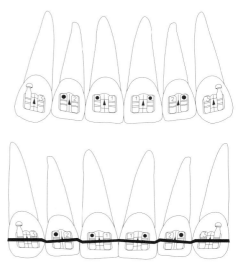

Artistic bends

Bayonet bends See Bends, First-order.

Distal-end bends (Cinching bends, Distal-end stops) Bends (usually in a gingival and/or medial direction) made on the archwire (after it is placed in all the brackets), distal to the terminal attachment, to

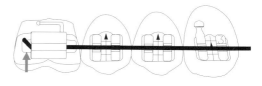

Distal-end bend

secure the archwire in place and prevent it from shifting through the brackets and causing soft tissue impingement during the time interval between patient visits. Distal-end bends are also useful in avoiding excessive proclination of the anterior teeth during leveling. [Also see Cinching.]

First-order bends (Offsets, In-out bends, Bayonet bends) Labiolingual offsets (step bends) in the archwire in the horizontal plane (in the plane of the wire), to accommodate for variations in the prominence and contour of labial/buccal surfaces of individual teeth. Typical locations along the archwire in which first-order bends were placed with the standard edgewise appliance were mesial to the maxillary lateral incisors (*insets* or *step-in bends*), canines (*offsets, canine eminence bends, curvature* or *step-out bends*) and first molars (*offsets, step-out* or *molar bayonet bends*). [Note: Vertical step bends that do not change the angulation of a tooth (e.g. step-up mesial and equal step-down distal to a bracket) are also considered first-order bends.]

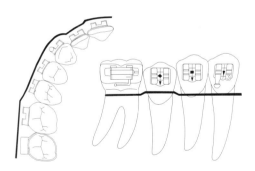

First-order bends

Gable bends See Bends, V-bends.

Second-order bends (Tip bends) Offsets in the archwire in the vertical plane, to change the angulation (mesiodistal tipping) of a tooth.

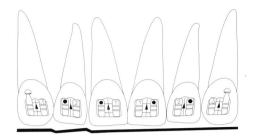

Second-order bends

Step bends Labiolingual or occlusogingival offsets in an archwire, in such a way that the segments of the wire on either side of the bend remain parallel to each other. A step bend generates equal and opposite forces and moments of equal magnitude and identical sense between the two teeth adjacent to it (corresponding to Burstone's geometry I). The magnitude of these forces and moments depends on the size of the step, the type and size of wire and the interbracket distance. Unlike V-bends, the force system created by a step bend remains practically unaffected by changing the location (mesiodistal position) of the step bend along the span between the two brackets. [Compare with Bends, V-bends.]

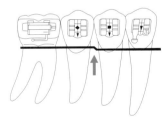

Step bend

Stop bends Bends that serve as archwire stops to keep the arch length constant, or to maintain the actual position of certain teeth

Third-order bends (Torquing bends) Twists in a rectangular archwire, placed when a change of the buccolingual or labiolingual inclination of specific teeth is desired. *See illustration next page.*

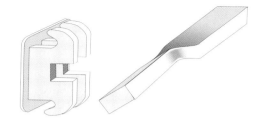

Third-order bend

Tip bends See Bends, Second-order.

Tip-back bends V-bends placed to tip teeth distally (as is typically done during the anchorage preparation stage of the Tweed technique).

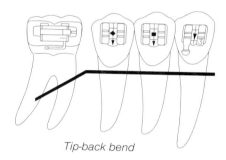

Tip-back bend

Tip-forward bends V-bends placed to tip teeth mesially. [Compare with Tip-back bends.]

Toe-in bends V-bends in the horizontal plane, typically placed at the ends of an

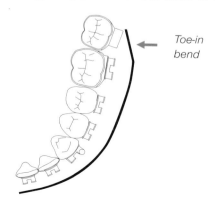

Toe-in bend

archwire, to achieve derotation or constriction of the terminal molars.

V-bends (Gable bends) 1. "V"-shaped bends with multiple applications, such as to avoid tipping of teeth into extraction sites during space closure. V-bends generate different force systems between two teeth, or two segments of teeth, depending on the location of the "V" along the wire (in relation to the two brackets). When the V-bend is in the center of the interbracket distance, the created force system involves equal and opposite moments between the teeth (corresponding to Burstone's geometry VI). [Also see Burstone's geometry classes.] [Note: According to the above definition, a V-bend changes the orientation of the long axis of the wire (i.e. the segment of the wire distal to the bend is no longer parallel with that mesial to it)].

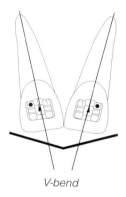

V-bend

2. The term V-bend occasionally is mentioned to denote a V-shaped stop (lug) bent into the archwire, maintaining the original wire orientation distal to it, as it is mesial to the bend. [Also see Archwire stop.]

Bennett angle On a lateral mandibular excursion, the non-working side condyle moves inferiorly, anteriorly and medially. The projection of this trajectory on the horizontal plane creates an angle with the sagittal plane, called the Bennett angle.

Bennett movement Lateral translation (side-shift) of the working side condyle during a lateral mandibular excursion. [Also see Bennett angle.]

Beta position The posterior component of an orthodontic spring, or the posterior point of attachment of a spring. [Compare with Alpha position.]

Beta-titanium alloy (TMA, β-Ti, Titanium-molybdenum alloy) A group of titanium-based alloys in which the elevated temperature body-centered cubic beta phase (crystalline structure) is stable at room temperature, rather than the hexagonal close-packed alpha phase. One such alloy, made of 77.8% titanium, 11.3% molybdenum, 6.6% zirconium, and 4.3% tin, was introduced to orthodontics in 1980 by C.J. Burstone and J.A. Goldberg, under the commercial name TMA (Ormco/Sybron).
TMA has a modulus of elasticity which is approximately 40% of that of stainless steel and double that of Nitinol. As well, it has excellent resilience and reasonably good formability, which allows stops and loops to be bent into the wire. In addition, beta-titanium wires can be spot-welded. However, its drawback is its high friction coefficient. The properties of TMA make it a good choice for fabrication of auxiliary springs and for intermediate and finishing archwires.

Bialveolar protrusion See Protrusion, Bimaxillary dentoalveolar.

Bialveolar retrusion See Retrusion, Bimaxillary dentoalveolar.

Bicortical screw See Fixation screws, Bicortical screw.

Bidimensional technique A fixed-appliance orthodontic treatment approach, developed by A.A. Gianelly, that is aimed at retraction of maxillary incisors by means of sliding mechanics, with good control of their inclination. This is attempted by using a 0.022-inch (0.56-mm) non-torqued bracket setup and a 0.016 x 0.022-inch (0.41 x 0.56-mm) stainless steel archwire, which has ninety-degree bends immediately distal to the lateral incisors, so as to fit into the incisor slots in a "ribbonwise" fashion. Alternatively, the incisors are bonded with 0.018-inch (0.46-mm) brackets and the canines, premolars and molars with 0.022-inch (0.56-mm) brackets, while an edgewise 0.018 x 0.025-inch (0.46 x 0.64-mm) stainless steel wire is used for retraction with sliding mechanics. The filling of the slot of the incisor brackets by the full-dimension archwire is supposed to result in good control of their root position and minimal lingual tipping as a side effect of retraction.

Bifid uvula A congenitally "split" uvula; a mild form of cleft palate.

Bilateral Occurring on both sides. [Compare with Unilateral.]

Bilateral sagittal split osteotomy (BSSO) See Osteotomy, Bilateral sagittal split.

Bi-level pin See Pin, Bi-level.

Bimaxillary dentoalveolar protrusion See Protrusion, Bimaxillary dentoalveolar.

Bimaxillary dentoalveolar retrusion See Retrusion, Bimaxillary dentoalveolar.

Bimaxillary prognathism See Prognathism, Bimaxillary.

Bimaxillary protrusion See Prognathism, Bimaxillary.

Bimaxillary retrognathism See Retrognathism, Bimaxillary.

Bimaxillary retrusion See Retrognathism, Bimaxillary.

Bimaxillary surgery See Orthognathic surgery, Bimaxillary.

Bimler appliance See Appliance, Bimler.

imler stimulator See Appliance, Bimler.

iocompatibility The ability to exist in harmony with the surrounding biological environment. The absence of all material properties that can harm biological tissues. In general, biocompatibility is measured on the basis of localized cytotoxicity (such as pulpal or mucosal response), systemic responses, allergenicity and carcinogenicity.

iofeedback A method of behavioral modification in which signals are relayed to the patient regarding the status of certain physiologic functions such as muscle activity, heart rate and blood pressure.

iomaterial Any substance other than medication that can be used for any period as a part of a system that treats, augments or replaces any tissue, organ or function of the body.

iomechanics Branch of science that deals with the mechanical properties of biologic structures as well as the interaction between mechanical devices and living tissues, organs and organisms. The implementation of engineering principles in living organisms.

iomechanics of tooth movement The field of study that seeks to relate force systems applied to the teeth, with the resulting quantitative and qualitative biological changes in the teeth and their surrounding structures.

ionator See Appliance, Bionator.

ird-beak pliers See Orthodontic instruments, Bird-beak pliers.

isected occlusal plane See Cephalometric lines, Occlusal plane.

ite See Occlusion.

ite block An interocclusal acrylic shelf that can be incorporated in a functional or other removable appliance to contact the occlusal surfaces of (usually) the posterior teeth.

Posterior bite blocks that are high enough to impinge into the freeway space are advocated by some clinicians for the treatment of patients with a long anterior lower facial height and an anterior open bite tendency. [Also see Appliance, Harvold-Woodside activator.]

Bite collapse (Posterior bite collapse) Reduction of the occlusal vertical dimension through (partial) loss or drifting of the posterior supporting dentition, often resulting in protrusion (flaring) of the maxillary anterior teeth.

Bite, Dual See Dual bite.

Bite force The force exerted by the masticatory musculature during biting, measured between particular occluding teeth—a parameter that is difficult to control. For standardization purposes, research attempts sometimes have turned to measuring "maximum bite force," a concept of relatively little value as it is rarely attained in everyday human masticatory function.

Bite former See Appliance, Bimler.

Bite-jumping appliance See Appliance, Kingsley.

Bite opening See Opening of the bite.

Bite plane The horizontal shelf-like part of a bite plate, on which the teeth touch. Bite planes also can be used in a fixed design (i.e. bonded to the teeth, or attached to a palatal arch).

Bite plate A removable orthodontic appliance designed to (temporarily) disengage the teeth and/or prevent selected teeth from occluding. A posterior bite plate commonly is used to disclude the anterior teeth and thus facilitate correction of an anterior crossbite. Anterior bite plates can be used to increase the lower anterior face height, to facilitate tooth movement and to correct a deep bite by extrusion of posterior teeth. *See illustration next page.*

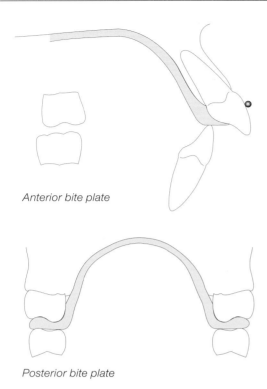

Anterior bite plate

Posterior bite plate

Bite raising The increase of lower face height by extrusion of the posterior teeth, as can be accomplished, for example, by a maxillary anterior bite plate contacting the incisal edges of the mandibular anterior teeth, while the opposing posterior teeth are kept apart and are free to erupt. Alternatively, extrusion of the posterior teeth can be obtained by using an anterior bite plane and fixed appliances, in combination with vertical posterior elastics. [Also see Opening of the bite.]

Bite registration (Wax bite) A wax record of an occlusal relationship between the maxilla and mandible, used in the trimming of orthodontic casts or in the mounting of casts on an articulator. A wax bite usually is taken in centric occlusion, or in centric relation (if there is a large mandibular CR-CO shift). [Also see Construction bite.]

Bite, "Sunday" See "Sunday" bite.

Bo See Cephalometric landmarks (Hard tissue Bolton.

Board-certified See ABO diplomate.

Board diplomate See ABO diplomate.

Board-eligible See ABO-eligible.

Board, Orthodontic A specialty certifying body whose main function is to establish the clinical proficiency and theoretical knowledge of an orthodontic specialist.

American Board of Orthodontic (ABO) The first specialty Board in dentistry, established in 1929 by the American Society of Orthodontia (former name of the American Association of Orthodontists). The ABO is the official certifying agency in orthodontics in the USA, recognized by the Council on Dental Education of the American Dental Association.
The Board continues to be sponsored by the American Association of Orthodontists but it is autonomous in organization. The eight directors of the ABO are nominated by the constituent organizations and elected by the House of Delegates of the American Association of Orthodontists.
ABO certification, which is a voluntary process, provides an extensive review of the orthodontist's basic education, as well as an intensive assessment of the orthodontist's clinical experience. Orthodontists may become certified as a Diplomate of the American Board of Orthodontics upon completion of three steps:
Phase I: Application
Phase II: Written Examination, and
Phase III: Clinical Examination.
[Also see ABO diplomate; ABO-eligible.]

Other Orthodontic Boards A number of other National or regional Boards exist worldwide, such as the Australian Orthodontic Board (AOB), the European Board of Orthodontists (EBO), the Mexican Orthodontic Board (Consejo Mexicano de

Ortodoncia—CMO), and the Philippines Board of Orthodontics (PBO).

odily movement (of a tooth) See Orthodontic tooth movement, Translation.

olton (Bo) See Cephalometric landmarks (Hard tissue), Bolton.

olton analysis A method developed by W. Bolton (1958) for the evaluation of mesiodistal tooth size discrepancies between sets of corresponding maxillary and mandibular teeth. The analysis distinguishes between the "overall ratio," which involves all permanent teeth except the second and third molars, and the "anterior ratio," which encompasses only the six anterior teeth of each jaw. For this analysis it is assumed that the relatively smaller tooth material is the correct one. A table of standard values lists the tooth width value in the opposing arch that is ideally related to this given correct value. The difference between the ideal and actual dental width in the arch with the excess value gives an estimate in millimeters of the severity of tooth size discrepancy between the arches. [See also Tooth size discrepancy.]

olton-Brush Growth Study The Bolton Growth Study is a longitudinal study of over 4,000 subjects from birth to adulthood, which was started in 1929 under the direction of B.H. Broadbent, Sr., at Case Western Reserve University in Ohio. The records that were obtained included lateral and P-A cephalometric radiographs, hand-wrist radiographs and dental casts, as well as nutritional, dental and medical health status data. Approximately 2,900 of the subjects of the Bolton study were also enrolled in the Brush study, which involved radiographs of the entire skeleton taken on a yearly basis, as well as extensive anthropometric, nutritional, health and psychological data, also recorded annually. All records of subjects in both studies are currently housed and curated through the Bolton-Brush Growth Study Center at Case Western Reserve University.

Bolton discrepancy See Tooth size discrepancy.

Bolton plane See Cephalometric lines, Bolton plane.

Bolton triangle See Cephalometric measurements (Hard tissue), Bolton triangle.

Bonded lingual retainer See Retainer, Bonded lingual.

Bonding The attachment (adhesion) of a material directly onto a tooth by means of a bonding agent. In common orthodontic use the term denotes the process by which orthodontic attachments are affixed to the teeth, which has become a routine part of fixed appliance therapy. The most commonly used bonding techniques involve acid etching and composite resin, or conditioning and glass-ionomer cement.

Direct bonding An intraoral procedure in which orthodontic attachments are oriented by inspection and bonded on each tooth individually. Direct bonding does not require a laboratory stage.

Indirect bonding A two-step procedure for bracket placement. Brackets are first placed temporarily on a plaster cast and subsequently transferred "en masse" to the mouth by means of a transfer tray (template). The transfer tray preserves the pre-determined orientation of the brackets and allows them to be bonded simultaneously. Indirect bonding is particularly useful for lingual attachments, due to the difficulties encountered in positioning them using a direct technique and the anatomical variability of the lingual surfaces of the teeth.

Sequential bonding Initial partial bonding of the teeth within an arch, bypassing certain teeth to avoid potential detrimental effects to the remaining teeth, as a consequence of the malposition of the former. An example is the exclusion of distally tipped maxillary canines from the initial archwire in a patient with deep overbite, for fear of causing extrusion of the incisors. The teeth that were omitted initially can be bonded and included in the archwire at a later time, once their position is improved spontaneously or by other intervention (e.g. segmental mechanics).

Bonding agent (Adhesive system) A material that, when applied to surfaces of substances, can join them together, resist separation, and transmit loads across the bond. Available bonding agents for orthodontic use include, in addition to the conventional autocuring composite resins, light-curing composite resins and glass-ionomer cements, as well as hybrid materials comprising glass-ionomer and composite components (*resin-modified glass-ionomers*). [Also see Bonding; Orthodontic cement, Glass-ionomer; Compomers.]

Bone A dense type of connective tissue, consisting of cells in a matrix of intercellular ground substance and collagen fibers. This organic matrix is impregnated with the mineral component of bone, consisting mainly of calcium phosphate and hydroxyapatite, which imparts rigidity to bone. Bone is a highly dynamic type of tissue that constantly remodels. Modeling and remodeling of bone constitutes the basis of orthodontic tooth movement.

Alveolar bone The bone making up the alveolar process. [Sometimes this term is used—strictly speaking, incorrectly—to refer to the bone lining the alveolus (what radiologists call *lamina dura* and histologists name *bundle bone*, because of the bundles of PDL fibers that are embedded in it).]

Basal bone The bone that underlies, supports, and is continuous with the alveolar process. [Also see Apical base.]

Bundle bone Immature bone that develops directly in uncalcified connective tissue and is only partially mineralized. Bundle bone is commonly found in areas of attach-

ments of ligaments and tendons, as we as adjacent to the periodontal ligament (li ing the alveolus). It contains characterist perpendicular striations created by Sha pey's fibers.

Cancellous bone Spongy bone foun adjacent to compact bone, forming labyrinthine system of trabeculae and inte communicating spaces, occupied by bon marrow. In younger individuals the space are filled by red (hematopoietic) marro and in adults by yellow marrow, with a hig fat cell content.

Cartilaginous bone (Endochondr bone) Any bone that develops through ca tilaginous (endochondral) ossification.

Compact bone (Dense bone) The har external portion of bone which, althoug it appears solid, microscopically exhibit spaces (*lacunae*) and intercommunicatin tunnels (*canaliculi*), occupied by the ostec cytes and their processes, respectivel The matrix consists of layers (*lamellae*), sep arated by cementing substance. Lamella occur as the result of differences in fibr orientation in adjacent layers. Rest perio in bone formation or destruction may b recorded as resting and resorption lines.

Cortical bone The external compact bon tissue covering any given bone.

(Intra)membranous bone Any bon that develops by intramembranous ossifica tion.

Lamellar bone A strong, highly organize and well-mineralized tissue, that compose 90% of the adult human skeleton. When ne lamellar bone is formed, a portion of the tot mineral content is deposited by osteoblast during primary mineralization. Secondar mineralization (to complete the process) a physiochemical process requiring mar months. Within physiological limits, strengt of bone is directly related to its miner content. In ascending order, the relativ strengths for different histological types of bone are woven bone < new lamellar bone < mature lamellar bone.

Woven bone A highly variable in structure, relatively weak, disorganized and poorly mineralized type of bone. It serves a critical wound healing role by 1) rapidly filling osseous defects, 2) providing initial continuity for fractures and osteotomy segments, and 3) strengthening a bone weakened by surgery or trauma. The first bone laid down as a consequence of orthodontic tooth movement is usually of the woven type. Woven bone is not found in the adult skeleton under normal, steady-state conditions. It either is compacted to form composite bone or is remodeled to lamellar bone.

ne apposition Addition of new bone to bony surfaces by osteoblastic activity.

ne graft See Graft, Alveolar bone.

ne modeling See Modeling (of bone).

ne plate See Fixation plate.

ne remodeling See Remodeling (of bone).

ne resorption The removal of bone by osteoclastic activity.

Direct resorption (Frontal resorption) The resorption of bone on the pressure side of the periodontal ligament (PDL) by osteoclasts that arrive at the site by the blood flow. Direct resorption occurs as a response to the application of sustained orthodontic force of relatively low magnitude. Despite the desirability of producing tooth movement by direct resorption, this can be difficult to perform in clinical practice. Even with very light forces, small avascular areas are likely to develop in the PDL and tooth movement will be delayed until these can be removed by undermining resorption. [Compare with Bone resorption, Undermining.]

Undermining resorption (Indirect resorption) If the magnitude of the applied force is high enough to totally occlude the blood vessels on the pressure side and cut off the blood supply to an area within the PDL, a sterile necrosis occurs. Because of its glass-like histologic appearance due to the disappearance of cells, such an avascular area is referred to as *hyalinized*. In such a situation, remodeling of bone adjacent to the necrotic area must be accomplished by cells derived from adjacent undamaged areas (since the blood supply is completely cut off), which does take place eventually, but only after the lapse of considerable time. Osteoclasts appear on the endosteal side of the lamina dura and begin to resorb the bone immediately adjacent to the necrotic PDL area. Since the osteoclastic attack is on the underside of the lamina dura, this process is described as undermining resorption. When hyalinization and undermining resorption occur, an inevitable delay (several days or weeks) in tooth movement results. [Also see Hyalinization.]

Bone scan See Emission scintigraphy.

Bonwill triangle An equilateral triangle, each side of which is supposed to be 4 inches (102 mm) long, as advocated by W.G.A. Bonwill in 1858. The triangle is formed by connecting the medial contact point of the mandibular central incisors (or the midline of the residual mandibular alveolar ridge) to the centers of the condyles.

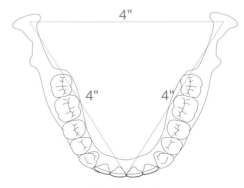

Bonwill triangle

Boot loop See Loop.

Border movements (of the mandible)
Movements of the mandible at the boundary or margin of the envelope of movement, as determined by the joint anatomy and function. All other mandibular movements take place within the limits of the border movements.

Box elastics See Orthodontic elastics, Vertical.

Box loop See Loop, Box.

Braces See Appliance, Fixed.

Brachycephalic Anthropometric term used to denote an individual with a larger than average cranial width; having a cephalic index greater than 81. Brachycephaly may result from premature synostosis of the coronal suture. [Compare with Dolichocephalic.]

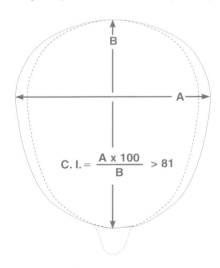

$$C.\ I. = \frac{A \times 100}{B} > 81$$

Brachycephaly

Brachyfacial (Brachyprosopic) A facial pattern characterized by a broad, square face. [Compare with Dolichofacial.]

Bracket Precisely fabricated orthodontic attachment made of metal, plastic or ceramic material, which can be bonded to a tooth or welded to a band. It carries a horizont and/or a vertical channel of standard siz called a "slot," that can receive an archwi or other orthodontic spring as part of a fixe orthodontic appliance. The size and shap of the slot vary with the orthodontic tec nique practiced and the type of applian used. The base of the bracket usually co tains a welded mesh or other retentive stru ture to increase bonding strength. [Also se Bracket slot; Bracket wings; Bracket setu

Begg bracket See Appliance, Begg.

Broussard bracket An edgewise brac et with an extra 0.0185 x 0.046-inch vertic slot, introduced by G.J. Broussard. The ve tical slot was designed to receive a doubl 0.018-inch auxiliary wire, but it also may t used for insertion of uprighting springs other orthodontic auxiliaries.

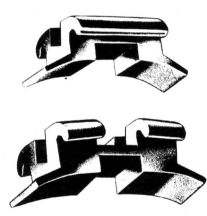

Broussard brackets

Ceramic bracket The esthetic alternati to plastic brackets [made of poly-monocrystalline alumina (sapphire)]. The brackets usually provide good color fidel and stain resistance. However, their frictic al resistance in sliding is increased whe compared to metal and plastic bracke Other potential drawbacks of ceram brackets include abrasion of antagonis teeth with which they come in conta proneness to fracture of wings, damac to enamel on debonding, difficulty of removal, discoloration, and increased thickness (bulk). These limitations call for caution in their use (for example, ceramic brackets may not be recommended for bonding onto teeth with cracks or signs of physical defects).

Clear bracket See Bracket, Esthetic.

Edgewise bracket See Appliance, Edgewise.

Esthetic bracket (Clear bracket) Type of bracket that is tooth-shaded and thus esthetically more attractive than conventional metal attachments (e.g. plastic and ceramic brackets).

Extraction series bracket Brackets designed with variations in tip, torque and rotation, as a further development of the straight-wire appliance, recommended by L.F. Andrews, to meet the needs of individual extraction cases. For example, extraction series canine brackets have increased angulation to counteract the tendency for distal tipping during canine retraction. Similarly, extraction series maxillary incisor brackets have extra torque to make up for the tendency of the incisors to tip lingually during retraction.

Fully programmed bracket The type of bracket used in the straight-wire appliance, which is pre-angulated, pre-torqued and has built-in offsets and insets to accommodate differences in morphology of various tooth types.

Lewis bracket A single bracket with a mesial and a distal extension wing, contacting the underside (lingual aspect) of the archwire. These extension wings are also available with anti-tip spurs at their ends that can be placed above or below the archwire to control the angulation of a tooth. Lewis brackets were designed to overcome the inefficiency of a single bracket to control the rotation and tipping of a tooth. By bending

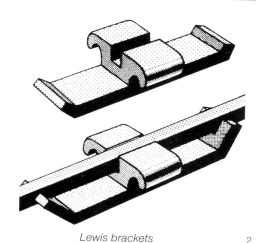

Lewis brackets 2

the extension wings of a Lewis bracket in the appropriate way, the force system required for derotation and uprighting of the tooth is created, by their interaction with the archwire.

Metal bracket The most widely used brackets, universally, for their superior qualities. They are typically made of stainless steel, but occasionally also of titanium and its alloys, or of Co-Cr alloys. The main drawback of metal brackets is their color and visibility, which may be objectionable to some patients. However, metal brackets have been miniaturized significantly through continuous redesigning by manufacturers. One additional limitation may be related to nickel hypersensitivity in some patients, when stainless steel brackets are used.

Plastic bracket The early plastic brackets were made of polycarbonate and plastic molding powder (Plexiglas). These brackets did not last long because of discoloration, fragility and softening with time (poor integrity of the bracket slot). Several improvements have been made to reinforce plastic brackets and to improve their color stability, including precision-made stainless steel slot inserts to reduce friction and ceramic material fillers (15% to 30%) to strengthen their matrix.

Pre-angulated bracket An orthodontic bracket having its slot inclined with respect to the plane of the archwire, permitting control of the mesiodistal (second-order) angulation of the tooth, by engaging a straight archwire.

Pre-torqued bracket An orthodontic bracket having its slot rotated with respect to its base (and the plane of the archwire), so that it permits control of the labiolingual (third-order) inclination of the tooth by engaging a straight rectangular archwire of suitable cross-sectional dimensions.

Self-ligating bracket A bracket which carries a special locking mechanism to engage the archwire in the slot, without the need of a ligature. [Also see Appliance, SPEED.]

Siamese bracket See Bracket, Twin.

Single bracket (Single-width bracket) Narrow bracket with one set of tie-wings, which is inferior to a twin bracket in terms of rotational and tipping control but offers lower load-deflection rate for the same arch-wire, due to increased interbracket distance.

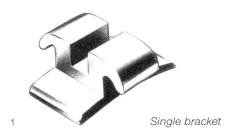

1   *Single bracket*

SPEED bracket See Appliance, SPEED.

Straight-wire bracket See Appliance, Straight-wire; Bracket, Pre-angulated; Bracket, Pre-torqued.

Twin bracket (Siamese bracket, Double-width bracket) A wide (double) bracket, with two sets of tie-wings, that allows better rotational control, as well as

better control of root position in the mes distal direction (angulation). However, whe a continuous archwire is used with tw brackets, the flexibility of the archwire decreased (compared to when single brac ets are used with the same archwire), due the reduced interbracket span.

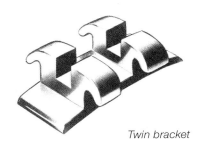

1   *Twin bracket*

Bracket-height gauge See Orthodon instruments, Bracket-positioning.

Bracket position indicator A disposab color-coded plastic attachment that is p vided by the manufacturer with some typ of brackets. It is meant to facilitate brack identification, as well as assist with the occ sogingival placement and axial orientati of the bracket during bonding.

Bracket-positioning instrument See Orth dontic instruments, Bracket-positionii instrument.

Bracket power arm See Power arm.

Bracket prescription See Appliance p scription.

Bracket-removing pliers See Orthodon instruments, Bracket-removing pliers.

Bracket setup Usually referring to the si of the bracket slot. The term *0.018-in (0.46-mm) setup* refers to a bracket slot s of 0.018 x 0.025 inch (0.46 x 0.64 mm) a the term *0.022-inch (0.56-mm) setup* refe to a slot size of 0.022 x 0.028 inch (0.56 0.70 mm). [Also see Appliance prescr tion.]

racket slot A standard component of an orthodontic bracket. A precisely fabricated horizontal and/or vertical channel, which can receive an archwire or other orthodontic mechanism as part of orthodontic treatment. The size and shape of the slot vary with the orthodontic technique practiced and the type of appliance used. The two bracket slot sizes most commonly used today, are 0.018 x 0.025 inch (0.46 x 0.64 mm) and 0.022 x 0.028 inch (0.56 x 0.70 mm).

Main slot The main horizontal slot of an edgewise or other bracket that receives the main archwire.

Vertical slot A standard part of a Begg bracket and an optional addition in an edgewise bracket. It is used for the insertion of various uprighting or rotation springs, or other segmental auxiliaries. [Also see Bracket, Broussard.]

racket slot engagement A measure of the play between the orthodontic archwire and bracket slot. [Also see "Play" of an orthodontic wire in the bracket slot; Second-order clearance; Third-order clearance.]

racket width The mesiodistal dimension of an orthodontic bracket.

racket wings Four projections (only two, in a single bracket) extending from the center of the bracket in a mesial-occlusal, distal-occlusal, mesiogingival and distogingival direction, creating undercuts that facilitate retention of the elastic or stainless steel ligatures that secure the archwire in the bracket slot.

raided wire See Orthodontic wire, Multistrand.

rass separator See Separator, Brass.

razing See Soldering.

Brittle A material exhibiting little or no permanent deformation before fracture. In other words, a brittle material fractures at or near its proportional limit.

Brittleness The relative inability of a material to sustain plastic deformation before it fractures.

Brodie syndrome See Crossbite, Complete maxillary buccal.

Broussard bracket See Bracket, Broussard.

Bruxism A diurnal or nocturnal parafunctional activity that includes clenching, bracing, gnashing and grinding of the teeth. Bruxism is a common cause of dental wear, muscle hypertrophy, pain and fatigue, and damage to the supporting tissues. It also is associated frequently with temporomandibular joint problems. Some consider occlusal interferences as a major factor in its etiology, whereas others believe that it is a centrally mediated phenomenon, related to emotional tension and stress. In absence of subjective awareness, bruxism can be diagnosed from the presence of shiny facets that are not generated by masticatory function. Bruxism can be observed through sleep laboratory recordings.

Bruxism appliance See Nightguard.

Bruxism splint See Nightguard.

BSSO See Osteotomy, Bilateral sagittal split.

Buccal crossbite See Crossbite, Buccal.

Buccal frenum See Frenum, Buccal.

Buccal overjet See Overjet, Buccal.

Buccal shield See Soft tissue shield.

Buccal stabilizing segment See Segment, Buccal stabilizing.

Buccally In the direction of the cheeks.

Buccinator muscle See Muscle, Buccinator.

Buccolingual tipping See Rotation, Third-order.

Buccolingually In a mediolateral direction, perpendicular to the sagittal plane (along the z-axis), for posterior teeth. When referring to anterior teeth, the term "labiolingually" is appropriate. [Also see Labiolingually; Global reference frame.]

Buccoversion Buccal inclination of a tooth or a group of teeth.

Bundle bone See Bone, Bundle.

Burlington cephalometric analysis See Cephalometric analysis, Burlington.

Burlington Growth Study A prospective longitudinal investigation that was started in 1952 in Burlington, Ontario, Canada, by R.E. Moyers of the Faculty of Dentistry, University of Toronto, under the responsibil-

ity of F. Popovitch. The 1,258 children i the Burlington sample represented 85% 90% of the children in Burlington, within th specified ages, at the time the study wა started. By the time the data collectio was completed in 1971, the population o Burlington had risen to 90,000 (from an ir tial 9,000 in 1952). Records were collecte annually from age 3 to 21 years. The recorc consisted of medical history, periodont: evaluation, six cephalometric radiograph one hand-wrist radiograph, impressions fc dental casts, intraoral radiographs (whei necessary), height and weight record: anthropometric data, social histories an electromyographic records for some sul jects. The entire material is currently house at the Burlington Growth Centre, Faculty c Dentistry, University of Toronto.

Burstone's geometry classes When tw teeth or two tooth-segments are connecte by a straight wire fully engaged in bot brackets, the generated force system varie depending on the relative angulation of th

Class	I	II	III	IV	V	VI
$\dfrac{\vartheta_A}{\vartheta_B}$	1.0	0.5	0	-0.5	-0.75	-1.0
$\dfrac{M_A}{M_B}$	1.0	0.8	0.5	0	-0.4	-1.0
$M_A \quad M_B$				0		
$F_A \quad F_B$	↓ ↑	↓ ↑	↓ ↑	↓ ↑	↓ ↑	0 0

Burstone's geometry classes

two brackets. There are six different possibilities (6 geometry classes) as described
by C.J. Burstone and H.A. Koenig (1974),
which are independent of the interbracket
distance. The geometries are based on the
ratio between the angles ϑ_A of the anterior
bracket and ϑ_B of the posterior bracket with
respect to a straight line passing through the
centers of the two brackets. In the description of the six geometries that follows, ϑ_A is
always (by convention) the smaller of the two
angles.

Geometry I In Class I geometry both brackets are angulated in the same direction and
by the same amount ($\vartheta_A/\vartheta_B = 1$). The same
situation is created when a straight wire is
inserted between two brackets, which lie at
different vertical heights, with parallel slots
(or equivalently, when a step bend is placed
on a wire between two aligned brackets).
The force system generated in this situation
consists of two equal and opposite forces
and two moments of equal magnitude and
the same sense. Since the moments at A
and B are equal in magnitude, the ratio
$M_A/M_B = 1$. Although the magnitude of the
moments may vary depending on the size
of the vertical discrepancy (step) and the
interbracket distance (assuming the material and size of the wire segment is constant),
the ratio M_A/M_B always remains +1 in Class
I geometry.

Geometry II In Class II geometry, both
brackets are angulated in the same direction
but the angle of the A bracket with the axis
connecting the centers of the two brackets
is half the size of that of the B bracket (ϑ_A/ϑ_B
= 0.5). As in geometry I, two equal and oppo-
site forces are created at the positions A and
B, as well as two moments of the same
sense. The magnitude of the moment at A
is 0.8 times that of the moment at B (M_A/M_B
= 0.8); thus it is reduced with respect to the
value developed in geometry I. Since the
ΣM is reduced, the magnitudes of the forces
are also reduced.

Geometry III This geometry is created
when the slot of the bracket A is parallel to
the line connecting the centers of the two
brackets ($\vartheta_A = 0$, and consequently ϑ_A/ϑ_B
= 0). A straight wire engaged in the bracket
slot at A would thus pass through the center of the bracket B. As in the first two geometries, two equal and opposite forces will be
produced at the brackets A and B, as well
as two moments of the same sense. In this
situation, the magnitude of the moment at
the bracket A is only half of that at the bracket B ($M_A/M_B = 0.5$). The magnitudes of
both forces and moments are reduced
with respect to those developed in geometry II.

Geometry IV In this situation the ratio
ϑ_A/ϑ_B is -0.5. In other words, the bracket at
position A is angled one-half of the
bracket at the position B (and in the opposite direction) relative to the axis connecting
the centers of the two brackets. The wire is
now said to be tied—to the A bracket—at the
point of dissociation. This means that forces
are independent from moments at position
A, where only a force is present and no
moment. The total force system that is produced by tying a straight wire into two brackets with this geometry includes equal and
opposite forces at the two brackets and a
moment at B, with no moment at A (M_A/M_B
= 0). The ΣM and the magnitudes of the
forces are further reduced in this geometry
compared to the previous ones.

Geometry V Class V geometry describes
a situation with a ratio ϑ_A/ϑ_B of -0.75. In
other words the two brackets still have oppo-
site angulation (as in geometry IV), but the
bracket A is now angulated 75% as much
as the bracket B relative to the axis connecting the centers of the two brackets. In
this situation the moment at bracket A is
opposite in sense to that of the moment generated at bracket B, and the ratio between
them is $M_A/M_B = -0.4$. The magnitude of
M_B is reduced further, as are the magnitudes of the forces acting on the two brackets.

Geometry VI In this geometry the two brackets are tipped towards each other by an equal amount ($\vartheta_A/\vartheta_B = -1$). The force system created consists of equal and opposite moments at the two brackets. No forces are generated. ΣM, the sum of all the moments, is equal to zero and the ratio M_A/M_B is equal to -1.

Button A small, mushroom-shaped orthodontic attachment that can be bonded directly onto a tooth or welded on a band. Buttons are mainly used as handles for elastic traction. [Also see Attachment, Orthodontic.]

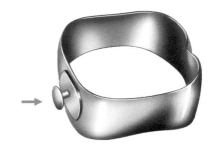

Button

Bypass arch See Arch, Bypass.

C

C See Cephalometric landmarks (Soft tissue), Cervical point.

C-clasp See Clasp, Circumferential.

Calculus (Tartar) Mineralized bacterial plaque, strongly attached to the tooth surface. According to its location there are two general types: supragingival and subgingival.

Callotasis See Distraction osteogenesis.

Callus The newly formed tissue (composed of varying amounts of fibrous tissue, cartilage and bone) that initially connects the bony fragments where a fracture has occurred.

Callus distraction See Distraction osteogenesis.

Camouflage orthodontic treatment The treatment of malocclusions with underlying mild to moderate skeletal jaw discrepancies, which achieves a good dental occlusion (Class I canine relationship and an ideal overjet and overbite), through extraction of certain teeth, to mask the skeletal problem. This type of treatment should be performed only if it will not have a harmful effect on facial esthetics, and if growth modification or orthognathic surgery are not applicable or not accepted by the patient. Extraction of teeth provides space for repositioning of the remaining teeth only in the anteroposterior plane of space. Patients with vertical or transverse skeletal problems would not benefit from extractions for camouflage. Similarly, if there is severe crowding, or excessive incisor protrusion in addition to a skeletal discrepancy (so that the extraction spaces will merely be used for alignment of the remaining teeth), camouflage treatment usually is contraindicated.

Camper's base plane See Cephalometric lines, Camper's base plane.

Cancellous bone See Bone, Cancellous.

Canine guidance (Canine-protected occlusion, Canine "rise") A particular scheme of disclusion of the dental arches during a lateral mandibular excursion. The labial (or distolabial) surface of the mandibular canine on the working side comes into contact with the lingual (or mesiolingual) surface of the maxillary canine, causing disarticulation of all other teeth.

Canine retraction Movement of the canine in a distal direction, usually into an extraction space. Individual retraction of the canines often is performed in an attempt to preserve posterior anchorage in patients with Class II malocclusions, and subsequently is followed by retraction of the incisors. Canine retraction can be performed by sliding or sectional mechanics.

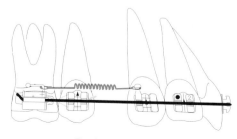

Canine retraction

Control of root position usually is critical, as bodily movement of the canines generally is required. [Also see Moment, Counter-moment.]

Canine rise See Canine guidance.

Canine-to-canine retainer See Retainer, Bonded lingual.

Cantilever See Orthodontic springs, Cantilever.

Cantilever mechanics See Mechanics, Cantilever.

Cantilever spring See Orthodontic springs, Cantilever.

Capitation dentistry A capitation dental program is one in which a dentist or dentists contract with the program's sponsor or administrator to provide all or most of the dental services covered under the program to subscribers in return for payment on a *per capita* basis. [Taken from the AAO Glossary of Dentofacial Orthopedic Terms, 1993.]

Capsular adhesion See Adhesion, Capsular.

Cartilage A semi-rigid specialized form of supporting/connective tissue, the characteristics of which mainly stem from the nature and predominance of ground substance in the extracellular matrix. Proteoglycans make up the ground substance and account for the solid, yet flexible, consistency of cartilage. Within the ground substance are embedded varying proportions of collagen and elastic fibers giving rise to three main types of cartilage: *hyaline cartilage, fibrocartilage* and *elastic cartilage.*
On completion of growth the cartilage mass consists of chondrocytes embedded in a large amount of extracellular matrix. At the periphery of mature cartilage is a zone of condensed supporting tissue called *perichondrium* containing chondroblasts with cartilage-forming potential. Growth of cartilage occurs by interstitial growth from with-

in and appositional growth at the periphery. Most cartilage is devoid of blood vessels and consequently the exchange of metabolites between chondrocytes and surrounding tissues depends on diffusion through the water of solvation of the ground substance. This limits the thickness to which cartilage may develop whilst maintaining viability of the innermost cells.

Elastic cartilage Elastic cartilage occurs in the external ear and external auditory canal, the epiglottis, part of the laryngeal cartilages and the walls of the Eustachian tubes. Its histological structure is similar to that of hyaline cartilage, with collagen as a major constituent. Its elasticity is derived from the presence of numerous bundles of elastic fibers in the cartilage matrix.

Fibrocartilage A type of cartilage which has features intermediate between cartilage and dense fibrous supporting tissue. It is found in the intervertebral discs, some articular cartilages, and in association with dense collagenous tissue in joint capsules, ligaments and the connections of some tendons to bone.

Hyaline cartilage The most common type of cartilage, found in the nasal septum, larynx, tracheal rings, most articular surfaces and the sternal ends of the ribs. It also forms the precursor of bone in the developing skeleton. Mature hyaline cartilage is characterized by small aggregations of chondrocytes embedded in an amorphous matrix of ground substance reinforced by collagen fibers.

Meckel's cartilage See Meckel's cartilage.

Primary cartilage See Primary cartilage.

Reichert's cartilage See Reichert's cartilage.

Secondary cartilage See Secondary cartilage.

artilaginous bone See Bone, Cartilaginous.

artilaginous joint See Joint, Cartilaginous.

asts See Orthodontic casts.

AT scan See Tomography, Computerized.

audal Inferior, towards the tail. [Compare with Cephalic.]

C See Chief complaint.

CD See Cleidocranial dysplasia.

ementation The attachment of bands or a fixed orthodontic appliance on the teeth by means of a dental cement.

enter of mass (CM) A point in a body where its entire mass can be considered concentrated for theoretical purposes. For homogeneous bodies with a regular geometrical shape, the CM is located at their geometric center (i.e. the center of a sphere, or the junction point of all three-dimensional diagonals of a cube).

enter of resistance (CRes) The point in a body at which resistance to movement can be considered concentrated, for mathematical analysis. For a free object in non-gravitational space, the center of resistance coincides with the center of mass. However, for a partially restrained object (as is the case for a tooth that is partially embedded in bone), the CRes is determined by the mass, shape and form of the tooth, as well as by the characteristics of the constraining elements (bone, PDL). [Other definition: CRes of a tooth is a point in the tooth on which the application of a single force will produce bodily movement of the tooth.] The location of the CRes is estimated to be between halfway and two thirds along the distance between the crest of the alveolar bone and the root apex in single-rooted teeth, and at the furcation area of multi-rooted teeth (assuming that the periodontal support is intact).

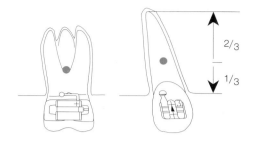

Center of resistance

Center of rotation (CRot) The point around which rotation actually occurs, when an object is being moved. The location of the CRot is variable and depends on the movement performed. The actual CRot of a tooth for a specific movement is almost impossible to determine and can be estimated only by the initial and final positions of the tooth. In orthodontics, the approximate location of the CRot can be controlled by varying the moment-to-force ratio at the bracket. The CRot during bodily movement is considered to lie at infinity. [For three-dimensional objects, the term *axis of rotation* is more accurate.]

Centric interference See Occlusal interference.

Centric occlusion (CO) See Occlusion, Centric.

Centric relation (CR) A gnathological term that has been used in dentistry for many years, especially in prosthodontics (as it was meant as a reproducible reference mandibular position, mainly in the construction of complete dentures). Although CR has had a variety of definitions (which has led to great confusion), it generally is considered to designate the relation of the mandible to the maxilla when the condyles are in a physiologically stable position, independent of tooth contacts. Centric relation has been described as:
1. The relation of the mandible to the maxilla when the mandible is in its most retrud-

ed, unstrained position from which lateral movements can be performed, at any given degree of jaw separation; also termed the "ligamentous" position, as it is determined mainly by the ligaments of the TMJ.

2. The maxillomandibular relationship in which the condyles articulate with the thinnest avascular portion of their discs, with the disc-condyle complex in the anterior-superior position against the slope of the articular eminence.

3. The most superoanterior position of the condyles in the articular fossae with the discs correctly interposed.

Centric relation may be impossible to record in the presence of dysfunction of the masticatory system.

Cephalic (Cranial)   Towards the head. [Compare with Caudal.]

Cephalic index See Index, Cephalic.

Cephalogram   See Cephalometric radiograph.

Cephalometer (Cephalostat) A head-holding device introduced in 1931 by B.H. Broadbent in the USA and by H. Hofrath in Germany. The original design included two ear rods for insertion into the external auditory canals, an infraorbital pointer and a forehead clamp, to achieve parallelism of the Frankfort plane with the floor. The cephalometer is used to obtain standardized and comparable craniofacial images on radiographic film.

Cephalometric analysis The process of evaluating skeletal, dental and soft tissue relationships of a patient, by comparing measurements performed on the patient's cephalometric tracing with population norms for the respective measurements, to come to a diagnosis of the patient's orthodontic problem. Refers also to the various standardized sets of cephalometric measurements (e.g. Downs' analysis, Steiner analysis) commonly used in the evaluation.

Burlington cephalometric analysis stepwise cephalometric appraisal, in whic the normative data has been incorporate in a set of templates, introduced by Popovich and G.W. Thompson in 1977. Th templates are constructed so that tw dimensional average growth increments f each landmark are depicted as a series X's, marked along the expected direction growth (there are separate templates f patients exhibiting a horizontal, a vertic and an average growth pattern). The ter plates (which have been developed for bo lateral and postero-anterior radiograph were derived from a sample of 120 boys ar 90 girls from the Burlington growth stud followed longitudinally for 16 years. Th analysis includes a static aspect (which aimed at diagnosing the degree of balanc or imbalance and its location) and a dynar ic aspect (which projects the direction ar amount of growth anticipated witho treatment for a certain patient). [Also se Burlington Growth Study.]

Di Paolo (Quadrilateral) cephalome ric analysis A cephalometric analys devised by R.J. Di Paolo in 1969. It consis of a number of ratios between linear me surements, with the addition of some ang lar measurements. Its norms are based a sample of 245 untreated adolescents (9 15 years of age), equally divided in terms gender and with "normal skeletal pattern.

Downs cephalometric analysis A set ten lateral cephalometric measuremen and their norms, developed by W.B. Dowr in 1948. It was based on a sample 20 Caucasian individuals 12–17 years ol with what Downs deemed as "clinica excellent occlusions." The analysis uses th Frankfort horizontal plane as its referenc plane. [Some of the individual measur ments of the Downs analysis are listed und Cephalometric measurements.]

Harvold cephalometric analysis A li ear assessment of maxillary and mandib lar unit length (and their difference), co ceived by E. Harvold, including linear measurement of the anterior lower face height. The data was derived from a serial sample of white children (6 to 16 years of age), from the Burlington Growth Centre at the University of Toronto, Canada.

McNamara cephalometric analysis An analysis introduced by J.A. McNamara, Jr., consisting of mostly linear measurements. It is based on some principles of the cephalometric analyses of Ricketts and Harvold, but also contains some original parts. The composite normative standards used in this analysis were derived from three sources: lateral cephalograms of the children comprising the Bolton standards, selected values from a group of untreated children from the Burlington Growth Centre and a sample of young adults from Ann Arbor, Michigan, having good-to-excellent facial configurations and a Class I occlusion, as selected by the author and coworkers. Five major sections are included in the analysis: assessing the relationship of the maxilla to the cranial base, that of the mandible to the cranial base, that of the maxilla to the mandible, the position of the maxillary and mandibular dentition and finally the (two-dimensional) size of the airway. The reference line in the sagittal plane is a line perpendicular to the Frankfort horizontal plane from Nasion (termed *Nasion-perpendicular*), extended inferiorly. Linear distances to the Nasion-perpendicular line are measured parallel to Frankfort horizontal to determine the anteroposterior position of the maxilla, mandible and chin.

Sassouni cephalometric analysis A method of evaluating vertical facial proportions, based on the convergence (or parallelism) of the mandibular plane, occlusal plane and palatal plane, as suggested by V. Sassouni. If these planes rapidly converge and intersect at a short distance behind the face, posterior vertical dimensions are relatively smaller than anterior ones, producing a skeletal open bite tendency. It also implies a relatively short ramus and an obtuse gonial

angle. On the other hand, when the palatal, occlusal and mandibular planes are almost parallel to each other, a skeletal predilection is present towards anterior deep bite. Individuals with this condition tend to have a longer ramus and a more acute gonial angle. [Also see Hyperdivergent; Hypodivergent.]

Steiner cephalometric analysis A series of angular and linear cephalometric measurements (including angles SNA, SNB and ANB) introduced by C.C. Steiner in 1953. The analysis uses the SN line as a reference plane. [For individual measurements of the Steiner analysis, see Cephalometric measurements.]

Tweed cephalometric analysis A set of three angular measurements (which constitute what has come to be known as the *Tweed triangle*), introduced by C.H. Tweed in 1946. The three angles that were originally described are the FMA (Frankfort-mandibular plane angle), the IMPA (Incisor-mandibular plane angle) and the FMIA (Frankfort-mandibular incisor angle). Their norms, as advocated by Tweed, were based on a sample of 95 individuals (some of whom were orthodontically treated) who according to him had good balance of facial outline, rather than ideal. The reference plane for the analysis is the Frankfort horizontal plane. Tweed's entire philosophy of diagnosis and treatment was built around the relationship of the mandibular incisors to the mandibular plane (IMPA angle). [For individual measurements of the Tweed analysis, see Cephalometric measurements.]

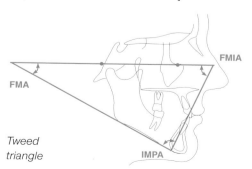

Tweed triangle

Wits cephalometric analysis See Cephalometric measurements, Wits appraisal.

Wylie cephalometric analysis A linear assessment of dysplasia in the sagittal plane, introduced by W.L. Wylie in 1947. The distances between the projections of a number of landmarks on the Frankfort horizontal plane were measured and their algebraic sum was calculated, to provide an indication of mandibular retrognathism or prognathism. The normative values were based on a sample (of unspecified size) of 10.5 to 13.5 year-old girls and boys.
The sagittal analysis described above was complemented later (1952) by a second set of linear and angular measurements for assessment of the vertical dimension. The sample on which the vertical assessment was based consisted of 57 children of the same age as the first sample mentioned, selected from the pretreatment records of the University of California on the basis of having "good facial balance."

Cephalometric landmarks Readily recognizable points on a cephalometric radiograph or tracing, representing certain hard or soft tissue anatomical structures (anatomical landmarks) or intersections of lines (constructed landmarks). Landmarks are used as reference points for the construction of various cephalometric lines or planes and for subsequent numerical determination of cephalometric measurements.
Following is a list of definitions of the most commonly encountered cephalometric landmarks. In these definitions, the following convention is used: *midsagittal* identifies landmarks lying on the midsagittal plane, *unilateral* identifies landmarks corresponding to unilateral structures and *bilateral* applies to landmarks corresponding to bilateral structures.

1. Hard tissue landmarks:

A-point (Point A, Subspinale, ss) The deepest (most posterior) midline point on the curvature between the ANS and

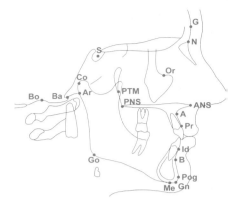

Hard tissue landmarks

prosthion. Its vertical coordinate is unreliable and therefore this point is used mainly for anteroposterior measurements. The location of A-point may change somewhat with root movement of the maxillary incisor teeth. (midsagittal)

Anterior nasal spine (ANS) The tip of the bony anterior nasal spine at the inferior margin of the piriform aperture, in the midsagittal plane. It corresponds to the anthropological point acanthion and often is used to define the anterior end of the palatal plane (nasal floor). (midsagittal)

Articulare (Ar) A constructed point representing the intersection of three radiographic images: the inferior surface of the cranial base and the posterior outlines of the ascending rami or mandibular condyles. It was meant to substitute condylion when the latter is not readily discernible. Any movement of the mandible (i.e. opening or closing) will change the location of articulare. (bilateral)

B-point (Point B, Supramentale, sm)
The deepest (most posterior) midline point on the bony curvature of the anterior mandible, between infradentale and pogonion. (midsagittal)

Basion (Ba) The most anterior inferior point on the margin of the foramen magnum.

in the midsagittal plane. It can be located by following the image of the slope of the inferior border of the basilar part of the occipital bone to its posterior limit, superior to the dens of the axis. (midsagittal)

Bolton (Bo) The highest points on the outlines of the retrocondylar fossae of the occipital bone, approximating the center of the foramen magnum. Named after C.B. Bolton. (bilateral)

Condylion (Co) The most superior posterior point on the head of the mandibular condyle. (bilateral)

Crista galli A vertically elongated, diamond-shaped radiopacity, appearing between the orbital outlines on postero-anterior cephalometric radiographs. Its location is used to establish a midsagittal reference plane. (midsagittal)

Dacryon The point of intersection of the frontomaxillary, lacrimomaxillary and fronto-lacrimal sutures. An anatomic reference point used to record interorbital distance. (bilateral) [Also see Orbital hypertelorism.]

Glabella (G) The most prominent point of the anterior contour of the frontal bone in the midsagittal plane. (midsagittal)

Gnathion (Gn) The most anterior inferior point on the bony chin in the midsagittal plane. (midsagittal)

Gonion (Go) The most posterior inferior point on the outline of the angle of the mandible. It may be determined by inspection or it can be constructed by bisecting the angle formed by the intersection of the mandibular plane and the ramal plane and by extending the bisector through the mandibular border. (bilateral)

Incision inferius (Ii) The incisal tip of the most labially placed mandibular incisor. (unilateral)

Incision superius (Is) The incisal tip of the most labially placed maxillary central incisor. (unilateral)

Infradentale (Id, Inferior prosthion) The most superior anterior point on the mandibular alveolar process, between the central incisors. (midsagittal)

L-point A point located in the anterior surface of the cortical plate, labial to the apices of the maxillary central incisors. Introduced by F.P.G.M. van der Linden, as a point representing the anterior border of the maxillary apical area. (midsagittal)

Menton (Me) The most inferior point of the mandibular symphysis, in the midsagittal plane. (midsagittal)

Nasion (N, Na) The intersection of the internasal and frontonasal sutures, in the midsagittal plane. (midsagittal)

Opisthion (Op) The most posterior inferior point on the margin of the foramen magnum, in the midsagittal plane. (midsagittal)

Orbitale (Or) The lowest point on the inferior orbital margin. (bilateral)

Pogonion (Pog, P, Pg) The most anterior point on the contour of the bony chin, in the midsagittal plane. Pogonion can be located by drawing a perpendicular to mandibular plane, tangent to the chin. (midsagittal)

Porion (Po) The most superior point of the outline of the external auditory meatus (*anatomic porion*). When the anatomic porion cannot be located reliably, the superior-most point of the image of the ear rods (*machine porion*) sometimes is used instead. (bilateral)

Posterior nasal spine (PNS) The most posterior point on the bony hard palate in the midsagittal plane; the meeting point between the inferior and the superior surfaces of the bony hard palate (nasal floor) at its posterior aspect. It can be located by extending the anterior wall of the ptery-gopalatine fossa inferiorly, until it intersects the floor of the nose. (midsagittal)

Prosthion (Pr, Superior prosthion, Supradentale) The most inferior anterior point on the maxillary alveolar process, between the central incisors. (midsagittal)

Pterygomaxillary fissure (PTM, Pterygomaxillare) A bilateral, inverted teardrop-shaped radiolucency, whose anterior border represents the posterior surfaces of the tuberosities of the maxilla. The landmark is taken at the most inferior point of the fissure, where the anterior and the posterior outline of the inverted teardrop merge with each other. (bilateral)

R-point (Registration point) A cephalometric reference point for registration of superimposed tracings, introduced by B.H. Broadbent, Sr., in his original presentation of the cephalometric technique. It is the midpoint on a perpendicular drawn from sella to the Bolton-nasion line. (midsagittal)

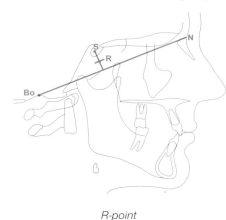

R-point

Sella (S) The geometric center of the pituitary fossa (sella turcica), determined by inspection—a constructed point in the midsagittal plane. (midsagittal)

2. Soft tissue landmarks

Cervical point (C) The innermost po[int] between the submental area and the ne[ck] in the midsagittal plane. Located at the int[er]section of lines drawn tangent to the ne[ck] and submental areas. (midsagittal)

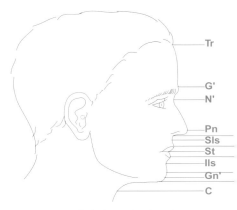

Soft tissue landmarks

Inferior labial sulcus (Ils) The point [of] greatest concavity on the contour of t[he] lower lip between labrale inferius and me[n]ton, in the midsagittal plane. (midsagittal)

Labrale inferior (Li) The point denot[ing] the vermilion border of the lower lip, in t[he] midsagittal plane. (midsagittal)

Labrale superior (Ls) The point denot[ing] the vermilion border of the upper lip, in t[he] midsagittal plane. (midsagittal)

Pronasale (Pn) The most prominent poi[nt] of the tip of the nose, in the midsagittal plan[e] (midsagittal)

Soft tissue glabella (G') The most prom[i]nent point of the soft tissue drape of the for[e]head, in the midsagittal plane. (midsagitt[al]

Soft tissue menton (Me') The most inf[e]rior point of the soft tissue chin, in the mi[d]sagittal plane. (midsagittal)

Soft tissue nasion (N', Na') The deepest point of the concavity between the forehead and the soft tissue contour of the nose in the midsagittal plane. (midsagittal)

Soft tissue pogonion (Pg', Pog') The most prominent point on the soft tissue contour of the chin, in the midsagittal plane. (midsagittal)

Stomion (St) The most anterior point of contact between the upper and lower lip in the midsagittal plane. When the lips are apart at rest, a superior and an inferior stomion point can be distinguished. (midsagittal)

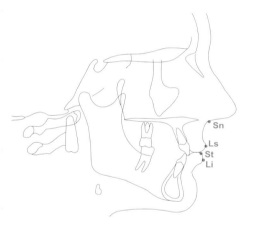

Stomion inferius (Sti) The highest midline point of the lower lip. (midsagittal)

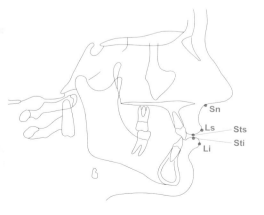

Stomion superius (Sts) The lowest midline point of the upper lip. (midsagittal)

Subnasale (Sn) The point in the midsagittal plane where the base of the columella of the nose meets the upper lip. (midsagittal)

Superior labial sulcus (Sls) The point of greatest concavity on the contour of the upper lip between subnasale and labrale superius, in the midsagittal plane. (midsagittal)

Trichion (Tr) An anthropometric landmark, defined as the demarcation point of the hairline in the midline of the forehead. (midsagittal)

Cephalometric lines (planes) Most analyses utilize one or more cephalometric lines that are joining two landmarks, are tangent to an outline from a landmark, or are perpendicular to another line from a landmark.
Listed below are some commonly used cephalometric lines:

A-B plane A line joining points A and B. As part of the Downs analysis, the superior angle formed by the intersection of the A-B plane and the facial line (N-Pog) is measured to evaluate the relation of the anterior limit of the apical bases to each other, relative to the facial line. This angle is negative in patients with skeletal Class II and positive in patients with skeletal Class III malocclusions.

Basion-Nasion line (Ba-N) A line considered by some to represent the cranial base more accurately than the SN line or the Bolton plane.

Bolton plane A line connecting points Bolton and nasion; an alternate representation of the cranial base.

Camper's base plane An anthropometric line connecting the center of the bony external auditory meatus and the anterior nasal spine. It was used as a horizontal reference line for evaluation of prognathism on dry skulls, prior to establishment of the Frankfort horizontal plane.

De Coster line A reference line proposed by L. De Coster as a stable area for cephalometric superimposition. It extends from the image of the anterior clinoid process along the planum sphenoidale and the anterior cranial edge of the sphenoethmoidal synchondrosis to the cranial aspect of the cribriform plate, terminating at the internal osseous line of the frontal bone above the crista frontalis.

E-line (E-plane, Esthetic line of Ricketts) A line tangent to the chin and nose, introduced by R.M. Ricketts for assessment of lip fullness. According to him, the lower lip should fall slightly ahead of the upper lip when related to this line.

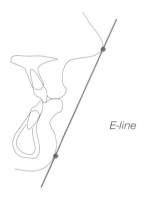

E-line

Esthetic plane of Rees See Cephalometric lines, Rees esthetic plane.

Esthetic plane of Steiner (S-line) See Cephalometric lines, S-line.

Facial axis of Ricketts A line connecting gnathion with cranial point "Pt," defined as the lower border of the foramen rotundum and approximated by the most posterosuperior point of the outline of the pterygomaxillary fissure. [Also see Cephalometric measurements (Hard tissue), Facial axis angle of Ricketts.]

Facial plane (FP, Facial line) A l extending from nasion to pogonion.

Frankfort horizontal plane (F Frankfort horizontal line, Auricu orbital plane, Eye-ear plane) An anth pological horizontal plane described dry skulls as passing through the low point in the floor of the left orbit and the hi est point on the margins of the exter auditory meati. The plane was adopted the 13th General Congress of Germ Anthropologists in Frankfort, Germany 1882 and later was endorsed by t International Agreement for the Unificati of Craniometric Measurements in Mona (1906) as a plane approximating the tr horizontal line when the head is in an uprig position. On a lateral cephalometric ra ograph, the Frankfort horizontal plane is re resented by a line connecting the cepha metric landmarks porion and orbitale.

H-line (Harmony line of Holdaway) line tangent to the soft tissue chin and t upper lip, introduced by R.A. Holdaway assessment of the soft tissue profile.

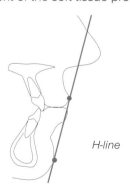

H-line

Intergonial line A line on a P-A cepha gram or tracing, connecting the goni points to each other.

Mandibular plane (MP, Mandibul line, ML) A line representing the pla passing through the mandibular borde (bilaterally). It can be drawn in two differe ways: by joining points gonion and gnathio or by drawing a tangent to the posterior aspect of the lower mandibular border from menton.

Nasion-perpendicular A line drawn perpendicular to the Frankfort horizontal from nasion. A reference line for anteroposterior measurements in the McNamara analysis.

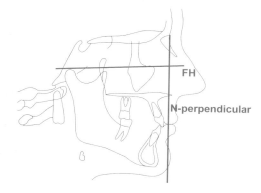

Occlusal plane (OP) A line on the cephalometric radiograph representing an imaginary plane at the level of the occlusion. [See also Occlusal plane.] There are various different definitions:

1. Bisected occlusal plane A line passing through the cusp tips of the maxillary and mandibular first permanent molars and midway between the incisal edges of the maxillary and mandibular central incisors (bisecting the overbite).

2. Functional occlusal plane A line drawn through the occlusal surfaces of the maxillary and mandibular first permanent molars and first and second premolars (or first and second deciduous molars).

3. Mandibular occlusal plane A line joining the cusp tips of the mandibular first permanent molars to the incisal edge of the mandibular central incisors.

4. Maxillary occlusal plane A line joining the cusp tips of the maxillary first permanent molars to the incisal edge of the maxillary central incisors.

Palatal plane (ANS-PNS, PP, Nasal line, Nasal floor, Spinal plane) A line joining PNS and ANS.

Rees esthetic plane A line tangent to the nasal tip and upper lip, introduced by T.D. Rees for assessment of the soft tissue profile. According to him, it should pass near the bony pogonion when the face is well balanced.

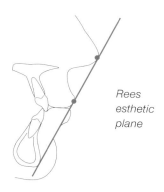

Rees esthetic plane

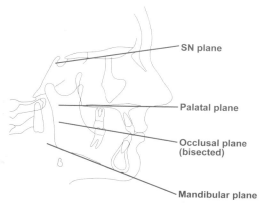

SN plane

Palatal plane

Occlusal plane (bisected)

Mandibular plane

Cephalometric planes

Reference line A line that is used as a basis for superimposition, or for comparison when several measurements are performed. Reference lines ideally should be stable with time and should not be affected by treatment. Because the cant or inclination of all intracranial reference lines is subject to biologic variation, it often is claimed that they are unsuitable for meaningful cephalometric analysis. Registration of the head in its natural position has the advantage that an extracranial "true" vertical or horizontal line can be used as a reference line for cephalometric analysis. [Also see Cephalometric lines, True vertical.]

Riedel plane A line on which the upper lip, lower lip and chin should fall in esthetic profiles, according to R.A. Riedel. A concept similar to the esthetic plane of Steiner, although not taking into account the nasal prominence.

S-line (Esthetic plane of Steiner) A line connecting the midpoint of the columella of the nose to the soft tissue pogonion. According to C.C. Steiner, the lips should fall on this line and any deviation shows prominence or flatness of the lips.

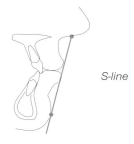

S-line

Sella-Nasion line (SN, Nasion-Sella line, NSL) A frequently used cephalometric reference line representing the anterior cranial base. A line joining points S and Na. [See also Cephalometric lines, Basion-Nasion; Cephalometric lines, Bolton plane.]

True horizontal line An external reference line constructed by drawing a perpendicular to the true vertical. [Also see Cephalometric lines, True vertical.]

True vertical line An external reference line, commonly provided by the image of a free-hanging metal chain taped on the film cassette during exposure. The true vertical line offers the advantage of no variation (since it is generated by gravity) and is used with radiographs obtained in natural head position. [Also see Natural head position.]

Y-axis (Growth axis) A line connecti[ng] points sella and gnathion. In the Dow[ns] analysis, the anteroinferior angle betwee[n] the Y-axis and the Frankfort horizontal (F[H) plane is measured as an indication of th[e] direction of mandibular growth.

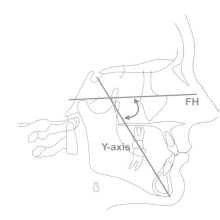

Z-line (Profile line of Merrifield) A li[ne] tangent to pogonion from the most prom[i]nent of the lips, introduced by L.L. Merrifie[ld] for soft tissue profile assessment. Accordin[g] to him, in well-balanced faces the upper [lip] should fall on the line and the lower [lip] should be slightly behind.

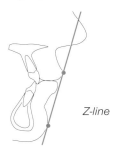

Z-line

Cephalometric measurements

1. Hard tissue measurements

A-B plane See Cephalometric lines, A[-B] plane.

ANB angle The difference between angl[es] SNA and SNB, as introduced by R.A. Ried[el] aiming at providing an evaluation of the anteroposterior relationship between the maxillary and mandibular apical bases. The measurement is not specific as to the location of the deformity.

Angle of convexity (NAPog) One of the measurements of the Downs cephalometric analysis, assessing the degree of convexity (or concavity) of the skeletal profile. The angle is formed by the lines NA and A-Pog and has a positive value in convex and negative value in concave profiles, whereas in patients with a straight profile the angle is approximately 0°.

Bolton triangle A triangle formed by connecting points Bolton, nasion and sella, representing the area of the cranial base to which the face is joined. It was believed by B.H. Broadbent, Sr. to be the most stable reference for superimposition of serial cephalograms.

Cranial base angle (NSBa, Saddle angle, Angle of flexure) The angle between the anterior and posterior cranial base, recorded as the inferior angle formed by the intersection of the lines BaS and SN. A large cranial base angle is thought to signify a posterior condylar and glenoid fossa position and a mandible that is positioned posteriorly with respect to the cranial base and the maxilla, unless it is compensated by a larger gonial angle and an increased mandibular length.

Facial angle (FH-NPog) The inferior posterior angle formed by the intersection of the Frankfort horizontal and the facial plane (N-Pog). Introduced by W.B. Downs to provide an assessment of the anteroposterior position of the chin in relation to the Frankfort horizontal plane.

Facial axis angle of Ricketts (Ba-Pt-Gn) The inferior angle formed by the intersection of the facial axis of Ricketts and the Ba-N line. This angle on the average approximates 90°. A value smaller than 90° indicates facial

growth primarily in the vertical direction and/or a Class II pattern, whereas a value greater than 90° indicates a horizontal growth pattern and/or a Class III tendency. [Also see Cephalometric lines, Facial axis of Ricketts.]

Facial height, Anterior; Posterior; and Total An appraisal of the face in the vertical dimension. The anterior lower facial height is expressed by the linear millimetric distance between the ANS and menton, measured directly, or along the true vertical line. The percent ratio of the previous linear measurement (ANS-Me) over the total anterior facial height (N-Me)—measured in the same way—provides an assessment of the relative proportionality of the anterior face in the vertical dimension. The measurement is obviously not specific as to the location of the deformity. Similarly, the linear measurement from S to Go on the lateral cephalometric radiograph provides an assessment of posterior facial height. The ratio of posterior face height x 100/anterior face height, according to the recommendations of J.R. Jarabak and J.A. Fizzel, can give an estimate of growth direction.

Frankfort-mandibular incisor angle (FMIA) The inferior posterior angle formed by the intersection of the long axis of the mandibular central incisor and the Frankfort horizontal plane. One of the angles of the "Tweed triangle." [Also see Cephalometric analysis, Tweed.]

Frankfort-mandibular plane angle (FMA) The anterior angle formed by the intersection of the mandibular and the Frankfort horizontal planes. One of the angles of the "Tweed triangle." [Also see Cephalometric analysis, Tweed.]

Gonial angle (Angle of the mandible, Condylar angle) The anterior angle formed by the intersection of a line tangent to the posterior border of the ramus and the mandibular plane. It determines the degree of inclination of the ramus to the mandibular plane and may give an indication about mandibular growth direction. (Alternatively measured as the angle between Ar-Go and Go-Gn.)

Holdaway ratio (LI-NB/Pg-NB) A measurement introduced by R.A. Holdaway to evaluate the relative prominence of the mandibular incisors, as compared to the size of the bony chin. It is calculated as the ratio of the linear distance from the labial surface of the mandibular central incisor to the NB line, over the linear distance of the chin to the same line.

Incisor-mandibular plane angle (IMPA) The posterior superior angle, formed by the intersection of the long axis of the mandibular central incisor and the mandibular plane. One of the angles of the "Tweed triangle" and a key measurement in the Tweed cephalometric analysis and treatment planning. [Also see Cephalometric analysis, Tweed.]

Interincisal angle A measurement of the degree of procumbency of the incisor teeth, introduced by W.B. Downs as the (posterior) angle formed by the intersection of the long axes of the maxillary and mandibular central incisors.

LI-to-AP distance The perpendicular distance (in mm) of the incisal edge of the mandibular central incisors to the A-Pog line. A measurement of the Downs analysis, expressing the degree of protrusion of the mandibular incisors.

Mandibular plane angle A measurement introduced by C.C. Steiner for assessment of the steepness of the mandibular plane in relation to the cranial base. The anterior angle formed by the intersection of SN and GoGn is measured. W.B. Downs defined the mandibular plane angle as the anterior angle formed by the intersection of the Frankfort horizontal plane and a tangent to the lower border of the mandible and symphysis.

SNA angle A commonly used measurement (of the Steiner analysis) introduced by R.A. Riedel for assessment of the anteroposterior position of the maxilla with regard to the cranial base. The inferior posterior angle formed by the intersection of lines SN and NA is measured.

SNB angle A measurement introduced by R.A. Riedel to evaluate the anteroposterior position of the mandible in relation to the cranial base (also part of the Steiner analysis). The inferior posterior angle formed by the intersection of lines NA and NB is measured.

UI-to-AP distance The perpendicular distance (in mm) of the incisal edge of the maxillary central incisors to the A-Pog line. A measurement of the Downs analysis expressing the degree of protrusion of the maxillary central incisors.

Wits appraisal A measurement introduced by A. Jacobson, designed to avoid the shortcomings of the ANB angle in evaluating anteroposterior jaw disharmonies. The method entails drawing perpendicular lines on a tracing of a lateral cephalogram from points A and B, onto the functional occlusal plane (which is drawn through the region of the overlapping cusps of the first premolars and molars) and subsequently measuring the distance between the two points of intersection of the two perpendicular lines with the functional occlusal plane, along the latter. The greater the deviation of this reading from 0 mm females and –1.0 mm in males, the greater the degree of sagittal discrepancy between the maxilla and mandible.
The Wits appraisal is a linear measurement and not an analysis, per se. It is simply a adjunctive diagnostic aid that can be useful in assessing the extent of anteroposterior skeletal dysplasia and in determining the reliability of the ANB angle. [The name is an abbreviation for "University of Witwatersrand," in Johannesburg, South Africa, where this appraisal was developed.]

Y-axis See Cephalometric lines, Y-axis.

2. Soft tissue measurements

Angle of facial convexity (G'Sn-SnPg')
A measurement developed by H.L. Legan to describe the overall convexity (or concavity) of the soft tissue profile. The inferior angle formed by the intersection of lines G'Sn and SnPg' is measured. The measurement does not take nasal projection into account.

H-angle (of Holdaway) The superior angle formed by the intersection of the H-line of Holdaway and the (bony) NB line. It provides a measurement of soft tissue protrusion or retrusion and is evaluated in conjunction with the ANB angle. The amount of deviation of the ANB angle from the average (1° to 3°) is added or subtracted from the H-angle for appropriate assessment of the lip and chin projection. The H-angle takes the skeletal relationship into account, but does not consider nasal contour and projection.

Interlabial gap The vertical distance between the upper and lower lip, measured with the lips at rest.

Lower face-throat angle (SnPg-CMe)
The posterior superior angle formed by the intersection of the subnasale-pogonion line and the menton-cervical line, as described by H.L. Legan. This measurement is used when mandibular surgery is contemplated to evaluate the potential esthetic impact of the procedure on the profile.

Lower lip length A linear measurement from soft tissue menton to stomion inferius, measured along the true vertical line.

Nasolabial angle (NLA) The anterior inferior angle formed by the intersection of a line tangent to the columella of the nose and a line drawn from subnasale to the mucocutaneous border of the upper lip. It evaluates the degree of protrusion or retrusion of the upper lip, in reference to the columella of the nose.

The nasolabial angle can influence the decision for extractions as part of the orthodontic treatment plan, as it is partially dependent on the anteroposterior position of the maxillary incisors.

Upper lip length A linear measurement (in mm) from subnasale to stomion superius, measured along the true vertical line.

Z-angle (of Merrifield) The inferior posterior angle formed by the intersection of the profile line of Merrifield (Z-line) and the Frankfort horizontal plane.

Cephalometric radiograph (Cephalogram) A radiograph of the head obtained under standardized conditions, introduced simultaneously in the United States and Germany (1931), by B.H. Broadbent and H. Hofrath, respectively.
Cephalometric radiographs are taken on a cephalometer, which dictates a standardized orientation of the head and a precisely defined relationship among x-ray source, subject and film. By convention, the distance between x-ray source and the midsagittal plane of the subject is either 5 feet (152.4 cm) or 150 cm. The distance between the midsagittal plane of the subject and the film may vary between 10 cm and 18 cm, depending on head size. Measurement of the subject-film distance and the source-subject distance allows calculation of the image magnification. The standard projections are lateral (profile), posteroanterior (P-A) and oblique projections.

Lateral cephalometric radiograph A radiograph of the head taken with the x-ray beam perpendicular to the patient's sagittal plane. The beam most commonly enters on the patient's right side, with the film cassette adjacent to the patient's left side (so that the patient's head is oriented to the right on the radiograph), but the reverse convention also is used.

Oblique cephalometric radiograph
Radiograph of the head usually taken at 45°

and 135° to the patient's midsagittal plane (or at any other angular projection that is required), usually to perform direct mandibular length measurements on either side in patients with facial asymmetry.

Posteroanterior (P-A) cephalometric radiograph A radiograph of the head taken with the x-ray beam perpendicular to the patient's coronal plane with the x-ray source behind the head and the film cassette in front of the patient's face. P-A cephalograms are usually taken for evaluation and treatment planning of patients with facial asymmetry.

Cephalometric superimposition See Superimposition.

Cephalometric tracing An overlay drawing produced from a cephalometric radiograph by copying specific outlines from it with a

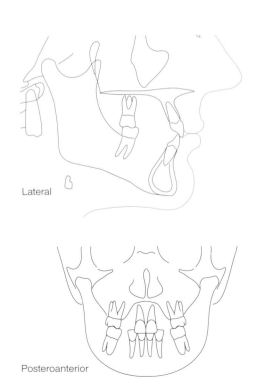

Lateral

Posteroanterior

Cephalometric tracing

lead pencil onto acetate paper, using a illuminated view-box. Tracings are used t facilitate cephalometric analysis, as well a in superimpositions, to evaluate treatmer and growth changes.

Cephalometrics, Computerized See Com puterized cephalometrics.

Cephalostat See Cephalometer.

Ceramic bracket See Bracket, Ceramic.

Cervical anchorage See Anchorage, Ce vical.

Cervical headgear See Headgear, Cervical

Cervical point (C) See Cephalometric lanc marks (Soft tissue), Cervical point.

Cheek bone See Zygomatic bone.

Chief complaint (CC) The patient's statemer of the main problem or primary concern.

Chin cap (Chin cup) See Appliance, Chin cap

Chromium-cobalt alloy See Cobalt-chrom um alloy.

Chronic pain disorders Persistent pain tha lasts more than six months, with associate behavioral and psychosocial factors.

Cinching (of the archwire) Placing a shar bend on the archwire distal to the termina attachments in an arch. Cinching is done t avoid excessive proclination of the anteric teeth during leveling or to prevent the arch wire from sliding in an anterior direction du ing the interval between patient visits. [Als see Bends, Distal-end.]

Cinching bends See Bends, Distal-end.

Circular fibers See Gingival fibers.

Circumferential clasp (C-clasp) See Clas| Circumferential.

Circumferential retainer See Retainer, Wrap-around.

Circumferential supracrestal fibrotomy (Edwards' procedure) An adjunctive periodontal surgical procedure developed by J.G. Edwards to reduce the relapse tendency of corrected individual tooth rotations. The procedure consists of inserting the sharp point of a fine blade into the gingival sulcus, down to the crest of the alveolar bone, to sever the gingival fibers around the tooth (including the transseptal fibers between it and the adjacent teeth).

Clasp (Retention clasp) An element of a removable appliance made of metal that serves to secure the appliance in place by engaging on undercuts provided by the morphology and inclination of the teeth.

Adams clasp (Modified arrowhead clasp) A clasp made of stainless steel wire, which was designed by C.P. Adams to retain removable appliances, by means of point contact with the mesio- and distobuccal undercuts of individual posterior teeth. The clasp is bent from a single piece of round wire and crosses the occlusal table at the mesial and distal embrasures of a posterior tooth (typically first permanent molar). It consists of a mesial and a distal retentive U- or V-shaped loops, which are pointed in a gingival direction and joined by a buccal bridge.

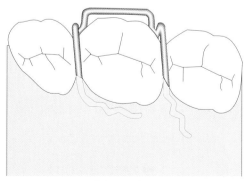

Adams clasp

Arrowhead clasp (Arrow clasp) Clasp made from stainless steel wire, bent in the shape of an arrowhead. It is meant to engage the distobuccal and mesiobuccal undercuts of adjacent teeth (in a fashion similar to a ball clasp). Two or more arrowhead clasps may be combined, joined by a buccal bridge.

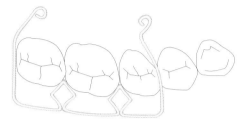

Arrowhead clasp

Ball clasp Clasp bent from round stainless steel wire, with a ball-shaped end. The clasp crosses the occlusal table at the embrasure between two adjacent teeth and engages their mesiobuccal and distobuccal undercuts.

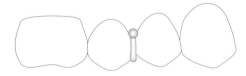

Ball clasp

Circumferential clasp (Three-quarter clasp, C-clasp) A single-tooth cast or bent stainless steel wire clasp that engages the cervical region of the canines and posterior teeth. The clasp usually crosses the occlusal table at an interproximal embrasure between two teeth, then progresses gingivally toward the other interproximal surface, engaging in the interproximal gingival undercut, thus traversing three surfaces of the tooth.

The diameter of the wire used for its fabrication typically is 0.024 inch (0.60 mm) for deciduous canines; 0.028 inch (0.70 mm) for deciduous molars, premolars and permanent canines; and 0.032 inch (0.80 mm) for permanent molars. Circumferential clasps function well on maxillary teeth as the morphology and the inclination of the posterior teeth provide adequate undercuts.

In the mandibular dental arch this is not always the case. By creating artificial undercuts with composite, circumferential clasps can provide firm retention of mandibular removable appliances. An advantage of the circumferential clasp is the possibility of avoiding occlusal interference of the part of the clasp that crosses the occlusal table.

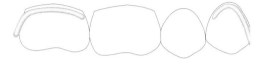

Circumferential clasp

Claw clasp A clasp introduced by F.P.G.M. van der Linden for retention on maxillar incisors. It is made of a 0.024-inch (0.60-mm) stainless steel spring-hard wire crossing the incisal edge and forming a small rectangular box on the labial surface of those teeth. The addition of composite at that point, to create an artificial undercut, greatly enhances retention.

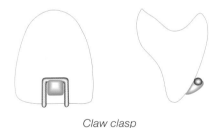

Claw clasp

Delta clasp A modification of the standard Adams clasp by W.J. Clark, for retention of the twin block appliance. The major difference is the shape of the retentive loops, which in the case of the delta clasp are shaped in a closed triangle, unlike the open V- or U-shaped loops, of the Adams clasp. Subsequent modification of the delta clasp produced circular loops, which are easier

to construct and have similar retentive properties.

The advantage of the delta clasp, according to its designer, is that the loops do not open with repeated insertion and removal of the appliance. Delta clasps, which are constructed from 0.028-inch (0.70-mm) or 0.030-inch (0.75-mm) stainless steel wire, can provide good retention on mandibular premolars and can be used on most posterior teeth. [Also see Appliance, Twin block.]

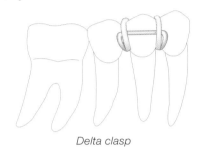

Delta clasp

Three-quarter clasp See Clasp Circumferential.

Clasp-adjusting pliers See Orthodontic instruments, Triple-beaked pliers.

Class I elastics See Orthodontic elastics Intramaxillary.

Class I mechanics See Mechanics, Class I.

Class I, II, III malocclusion See Angle classification.

Class II elastics See Orthodontic elastics Class II.

Class II mechanics See Mechanics, Class

Class III elastics See Orthodontic elastics Class III.

Class III functional appliances See Appliance, Class III Functional.

Class III mechanics See Mechanics, Class

Classification of gingival recession See Miller classification.

Classification of malocclusion See Angle classification.

Claw clasp See Clasp, Claw.

Clear bracket See Bracket, Esthetic.

Cleat, Lingual See Lingual cleat.

Cleft lip and/or palate (CLP) The most common craniofacial anomaly (approximately 1 in 600 to 1 in 700 live births—higher in some populations), characterized by failure of fusion between certain embryological processes (swellings) during facial morphogenesis. Failure of fusion between the medial and lateral nasal and the maxillary swellings results in a cleft of the lip and/or alveolar process. Failure of fusion between the lateral palatine swellings results in a cleft of the palate. These problems are thought to result from a deficiency of mesenchyme in the facial region, brought about by failure of neural crest cells to migrate or failure of the facial mesenchyme to proliferate. A cleft can be complete or incomplete, and it can occur unilaterally or bilaterally. Cleft lip may occur without clefting of the alveolar process or the palate, and cleft palate also can occur as an isolated phenomenon. A useful classification divides the anatomy into primary and secondary palates. [Also see Palate, Primary; Palate, Secondary.] An individual thus may have clefting of the primary palate, the secondary palate, or both. In addition, a CLP may be an isolated phenomenon, or may occur as part of a syndrome.

The etiology of cleft lip and palate is thought to be multifactorial. Genetics is implicated in 20% to 30% of patients. Even in those individuals whose genetic background may verify familial tendencies for clefting, the mode of inheritance is not understood completely. Environmental factors that have been shown in experimental animals to result in clefting include nutritional deficiencies, radiation, several drugs, hypoxia, viruses, and vitamin excesses or deficiencies.

In complete unilateral or bilateral clefts of the lip, alveolus and palate, the maxillary arch typically is collapsed in the transverse direction, especially in the area of the cleft. The maxillary permanent lateral incisors may be congenitally missing or malformed, and many atypically shaped supernumerary teeth may be present in the area of the cleft. The treatment of patients with cleft lip and/or palate is a long and involved process, requiring many stages of intervention by many different specialists, forming a "cleft lip and palate team." The involvement of the team orthodontist starts a few days after the baby is born, with presurgical infant orthopedic treatment (if applicable), in preparation for the initial repair.

Repair of the lip usually is performed within the first three months after birth, and the palate subsequently is repaired within the first year. The scar tissue created from these and other surgical procedures is considered responsible for variable degrees of maxillary growth inhibition which is commonly seen during subsequent growth.

When the cleft involves the alveolar process, a bone graft may be necessary to restore the alveolar anatomy. Alveolar bone grafting usually is performed prior to the eruption of the permanent maxillary canine on the side of the cleft.

Phase I of orthodontic treatment, in preparation for the alveolar bone graft, may consist of expansion of the constricted maxilla and correction of any crossbites.

Following alveolar bone grafting, and when the patient is in the permanent dentition, phase II of orthodontic treatment is performed to idealize the occlusion, or if a severe skeletal discrepancy is present, to prepare the arches for orthognathic surgery. [Also see Graft, Alveolar bone.]

Cleidocranial dysplasia (Cleidocranial dysostosis, CCD) Inheritable disorder (autosomal dominant) affecting both intramembranous and endochondral bone formation.

The clinical features include a characteristic brachycephalic skull (cephalic index commonly in excess of 81), with frontal and parietal bossing and the appearance of a small face. Paranasal sinuses and mastoids often are underdeveloped or absent. Clavicles are hypoplastic or aplastic, and closure of fontanels and cranial sutures is delayed, sometimes for life.

The palate is highly arched, and there may be a submucous or complete cleft palate. The maxilla is underdeveloped and a skeletal Class III malocclusion usually is present. The dentition often presents a chaotic appearance with multiple supernumerary teeth, multiple crown and root abnormalities, ectopic development, retention of deciduous teeth and failure of eruption of permanent teeth. Extraction of retained deciduous teeth usually does not facilitate the eruption of their permanent successors. The molecular pathology of this condition was shown to be associated with mutations of a gene called CBFA. This gene is a transcription factor essential for osteoblast differentiation and bone formation, which explains the general bone dysplasia in the condition.

Clenching Parafunctional activity characterized by hyperactivity of the elevator masticatory muscles, with the teeth in contact. Clenching is considered to be stress-related and, together with bruxism, is thought to be part of the predisposing/initiating/perpetuating factors in the development of temporomandibular joint disorders.

Clicking Brief, sharp sound (distinct snapping or cracking), audible with or without a stethoscope, or detectable by palpation, emanating from one or both temporomandibular joints during mandibular movements. The most common cause for clicking is anterior or antero-medial displacement of the articular disc. Clicking may or may not be associated with internal derangement of the TMJ, and it may occur only during the opening or closing movement of the mandible (single click), or during both (reciprocal click).

Early closing clicking A clicking noise that occurs at the initiation of retrusive condylar translation.

Early opening clicking A clicking sound from the TMJ that occurs at the initiation of protrusive condylar translation.

Late closing clicking (Terminal closing clicking) A click that occurs before the end of retrusive condylar translation.

Late opening clicking (Terminal opening clicking) A click that occurs just before the end of protrusive condylar translation.

Mid-closing clicking A clicking noise that occurs midway along the condylar translatory path during closing.

Mid-opening clicking A clicking noise that occurs midway along the condylar translatory path during opening.

Reciprocal clicking A pair of clicking noises from the temporomandibular joint heard during the mandibular opening movement and again just before the teeth occlude during the closing movement. Reciprocal clicking is a common characteristic of disc displacement with reduction. From a closed mouth position, the temporarily misaligned disc reduces or improves its structural relation with the condyle when mandibular translation occurs, which produces the first clicking noise. The closing noise is usually of less magnitude and is thought to be produced by a displacement of the disc to its previous position. [Compare with Clicking, Single.]

Single clicking An individual clicking noise, occurring either during the opening or during the closing stage of mandibular movement. [Compare with Clicking, Reciprocal.]

Clockwise rotation of the mandible (Posterior rotation of the mandible) See Mandibular rotation, Clockwise.

Closed bite Excessive vertical overlap of the anterior teeth; extremely deep bite.

Closed coil spring See Orthodontic springs, Coil spring, Closed.

Closed curettage See Curettage, Closed.

Closed lock See Disc displacement without reduction.

Closed loop See Loop, Closed.

Closed spring See Orthodontic springs, Closed.

Closing coil spring See Orthodontic springs, Coil spring, Retraction.

Closing loop See Loop, Closing.

Closing loop arch See Arch, Closing-loop.

CLP See Cleft lip and/or palate.

CM See Center of mass.

CMD See Temporomandibular disorders.

CO See Occlusion, Centric.

Co See Cephalometric landmarks (Hard tissue), Condylion.

Co-Cr See Cobalt-chromium alloy.

Coated abrasive strips See Abrasive strips.

Coaxial wire See Orthodontic wire, Multistrand.

Cobalt-chromium alloy (Co-Cr, Cobalt-chromium-nickel alloy, Chromium-cobalt alloy) Highly corrosion-resistant alloys based on cobalt and chromium, used for fabrication of orthodontic wires or clasps. Cobalt-chromium orthodontic wires are very similar in appearance, mechanical properties, and joining characteristics to stainless steel wires, but have a significantly different composition and considerably greater heat treatment response.

One of the most widely known alloys, introduced to orthodontics under the trademark "Elgiloy" (Rocky Mountain Orthodontics), consists of approximately 40% cobalt, 20% chromium, 15% nickel, 15.8% iron, 7% molybdenum, 2% manganese, 0.15% carbon, and 0.04% beryllium. Concerns about the toxicity of beryllium have led to the development of beryllium-free cobalt-chromium alloys such as "Remaloy" (Dentaurum).

Cobalt-chromium wires are available in different tempers. The soft-temper wires are popular with clinicians because they are more easily formable and subsequently they can be hardened by heat treatment. Cobalt-chromium alloys have a modulus of elasticity (E) equivalent to that of stainless steel. However, they "feel" softer in the not-hardened state, as their yield strength and elastic range are lower compared to the more resilient stainless steel alloys.

Coefficient of friction (μ) See Frictional coefficient.

Coffin spring See Orthodontic springs, Coffin spring.

Cohesion The property of a material by which its constituent molecules are attracted to each other, resisting separation. [Compare with Adhesion.]

Coil eyelet See "Pigtail" attachment.

Coil spring See Orthodontic springs, Coil spring.

Coil-spring space regainer See Space regainer, Coil-spring.

Col See Gingival col.

Cold working See Hardening, Work.

Collagen A large family of structural and regulatory fibrous proteins composed of three polypeptide chains (α-chains) coiled around each other to form a typical triple helix. There are many different types of collagens found in connective tissue, Type I being by far the most common.

Type I collagen is the major structural component of many connective tissues, including gingiva, periodontal ligament, dentin, cementum and bone.

Type II has been found in cartilage and intervertebral discs.

Types III and V are also abundant in the skin, periodontal ligament and gingiva and are thought to be involved in inflammation and tissue regeneration.

Type IV collagen typically is found in epithelial and endothelial cells and is a major component of basement membranes.

Type VI collagen is widely distributed in most soft and mineralized connective tissues, including the skin, whereas Type XII is also found in association with Type I collagen, and is synthesized in several tissues, including the periodontal ligament.

Type VIII collagen was originally isolated in endothelial cells, but later was identified also in corneal basement membrane, perichondrium, periosteum and several carcinoma cells.

Type XIII collagen has been found to be synthesized in epidermis, intestinal mucosa, periosteum, cartilage, muscle, and in bone marrow cells.

After being secreted into the extracellular space collagen molecules assemble into ordered polymers called *collagen fibrils.* The strength of collagen fibrils is increased by formation of cross-links between them, which enables them to better withstand tensile loads. Collagen fibrils often aggregate into larger bundles called *collagen fibers.*

Collapsed bite See Bite collapse.

Collateral ligaments Ligaments attaching the medial and lateral borders of the articular disc of the temporomandibular joint to the respective poles of the condyle. These ligaments permit the disc to rotate anteriorly and posteriorly on the articular surface of the condyle during mandibular movements.

Collimator A diaphragm, cone or tube containing a lead disk with an aperture designed to fit on an x-ray source so as restrict the size and shape of the primary beam, by eliminating its peripheral (most divergent) portion. The aperture of the collimator may be circular or rectangular.

Coloboma A congenitally occurring lack continuity ("cleft") in the orbital region. The defect may be restricted to the eyelid or extend into the globe from the iris to the retina. Lower lid and/or lateral canthus colobomas are commonly seen in patients with Treacher Collins syndrome. [Also see Treacher Collins syndrome.]

Columella The small fleshy column connecting the upper lip and the tip of the nose between the nares; a continuation of the nasal septum.

Combination headgear See Headgear, Straight-pull.

Combination of forces See Force composition.

Combined functional/extraoral traction appliance See Appliance, Combined functional/extraoral traction.

Comminuted fracture See Fracture, Comminuted.

Compact bone See Bone, Compact.

Compensating curve See Curve of Spee.

Compensation, Dental See Dentoalveolar compensation.

Complete mandibular buccal crossbite See Crossbite, Complete mandibular buccal.

Complete mandibular lingual crossbite See Crossbite, Complete mandibular lingual.

omplete maxillary buccal crossbite (Brodie syndrome) See Crossbite, Complete maxillary buccal.

omplete maxillary palatal crossbite See Crossbite, Complete maxillary palatal.

omplete maxillary osteotomy See Osteotomy, Complete maxillary.

omplex fracture See Fracture, Complex.

ompomers A class of bonding agents formed by combining composite resin and fluoride silicate glass.

omponent forces See Force, Component forces.

ompound fracture See Fracture, Compound.

omprehensive orthodontic treatment Coordinated treatment aiming at improving a patient's craniofacial dysfunction and/or dentofacial deformity, taking into account anatomical, functional and esthetic factors. Treatment may incorporate several phases, with specific objectives at various stages of dentofacial development. Adjunctive procedures such as extractions, dentofacial orthopedic treatment, orthognathic surgery, myofunctional or speech therapy, and restorative or periodontal treatment may be performed concurrently to achieve the best attainable result. Typically, at the end of active comprehensive orthodontic treatment each tooth is in its ideal position and the achievable optimum in occlusion has been obtained. Long-term periodic reevaluation following active treatment is important for maintenance of the achieved result. [Compare with Limited orthodontic treatment.] [Modified from the AAO Glossary of Dentofacial Orthopedic Terms, 1993.]

ompressive deformation (Compressive strain) The shape change of a body when it is subjected to compressive stress (e.g. the shortening of an orthodontic open coil upon compression).

Compressive stress See Stress, Compressive.

Computer-assisted tomography See Tomography, Computerized.

Computerized cephalometrics The process of entering cephalometric data in digital format into a computer for cephalometric analysis. Depending on the software and hardware available, the incorporation of data can be performed by digitizing points on a tracing, by scanning a tracing or a conventional radiograph, or by originally obtaining computerized radiographic images that are already in digital format, instead of conventional radiographs.
Computerized cephalometrics offers the advantages of instant analysis; readily available race-, sex- and age-related norms for comparison; as well as ease of soft tissue change and surgical predictions.

Computerized tomography See Tomography, Computerized.

Concrescence Union of the cellular cementum of two teeth that have developed from two separate tooth buds. [Compare with Fusion; Gemination; Twinning.]

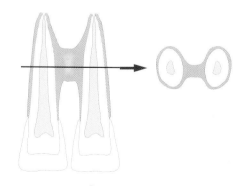

Concrescence

Concurrent forces See Force, Concurrent forces.

Condylar angle See Cephalometric measurements (Hard tissue), Gonial angle.

Condylar dislocation (Condylar displacement) See Dislocation of the condyle.

Condylar displacement See Dislocation of the condyle.

Condylar fracture See Fracture, Condylar.

Condylar gliding See Translation of the condyle.

Condylar growth Proliferation of condylar cartilage, followed by endochondral ossification. The condyle, the coronoid process and the ramus are the principal sites of growth of the mandible. As condylar growth occurs, the mandible is translated inferiorly and anteriorly, which can be visualized by inspection of cephalometric superimpositions using the cranial base as a reference. The upward and backward direction of condylar growth is seen clearly by mandibular superimposition. Condylar growth normally stops shortly after that of the rest of the face, although it may continue well beyond adolescence, particularly in males. [Also see Growth center; Growth site.]

Condylar guidance The functional guidance of the mandibular excursions, as determined by the relationship between the mandibular condyles and the contours of the glenoid fossae, articular eminences and articular discs.

Condylar hyperplasia Excessive growth of the condyle, usually unilateral, resulting in facial asymmetry and an associated malocclusion. Such malocclusions often are associated with an open bite on the affected side and/or a crossbite on the non-affected side, with a corresponding midline discrepancy. The condition typically appears in the late teens, but may begin at an earlier age. A bone scan (scintigram) with Tc^{99m}, an isotope that is concentrated in areas of active bone deposition, can be used to distinguish

between an actively growing ("hot") cond and an enlarged condyle that has ceas growing. The treatment for severe cases condylar hyperplasia is usually surgical.

Condylar process of the mandible S Condyle.

Condylar rotation See Rotation of t condyle.

Condylar translation See Translation of t condyle.

Condyle (Condylar process of the ma dible) The posterior process of t mandibular ramus. It is composed of tv parts: a superior part (the articular portic and an inferior part (the condylar nec The articular portion forms a rounded he covered with cartilage, which fits into the g noid fossa of the temporal bone. The co stricted portion below the articular pa forms the neck of the condyle.

Condylectomy Surgical removal of the ent mandibular condyle.

Condylion (Co) See Cephalometric landmar (Hard tissue), Condylion.

Condylysis Idiopathic resorption or dissoluti of the condyle.

"Cone-funnel" mechanism The mechanis by which it is theorized that interdigitation posterior teeth is achieved in the late stag of their eruption. Occlusal contacts betwee the maxillary and mandibular posterior tee dictate a series of adjustments in mesiod

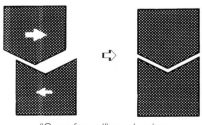

"Cone-funnel" mechanism

tal angulation and buccolingual inclination over a relatively short period of time, leading to their final interdigitation.

nnective tissue graft See Graft, Subepithelial connective tissue.

nsistent force system See Force system, Consistent.

nstant force See Force, Constant.

nstraint conditions See Load/deflection rate.

nstruction bite A bite registration at the desired occlusal relationship, to permit articulator mounting of the casts for fabrication of an (most commonly functional) appliance. The construction bite is sent to the orthodontic laboratory, together with the impressions (or casts) and a prescription with the required specifications of the appliance. [Also see Bite registration.]

nsultation 1. A joint deliberation between two or more medical or dental practitioners, aiming through the exchange of information to arrive at a decision with respect to the diagnosis or treatment of a particular patient.
2. A deliberation between a medical or dental practitioner and a patient (and his or her family) on the diagnosis and treatment plan.

ntinuous archwire See Archwire, Continuous.

ntinuous archwire mechanics See Mechanics, Continuous archwire.

ntinuous force See Force, Continuous.

ntinuous posterior torque See Torque, Continuous posterior.

ntralateral Referring to the side opposite to the one that is being considered. [Compare with Ipsilateral.]

Controlled tipping See Orthodontic tooth movement, Tipping (Controlled).

Conversion (of a tube into a bracket) The process of removing the buccal cap of a convertible tube of a molar attachment to transform the tube into a bracket. [Also see Orthodontic instruments, Conversion instrument; Tube, Convertible.]

Conversion instrument See Orthodontic instruments, Conversion instrument.

Convertible tube See Tube, Convertible.

Coon ligature-tying pliers See Orthodontic instruments, Coon ligature-tying pliers.

Coordinate system See Global reference frame.

Coordination of arches See Arch coordination.

Coordination of archwires See Archwire coordination.

Coplanar forces See Force, Coplanar forces.

Coronal plane See Frontal plane.

Corrosion A chemical or electrochemical degrading process, through which a material is attacked by corrosive agents, such as acids (but also air and saliva, in the case of the intraoral environment), resulting in partial or complete dissolution, deterioration, or weakening. Although glasses and other nonmetals also are susceptible to environmental degradation, metals generally are more prone to such an attack because of electrochemical reactions.

Galvanic corrosion An accelerated attack occurring on the least noble of two or more electrochemically dissimilar metals, in the presence of an electrolyte.

Pitting corrosion Sharply localized corrosion occurring on base metals such as iron, nickel and chromium, or some alloys, which are protected by a naturally forming, thin film of oxide. In the presence of chlorines in the environment of e.g. stainless steel, the film locally breaks down and rapid dissolution of the underlying material occurs, in the form of pits.

Stress corrosion Degradation by the combined effects of mechanical stress and a corrosive environment, usually in the form of cracking.

Cortical bone See Bone, Cortical.

Cortical drift All bone structures have one growth principle in common, which was termed *drift* by D.H. Enlow. The cortical plate can be relocated by simultaneous apposition and resorption processes on the opposing periosteal and endosteal surfaces (cortical drift). The bony cortical plate drifts by apposition and resorption of bone substance on its outer and inner surfaces, respectively, in the direction of growth. If resorption and deposition take place at the same rate, the thickness of the bone remains constant. Should more bone be deposited than resorbed, the thickness of the structure increases, as during growth. The teeth follow the drift of the alveolar processes while the jaw is growing, and thus they maintain their position within the surrounding bony structure, despite the displacement of the entire bone. [Also see Displacement (of a bone).]

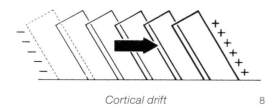

Cortical drift 8

Cortical osteotomy See Corticotomy.

Cortical plate The dense layer of cortical bone covering the buccal and lingual aspects of the alveolar process. [Also see Bon Cortical.]

Corticotomy (Cortical osteotomy) A part osteotomy, involving only the cortical plat to weaken the resistance of the bone to th application of forces. Such a procedu is routinely performed prior to distracti osteogenesis for elongation of the mandib or the maxilla. [Also see Distraction oste genesis.]

Costen's syndrome Condition involving diz ness, tinnitus, earache, stuffiness of the e dry mouth, burning in the tongue and thro sinus pain and headaches, described by t otolaryngologist J.B. Costen in 1934. H attributed the symptoms to overclosure the bite and posterior displacement of th mandibular condyle. [Term formerly used f "temporomandibular joint disorders."]

Costochondral graft See Graft, Cost chondral.

Counterclockwise rotation (of the ma dible) See Mandibular rotation, Count clockwise.

Counter-moment See Moment, Count moment.

Couple A pair of equal and opposite no collinear forces applied to a body. A coup always results in a pure moment, with a te dency to rotate around the center of res tance. [See also Moment of a couple.]

Couple-force ratio See Moment-to-force rat

CR See Centric relation.

CR-CO shift See Mandibular shift.

Cranial See Cephalic.

Cranial base The bones of endochondral o gin that form the antero-inferior aspect of th brain case. Because the bones of the cr nial base stop growing relatively early, th often are used in the superimposition of serial cephalograms or tracings as reference structures to assess growth of the jaws or treatment results.

anial base angle See Cephalometric measurements (Hard tissue), Cranial base angle.

anial index See Index, Cranial.

anial suture See Suture.

aniofacial clefts Rarely occurring clefts that are not limited to the lip and palate, but also involve the facial soft tissues and underlying bone. They result from problems in the migration of neural crest cells and failure of fusion between facial processes (swellings), or from differentiation defects of facial tissues of mesodermal origin in the first trimester of pregnancy. Some craniofacial clefts produce extensive facial defects with severe tissue deficits.

There are many kinds of craniofacial clefts, commonly classified under a system described by P. Tessier, which involves numbers from 0 to 14, centered around the eye.

aniometry A branch of anthropometry dealing with the measurements of dimensions and angles of the bony skull.

aniomandibular articulation See Joint, Temporomandibular.

aniomandibular disorders (CMD) See Temporomandibular disorders (TMD).

aniosynostosis A birth defect that may occur as an isolated phenomenon or as part of a syndrome, consisting of premature fusion of one or more skull sutures. Craniosynostosis results in craniofacial deformity and potentially in increased intercranial pressure, which can be deleterious to brain function. For this reason, surgical release of the fused sutures sometimes is undertaken quite early in life.

A number of craniofacial syndromes sharing the clinical feature of craniosynostosis (such as Crouzon syndrome, Pfeiffer syndrome and Apert syndrome) have been found to result from mutations in the genes for fibroblast growth factor receptors (FGFR gene mutations).

Creep See Viscoelastic behavior, Creep.

Crefcoeur appliance See Appliance, Crefcoeur.

Crefcoeur spring See Appliance, Crefcoeur.

Crepitus (Crepitation, Grating sound) Rough, sandy, diffuse noise or vibration, produced by the rubbing together of irregular bone or cartilage surfaces, usually identified with osteoarthritic changes when heard in joints.

CRes See Center of resistance.

Crib See Appliance, Crib.

Crimpable attachments A number of different orthodontic attachments (e.g. hooks, stops) that can be fixed on an archwire by squeezing their base with special sharp-beaked pliers or cutters.

Criss-cross elastics See Orthodontic elastics, Crossbite.

Crista galli See Cephalometric landmarks (Hard tissue), Crista galli.

Crossbite An abnormal relationship of one or more teeth to one or more teeth of the opposing arch, in the buccolingual or labiolingual direction. A crossbite can be *dental* or *skeletal* in etiology. [Note: The appropriate type of crossbite can be specified by identifying the teeth or jaws that deviate the most from their ideal position (e.g. when a crossbite is mainly due to a narrow maxillary arch the correct term is "maxillary posterior lingual crossbite" as opposed to "mandibular posterior buccal crossbite").]

Anterior crossbite Situation in which one or more primary or permanent mandibular incisors are labial to their antagonists (or one or more maxillary incisors are lingual to their antagonists) in habitual occlusion.

Buccal crossbite A crossbite due to buccal displacement of the affected tooth (or group of teeth) from its (their) ideal position relative to its (their) antagonist(s).

Complete mandibular buccal crossbite A situation in which the mandibular dental arch is wide and lies entirely buccal to (contains) the maxillary dental arch. This rare situation is sometimes seen in extreme Class III anomalies associated with mandibular hyperplasia. [Compare with Crossbite, Complete maxillary palatal.]

Complete mandibular lingual crossbite A situation in which the mandibular dental arch is narrow and lies entirely palatal to (contained within) the maxillary dental arch. This rare situation sometimes is seen in extreme Class II anomalies associated with mandibular hypoplasia. [Compare with Crossbite, Complete maxillary buccal.]

Complete maxillary buccal crossbite (Brodie syndrome) A situation in which the maxillary dental arch is wide and lies entirely buccal to (contains) the mandibular dental arch (named after A.G. Brodie). This rare situation sometimes is seen in extreme Class II anomalies associated with maxillary hyperplasia. [Compare with Crossbite, Complete mandibular lingual.]

Complete maxillary palatal crossbite A situation in which the maxillary dental arch is narrow and lies entirely lingual (contained within) the mandibular dental arch. This rare situation sometimes seen in extreme Class III anomalies associated with maxillary hypoplasia. [Compare

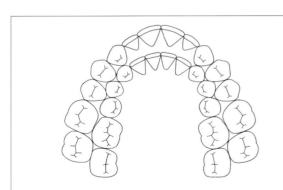

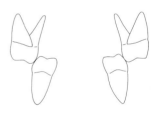

Complete maxillary buccal crossbite

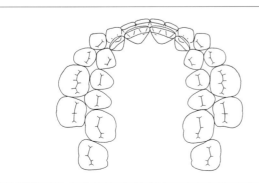

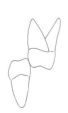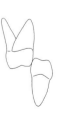

Complete maxillary palatal crossbite

with Crossbite, Complete mandibular buccal.]

Dental crossbite An abnormal relationship between antagonist teeth that is due to deviations in the position or inclination of one or a few teeth (i.e. the relationship between the maxilla and mandible is harmonious). Such crossbites usually are treatable by means of tooth movement alone. [Compare with Crossbite, Skeletal.]

Functional crossbite (Pseudo-crossbite) A crossbite that is due to a shift of the mandible (i.e. forced bite) into a faulty habitual occlusion (CO) because of a premature occlusal interference in centric relation (CR). The shift may occur in an anterior and/or in a lateral direction. Such crossbites often are seen in children, typically because of interferences caused by lack of wear of their deciduous canines. The treatment advocated for such problems may be enameloplas-

ty of the deciduous canines or expansion of the maxillary dental arch. [Also see Forced bite; Lateroclusion.]

Lingual crossbite A crossbite mainly due to lingual displacement of the affected mandibular tooth (or group of teeth) from its (their) ideal position relative to its (their) antagonist(s).

Palatal crossbite A crossbite mainly due to palatal displacement of the affected maxillary tooth (or group of teeth) from its (their) ideal position relative to its (their) antagonist(s).

Posterior crossbite A type of crossbite in which one or more deciduous or permanent posterior teeth occlude in an abnormal buccolingual relation with their antagonists. Posterior crossbites may occur unilaterally or bilaterally. They may be maxillary or mandibular, buccal or lingual, and may be

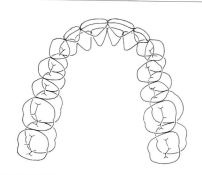 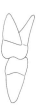 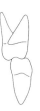

Unilateral posterior maxillary palatal crossbite 2

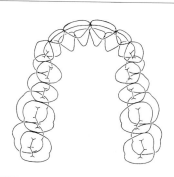 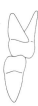 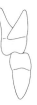

Bilateral posterior maxillary palatal crossbite 2

accompanied by a lateral functional shift of the mandible (especially in the case of unilateral posterior crossbites).

Scissors-bite Situation in which several adjacent posterior teeth overlap vertically in habitual occlusion with their antagonists, without contact of their occlusal surfaces. The deviation of the affected teeth from their ideal position could occur either in a buccal or a lingual direction.

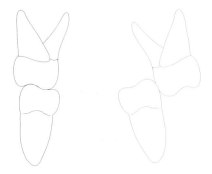

Scissors-bite

Skeletal crossbite Anterior or posterior (unilateral or bilateral) crossbite that is due to a sagittal or transverse incoordination in the size or shape of the maxilla and/or mandible. The treatment of such crossbites usually requires a skeletal expansion by means of rapid maxillary expansion or orthognathic surgery. [Compare with Crossbite, Dental; also see Laterognathia.]

Telescoping bite A term denoting either a complete mandibular lingual, or a complete maxillary buccal crossbite. The opposite (i.e. a complete maxillary palatal or a complete mandibular buccal crossbite) sometimes is called a *reverse telescoping bite.*

Crossbite elastics See Orthodontic elastics, Crossbite.

Cross-section of orthodontic wires See Archwire cross-section.

CRot See Center of rotation.

Crowding See Arch length discrepancy, Arch length deficiency.

Crown torque See Torque, Crown.

Crown movement See Orthodontic tooth movement, Pure crown movement.

Crozat appliance See Appliance, Crozat.

CT scan See Tomography, Computerized.

Curettage Soft tissue periodontal procedure aiming at removal of necrotic tissue lining the soft tissue wall of periodontal pockets by means of a curet.

Closed curettage Curettage that is performed via the gingival crevice, without an incision.

Open curettage Curettage facilitated by reflection of a gingival flap.

Curve of Monson A three-dimensional combination of the curves of Spee and Wilson. According to G.S. Monson, who introduced

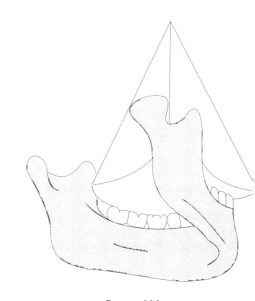

Curve of Monson

this concept (1920), all cusps and incisal edges in a natural dentition are tangent to a surface of a sphere, approximately 4 inches (10.2 cm) in radius, with its center in the area of the glabella.

Curve of Spee (Compensating curve) The curve displayed in the sagittal plane (or rather, in a plane parallel with the body of the mandible on either side) by the cusps and incisal edges of the mandibular teeth. The convex aspect of the curve of Spee is pointing inferiorly. The concept was first introduced by F. Graf von Spee in 1890, who theorized that the extension of this curve would be tangent to the anterior surface of the mandibular condyles, bilaterally.

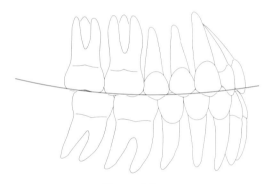

Curve of Spee

Reverse curve of Spee In many patients with a deep overbite, the curve formed by the cusps and incisal edges of the maxillary teeth is reverse to the curve of Spee, namely having its convex aspect pointing superiorly. When using continuous archwire mechanics for leveling of the mandibular arch, some clinicians incorporate a reverse curve of Spee in the mandibular archwire. Conversely, during leveling of the maxillary arch in a patient with a reverse curve of Spee, the opposite curve (i.e. accentuated curve of Spee) is incorporated into the maxillary archwire.

urve of Wilson When looking at a coronal section of the mandibular dentition one can

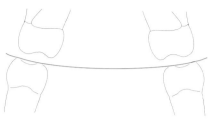

Curve of Wilson

see that the long axes of the mandibular molars and premolars converge towards the midline (i.e. they are tipped lingually). From this view the occlusal surfaces of these teeth bilaterally form a curve in a buccolingual direction. This imaginary curve that is defined by a line tangent to the buccal and lingual cusps of the mandibular posterior teeth bilaterally, is termed the *curve of Wilson*.

Cusp A conical-shaped, pointed or rounded eminence, on or near the occlusal surface of posterior teeth and on the lingual surface of anterior teeth, which may come into occlusal contact with a tooth of the opposing dental arch.

Functional cusps (Supporting cusps) The palatal cusps of the maxillary posterior teeth and the buccal cusps of the mandibular posterior teeth that come into occlusal contact in intercuspal position, maintaining the occlusal vertical dimension.

Non-functional cusps (Non-supporting cusps) The buccal cusps of the maxillary posterior teeth and the lingual cusps of the mandibular posterior teeth that do not directly contact the opposing teeth in intercuspal position. They act like the rim of a pestle to prevent food from escaping from the occlusal table, and they protect the buccal mucosa and the tongue by keeping them away from the functional cusps.

Plunger cusp A cusp that tends to forcibly wedge food into the interproximal area of two teeth of the opposing arch.

Cuspid See Canine.

Cutaneous Related to the skin.

Cyclosporine A pharmacological substance that can cause gingival hyperplasia. It is an immunosuppressant and antifungal agent, sometimes used to prevent rejection in recipients of organ transplants.

Cytokines A family of growth factors that mediate considerable roles in growth, differentiation and tissue damage by cellular receptors.

D

Dacryon See Cephalometric landmarks (Hard tissue), Dacryon.

De Coster line See Cephalometric lines, De Coster.

De la Rossa pliers See Orthodontic instruments, Arch-forming pliers.

Deactivation The process following the activation of an appliance (or an appliance part), during which the stored force is delivered to the dentition.

Debanding The removal of cemented orthodontic bands.

Debanding pliers See Orthodontic instruments, Band-removing pliers.

Debonding The removal of bonded orthodontic attachments.

Debonding pliers See Orthodontic instruments, Bracket-removing pliers.

Decalcification The removal of various minerals from a bone or tooth. [Also see White spot lesion.]

Deciduous dentition See Dentition, Deciduous.

Decompensation The process of removing the dentoalveolar compensations that may be present (by re-establishing the correct tooth position with regard to the skeletal base), usually prior to surgical correction

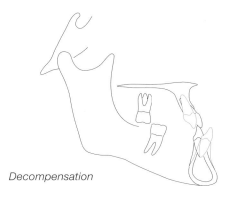

Decompensation

of a skeletal malocclusion. [Also see Dentoalveolar compensation.]

Decomposition of forces See Force resolution.

Decompression Force delivered by a component of an appliance that has been activated previously by elastically constricting its characteristic shape (e.g. the compression of an open coil spring). [Compare with Traction.]

Decompression of a joint (Unloading of a joint) Removal or release of pressure (stress) from a joint.

Deep bite Excessive overbite. Type of malocclusion in which the vertical overlap of the anterior teeth is increased beyond the ideal relationship; it is frequently associated with decreased vertical facial dimensions. Impingement of the mandibular incisors in the mucosa palatal to the maxillary incisors

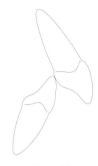

Deep bite

commonly is seen in malocclusions with extremely deep bite. As well, in some Class II, Division 2 malocclusions with minimal overjet the retroclined maxillary incisors may impinge in the keratinized tissue labial to the mandibular incisors, causing gingival recession.

Deflection A bending type of deformation, such as the deviation from the straight line (curving or arching) of a beam under an applied load.

Deflection (of the mandible on opening) Eccentric displacement of the mandible away from the midsagittal plane on mouth opening, without return to the centered position upon full opening. [Compare with Deviation.]

Deflective occlusal contact See Occlusal interference.

Deformable body A body that changes its shape when subjected to external forces, as opposed to a rigid body (an ideal concept).

Deformation A change in geometry (size and/or shape) of a body produced by the application of a mechanical force: an adaptive process of materials to stress.

Elastic deformation A temporary change of shape brought about on a body by the application of a mechanical force, within the elastic limit of the material from which the body is made. Upon removal of the deforming force there is full recovery to the original configuration, as the atoms in the crystalline structure of the body that were temporarily displaced resume their original position.

Permanent (Plastic, Inelastic) deformation A permanent change of shape or dimension brought about on a body by a mechanical force that exceeds the proportional limit of the material from which the body is made. The material will not recover its original shape on removal of the deforming force, as a permanent change has occurred in its crystalline structure.

Deformity A type of morphological defect involving an alteration in shape and/or structure of a previously normally formed part of the body, caused by nondisruptive mechanical forces (e.g. clubfoot, or congenital hip dislocation). Deformities arise most frequently during late fetal life. [Compare with Malformation; Disruption.]

Degeneration Deterioration of soft tissue, cartilage and bone into a tissue of inferior quality. When referring to a complex structure such as a joint or articulation, describes the failure to adapt to loading forces, resulting in impaired function.

Degenerative arthritis See Osteoarthritis.

Degenerative joint disease (DJD) See Osteoarthritis.

Deglutition See Swallow.

Degrees of freedom The number of independent coordinates required to specify the complete position of a body. For example, a body pivoting about a fixed axis has a single degree of freedom, reflecting the fact that motion is permitted in only one plane. A rigid body in space (such as a tooth) has six degrees of freedom, corresponding to its six possible motions: linear motion along the x-, y- and z- axes and angular motion (rotation) about the three axes x-, y- and z-.

ehiscence An isolated vertical soft tissue and bony defect, exposing a part of the root of a tooth. It occurs more commonly on the vestibular aspect of anterior teeth, especially mandibular incisors.

e-impaction Any process aiming at bringing an impacted tooth into the dental arch.

elaire face mask See Appliance, Face mask.

elta clasp See Clasp, Delta.

ens evaginatus (Leong's premolar) A dental anomaly characterized by a supernumerary cusp on the occlusal aspect of an otherwise normal tooth. It is thought to be the reverse of dens invaginatus and occurs in approximately 2% of the Asian and Native American population. Histologically, the extra cusp is composed of a thin pulpal extension surrounded by dentin and enamel. Dens evaginatus occurs most commonly in premolars as an extra cusp which may be large enough to cause occlusal interferences. Any attempt at occlusal equilibration, or simply occlusal wear or trauma, can result in pulpal degeneration and periapical inflammation. The teeth with the anomaly typically are caries-free, and may have an immature root. If extractions are indicated as part of the orthodontic treatment plan, the premolars with the anomaly typically are given preference, as endodontic treatment may have a poor prognosis due to the immature root or arrested root formation of these teeth.

ens in dente See Dens invaginatus.

ens invaginatus (Dens in dente) A developmental defect resulting in invagination of a pit or fissure in the crown, before it is calcified, into the future pulp space, giving the appearance of "a tooth within a tooth". The invagination is partially or completely lined with enamel and may extend all the way to the apex. Dens invaginatus is occasionally seen in (peg-shaped) maxillary lateral incisors. In the presence of caries an acute or chronic pulpal inflammation could rapidly occur, and thus these teeth should be preferred when extractions are indicated, especially since their crowns and/or roots typically are malformed.

Dental arch See Arch, Dental.

Dental casts See Orthodontic casts.

Dental compensation See Dentoalveolar compensation.

Dental crossbite See Crossbite, Dental.

Dental hygienist A dental auxiliary person who has been trained in an approved course in dental hygiene and is licensed to provide dental hygiene services. [Taken from the AAO Glossary of Dentofacial Orthopedic Terms, 1993.]

Dental mobility See Tooth mobility.

Dental plaque See Plaque.

Dental protrusion See Protrusion, Dental.

Dental retrusion See Retrusion, Dental.

Dental wear See Attrition.

Dentinogenesis imperfecta A hereditary disorder that can appear in several different types, which affects the development of dentin and may be accompanied by a similar disturbance of the bones. Clinically the teeth may appear opalescent or gray with bulbous crowns; attrition is rapid and enamel chips easily. Usually, extensive prosthetic restorations are indicated.

Dentition The complement of teeth.

Deciduous dentition (Primary dentition) The deciduous teeth.

Mixed dentition (Transitional dentition) The dentition in the period spanning from the eruption of the first permanent tooth until the shedding of the last deciduous tooth, during which both permanent and deciduous teeth are present in the mouth.

Permanent dentition The permanent teeth.

Dentoalveolar Concerning the teeth and the alveolar bone. [The term often is used to indicate a correction that is achieved by adaptation of the teeth and alveolar processes, without any skeletal effect.]

Dentoalveolar compensation The natural adaptive changes of the dentition, which tend to mask the severity of any skeletal discrepancy that may be present between the maxilla and mandible (e.g. proclination of the maxillary incisors and retroclination of the mandibular incisors resulting in a positive overjet in a skeletal Class III malocclusion).

Dentofacial deformity A malformation of the teeth, jaws and/or face characterized by disharmonies of size, form and/or function. The term encompasses problems such as malocclusion, cleft lip and palate and other skeletal or soft tissue anomalies, or syndromes that involve the face and the dentoalveolar complex.

Dentofacial orthopedics See Orthodontics and dentofacial orthopedics.

Dento-gingival fibers See Gingival fibers.

Dento-periosteal fibers See Gingival fibers.

Depression of the mandible See Arthrokinetics of the TMJ.

Deprogramming splint See Splint, Diagnostic.

Derotation of molars The term usually is meant to describe the procedure aimed at correction of the mesiolingual rotation (about the large palatal root) of the maxillary

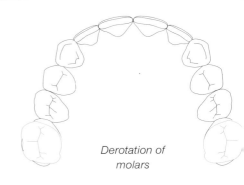

Derotation of molars

first permanent molars, a common finding in Class II malocclusions.
Derotation of molars can be achieved with various treatment modalities, e.g. by using transpalatal arch.

Development In the normal youngster, growth and development are processes that work in concert with one another and actually are inseparable. It is helpful, however in understanding the contributions that each one makes to the progress of individual change to divide them arbitrarily into their actual areas of manifestation. Therefore development is considered the area of differentiation and maturation that leads to increased skill, more comprehensive function and sexual dimorphism in progress toward maturity.
Growth, arbitrarily separated from development, relates to the changes in physical size which may be measured in increments weight or linear change.
Through this artificial separation of these two elements one is able to note individual changes that may exhibit an increase size but be lacking in maturational evolution whereas, on the other hand, one may observe conditions in which the natural maturational processes toward adulthood take place without a significant or measurable increase in size. [Also see Growth.]

Developmental guidance An orthodontic and orthopedic effort to influence change in the dentition, growth of the jaws, and functional conditions with the objective guiding abnormal development into a normal situation. This generally requires a combination of carefully timed interceptive procedures or appliance therapies based on supervisory examinations, involving radiographic and other diagnostic records at various stages of development. This may be required from the earliest date of detection of a developing malformation until the craniofacial skeleton is mature. [Modified from the AAO Glossary of Dentofacial Orthopedic Terms, 1993.]

Deviation (of the mandible on opening) Eccentric displacement of the mandible on mouth opening, away from the midsagittal plane, with correction to the centered position upon full opening. [Compare with Deflection (of the mandible on opening).]

Di Paolo cephalometric analysis See Cephalometric analysis, Di Paolo.

Diagnosis The determination of the nature of a disease or condition, by study and consideration of the patient's history, as well as the signs and symptoms and their manifestation.

Diagnostic casts See Orthodontic casts, Study casts.

Diagnostic imaging Any hard-record representation or visual reproduction of a body part or structure produced for diagnostic purposes (includes procedures such as conventional radiography, ultrasound, CT and MRI).

Diagnostic setup (Kesling setup) A laboratory procedure first described by H.D. Kesling. The teeth are cut from a duplicate study model and realigned in the desired position using wax to evaluate the predicted occlusal result of a specific orthodontic treatment plan or diagnose a tooth size discrepancy.

Diagnostic splint See Splint, Diagnostic.

Diagonal elastics, Anterior See Orthodontic elastics, Anterior diagonal.

Diagram, Free body See Free body diagram.

Diastema A space between two adjacent teeth in the same arch. [Also see Midline diastema.]

Differential force theory A theory proposed by P.R. Begg (1956), which constitutes the basic philosophy behind the Begg technique. According to this, the force applied for space closure should be light enough to exceed the "critical threshold of stress"

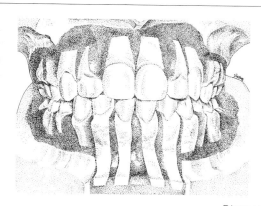 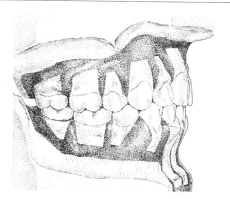

Diagnostic setup

2

necessary for tooth movement on the active segment of teeth, but still be below the "critical stress threshold" for movement of the anchorage segment, so that no anchorage loss occurs. The area of root surface over which the force is dissipated is a determining factor for the amount of movement that will be experienced by a specific tooth (or segment of teeth). Incorporating more teeth in the anchorage segment increases the root surface area, reducing the stress in the periodontal ligament for the same magnitude of force.

According to the same theory, it is hypothesized that there is a certain level of stress in the periodontal ligament beyond which hyalinization will occur. If a force of such a high magnitude is used during space closure, there may be no or little movement of the active segment because of hyalinization, but the resulting stress over the larger root surface area of the anchorage segment could exceed its threshold for tooth movement, resulting in anchorage loss. [Also see Appliance, Begg.]

Differential impaction (of the maxilla) See Impaction of the maxilla.

Differentiation The change from generalized cells or tissues to more specialized ones during development. It is a change in quality or kind.

Digastric muscle See Muscle, Digastric.

Digital subtraction radiography See Subtraction radiography.

Digitization (of radiographs) Conversion of landmarks on a radiograph or tracing to numerical values on a two- (or three-) dimensional coordinate system, usually for the purpose of computerized cephalometric analysis. The process allows for automatic measurement of landmark relationships. [See also Computerized cephalometrics.]

Dilaceration A developmental distortion of the form of a tooth, whereby the root or the apex forms an angle with the long axis of the tooth (i.e. the tooth appears sharply "curved" or "bent"). Dilacerations can occur as a result of trauma or mechanical impedance of tooth eruption. In the latter situation, the developing apical part of the erupting tooth is forced to move in a direction opposite to that of eruption, inducing resorption of bone in an area where it usually does not occur. Teeth with severe dilaceration may be impossible to align in an ideal way and in severe cases extraction may be indicated.

Dillon dimple A latching indentation on the palatal wall of a sheath, in which the doubled end of the palatal arch fits tightly, providing a "lock" to retain the palatal arch in position. Named after its innovator, C.F.S. Dillon. [Also see Sheath.]

Diplomate See ABO diplomate.

Direct bonding See Bonding, Direct.

Direct resorption (Frontal resorption) See Bone resorption, Direct.

Direction (Line of action) One of the four characteristics of vectorial quantities (the other three are point of application, sense and magnitude). Direction refers to the line on which the specific vector lies. It can be defined by specifying the angular deviation (in degrees) of the vector from a given reference line or axis.

Disarticulation See Disclusion.

Disc See Articular disc.

Disc-condyle complex The condyle and its disc articulation, which functions as a simple hinge joint.

Disc derangement See Disc displacement.

Disc displacement (Disc derangement, Disc prolapse, Disc interference disorder) The dislocation of the articular disc of the temporomandibular joint from its physiologic position on the head of the condyle. It most often occurs in an antero-medial direction. Disc displacements are a common etiologic factor for joint sounds (clicks or pops) and often result in an unusual opening and closing trajectory of the mandible, or in limitation of maximal opening.

Disc displacement with reduction A situation in which the articular disc of the temporomandibular joint is displaced (usually in an anteromedial direction) when the mandible is in the intercuspal position, but resumes a normal anatomic relationship with the condyle (is "re-captured" by the condyle) on mandibular movement. [Also see Clicking, Reciprocal.]

Disc displacement without reduction A situation in which the articular disc of the temporomandibular joint is displaced when the mandible is at the intercuspal position and does not resume a physiologic anatomic relationship with the condyle upon mandibular movement.

sc interference disorder See Disc displacement.

sc locking See Disc displacement without reduction.

sc perforation A circumscribed tear in the articular disc of the TMJ, usually as a result of a degenerative thinning in its central portion, permitting communication between the superior and inferior joint spaces and direct contact between the articular surfaces of the condyle and temporal bone.

sc prolapse See Disc displacement.

sc-repositioning surgery Arthrotomy of the TMJ with the purpose of reestablishing a physiologic anatomic disc-to-condyle relationship. [Also see Plication.]

scectomy (Meniscectomy) Surgical removal of the articular disc of a joint.

Disclusion (Disocclusion, Disarticulation) Separation of the mandible from the maxilla through tooth-guided contacts during mandibular excursive movements.

Discrepancy Inconsistency, incongruency or disagreement. [See Arch length discrepancy; Tooth size discrepancy; Midline discrepancy.]

"Dished-in" profile A profile with severely reduced lip prominence. The term originally referred to the side effect of early orthodontic treatment attempts to "camouflage" an underlying skeletal discrepancy (usually a Class II malocclusion) by removing premolar teeth (a routine treatment method up until the 1970's). More recently, the advancement of orthognathic surgical techniques as well as the rise in popularity of growth modification in North America have led to increased awareness of the esthetic facial changes brought upon by various orthodontic treatment options. [Also see "Camouflage" orthodontic treatment.]

Disjunction, Pterygomaxillary See Pterygomaxillary disjunction.

Disk See Articular disc.

Dislocation of the condyle (Luxation, Open lock) Non-reducible displacement of the mandibular condyle in an anterior direction, past the articular eminence.

Disocclusion See Disclusion.

Displaced fracture See Fracture, Displaced.

Displacement Movement away from a certain position or place.

Displacement (of a bone) In addition to direct bone growth due to apposition and resorption, a second characteristic mechanism of skull growth is the process of displacement, i.e. the translatory movement of the bone as a whole. The entire bone is carried away from its articular interfaces

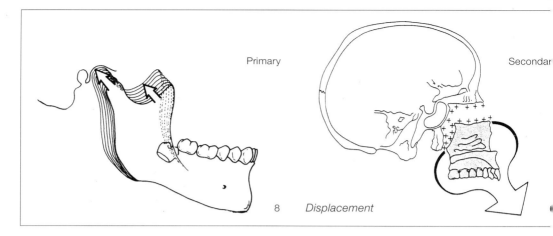

Primary   Secondar

8   *Displacement*

(sutures, synchondroses, condyles) with adjacent bones.

D.H. Enlow used the term *primary displacement (translation)* for that occurring in conjunction with a bone's own growth. Primary displacement always takes place in a direction opposite to that of the bone growth (e.g. the mandibular condyle grows upward and backward, but the result is downward and forward displacement of the mandible).

Bone displacement caused by enlargement of adjacent or remote bones or tissues but not of the bone itself, is termed *secondary displacement* (e.g. secondary displacement of the nasomaxillary complex is caused by growth of the middle cranial fossa and the brain, in a downward and forward direction).

Displacement (of a tooth)   See Orthodontic tooth movement.

Disruption   A morphological defect of an organ, part of an organ, or a larger region of the body resulting from a breakdown of, or interference with, an originally normal developmental process. An example is an amputation of a digit in utero, or a atypical facial cleft caused by an amniotic band. [Compare with Malformation; Deformity.]

Dissociation, Point of   See Burstone's geometry classes, Geometry IV.

Distal   Away from a point of reference. In t case of teeth, away from the dental midlir along the dental arch (in a right or left dire tion when referring to anterior teeth, or ir posterior direction when referring to pos rior teeth). [Compare with Mesial.]

Distal drift   See Drift (of teeth), Distal.

Distal-end bends   See Bends, Distal-end.

Distal-end cutter   See Orthodontic instr ments, Distal-end cutter.

Distal-end stops   See Bends, Distal-end.

Distal segment   See Segment, Distal.

"Distal shoe" space maintainer   See Spac maintainer, "Distal shoe."

Distal step   See Terminal plane, Distal step.

Distal tipping   Tipping of the crown of a too in the distal direction.

Distalization   The movement of teeth to the d tal.

Molar distalization   A treatment proc dure designed to provide space for alig ment of teeth and achievement of ide overjet and overbite, as an alternative

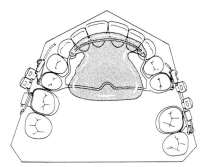

Molar distalization with repelling magnets 5

premolar extraction. The procedure can be performed with or without extraction of the second molars. Various appliances are designed for this purpose, including the ACCO and pendulum appliances, appliances with compressed coils or repelling magnets, and extraoral traction appliances.

istoclusion See Angle classification, Class II malocclusion.

istortion Deviation of a radiographic image from the true outline or shape of the object or structure.

istoversion Distal tipping (angulation) of a tooth or group of teeth.

istraction (of the condyle) Separation or forced downward movement of the condyle from the articular fossa.

istraction (of the mandible) See Arthro-kinetics of the TMJ.

istraction osteogenesis (Distraction osteosynthesis, Ilizarov technique, Callus distraction, Callotasis) A technique for lengthening of long bones of the extremities attributed to G.A. Ilizarov, although it was first described by A. Codivilla in 1905. Other applications of the method in orthopedics are in the treatment of fractures or malunions. It also is used in the craniofacial area for the correction of bone defects in the skull and for the treatment of hypoplasias of the maxilla or the mandible. It involves a corticotomy followed by gradual distraction of the segments, with formation of new bone (*regenerate* bone) between them. The distraction can be performed by an extraoral or an intraoral device containing some type of screw that can be wound gradually, in a manner similar to rapid maxillary expansion.

The advantage of the technique is that it allows simultaneous expansion of the surrounding soft tissue envelope and generates bone without the need for a graft.

The disadvantages include the facial scars and inconvenience in the case of an extraoral distraction appliance, as well as the lack of adequate control of the direction of movement (mainly in the case of the proximal segments in mandibular distraction). Furthermore, little is known about the potential implications of a mandibular distraction procedure on the TMJs.

DJD See Osteoarthritis.

Dolichocephalic Anthropometric term denoting an individual with a long, narrow cranial form; having a cephalic index smaller than 76. Severe dolichocephaly may result from premature synostosis of the sagittal suture. [Compare with Brachycephalic.]

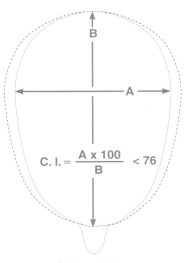

$$C.\,I. = \frac{A \times 100}{B} < 76$$

Dolichocephaly

Dolichofacial A facial pattern characterized by a long, narrow face. [Compare with Brachyfacial.]

Donor site The area of the body from which a graft is taken. [Compare with Recipient site.]

"Donut" See Separator, Elastic; Elastomeric modules, Elastomeric ligature.

Double-contrast arthrography See Arthrography of the TMJ, Double-contrast.

Double-space arthrography See Arthrography of the TMJ, Double-space.

Double-width bracket See Bracket, Twin.

Down-fracture (of the maxilla) An orthognathic procedure in which all or part of the maxillary alveolar and basal bone is separated from the more superior elements of the midfacial skeleton. The procedure usually involves a Le Fort I or sometimes a Le Fort II osteotomy.

Down-grafting (of the maxilla) Surgical repositioning of the maxilla in a direction inferior (occlusal) to its original position, usually after a Le Fort I osteotomy, with the use of an interpositional bone graft.

Down syndrome (Trisomy 21) Down syndrome is the most common and well known of all malformation syndromes of chromosomal etiology, and is characterized generalized physical and mental deficiencies. Its birth prevalence varies from 1 in 60 to 1 in 2000 live births. The condition was first described by J.L. Down in 1866.

Patients with Down syndrome typically present with a degree of brachycephaly, a small nose with flattening of the nasal bridge and hypoplasia of the midface. Upward slanting of the palpebral fissures and epicanthic folds are common.

The lips are fissured and dry. Perioral muscles are affected by characteristic muscle hypotonia, leading to descending angles the mouth and an everted lower lip. An open mouth with a protruding tongue is observed. The tongue often is fissured or scalloped and appears large either because of a relatively small oral cavity or because of true macroglossia. Mouth breathing common is seen, contributing to chronic periodontitis and xerostomia. A cleft of the lip and/palate is present in 0.5% of cases.

The midfacial hypoplasia commonly results in a Class III skeletal pattern with an anterior or posterior crossbite. The length, height and depth of the palate commonly are affected, but the width usually is not. An anterior open bite also is a frequent finding for which when true macroglossia is present, a partial glossectomy occasionally is advocated. Maxillary and mandibular incisors frequently are proclined.

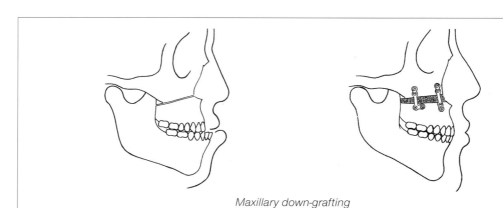

Maxillary down-grafting 4

Patients with Down syndrome exhibit proneness to periodontal disease (reportedly over 90% of patients), as well as a relatively low prevalence of dental caries.

Between 35% and 55% of affected individuals present with microdontia in both the primary and secondary dentition. Eruption of both deciduous and permanent teeth often is delayed. An irregular sequence of eruption also is common, deciduous first molars sometimes preceding incisors. Taurodontism is reported to occur with greater than expected frequency. [Also see Taurodontism.]

owns cephalometric analysis See Cephalometric analysis, Downs.

ownward and backward rotation (of the mandible) See Mandibular rotation, Clockwise.

rift (of bones) A term established by D.H. Enlow to signify the movement of a bony structure in relation to adjacent structures, caused by simultaneous bone apposition and resorption processes on opposing surfaces. [Also see Cortical drift.]

rift (of teeth) Spontaneous movement of teeth without the direct application of orthodontic forces.

Distal drift 1. The occasional tendency of teeth mesial to an edentulous space to move distally into it. **2.** The spontaneous distal movement of teeth associated with active distalization of adjacent teeth (e.g. the distal drift of the maxillary premolars following molar distalization.)

Mesial drift (Mesial migration, Approximal drift) A term applied to either a natural developmental phenomenon whereby the posterior teeth continually move in a mesial direction as a result of interproximal surface wear, or to the tendency of teeth distal to an edentulous space to move mesially into it. [See Physiologic tooth movement, Posteruptive].

Dual-cured glass-ionomer cement See Orthodontic cement, Resin-modified glass-ionomer.

Dual bite A situation in which a patient has two positions of habitual occlusion (intercuspal position) that differ by more than 2 mm.

Ductility The ability of a material to sustain a large permanent deformation under a tensile load without rupture. A metal that can be drawn readily into a wire is said to be ductile. Ductility is heavily dependent on strength. [Compare with Malleability.]

Dynamic fatigue failure See Fatigue failure, Dynamic.

Dynamic friction See Friction.

Dynamics The branch of mechanics that considers forces on bodies which are being accelerated positively or negatively. Dynamics plays a relatively minor role in orthodontics, where accelerations or decelerations are practically negligible. Dynamics is comprised further of *kinematics* and *kinetics*.

Kinematics The branch of dynamics that studies the motion of bodies without reference to the forces that cause the motion.

Kinetics The branch of dynamics that considers the forces acting on bodies in relation to the resulting motions.

Dysfunction Abnormal, impaired or altered function.

Dysostosis A pathological condition characterized by defective ossification, especially involving fetal cartilages.

Dysplasia Abnormality of development.

E

E See Modulus of elasticity.

E-arch See Arch, E-arch.

E-line (Esthetic line of Ricketts) See Cephalometric lines, E-line.

E-modulus See Modulus of elasticity.

E-plane See Cephalometric lines, E-line.

Early closing click See Clicking, Early closing.

Early opening click See Clicking, Early opening.

Eccentric extraoral traction See Headgear, Asymmetric.

Eccentric headgear See Headgear, Asymmetric.

Ectopic eruption The eruption of a tooth in an abnormal position. In the permanent dentition, this condition occurs most often in maxillary first molars and maxillary or mandibular incisors and canines. A typical example is the eruption of a maxillary fir permanent molar in a mesial position und the distal part of the crown of the adjace second deciduous molar.

Edentulous ridge See Ridge, Residual.

Edge bevel Rounding of the edges of orth dontic wires with square or rectangul cross section, as part of their manufacturir process. A certain amount of edge bevelir is desirable to prevent discomfort of the sc tissues and to facilitate engagement of th archwire in the bracket slot. If the amount rounding is excessive, it can be of clinic significance for control of the buccolingu inclination of the teeth provided by the arc wire-bracket combination.

Edge-to-edge bite (End-to-end bite) A sit ation in which the maxillary and mandibul incisors meet with contact of their incis edges. This type of occlusal relationship most commonly seen in malocclusions wi a Class III component.

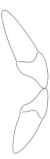

Edge-to-edge bite

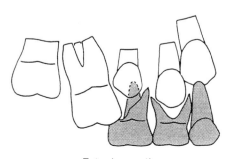

Ectopic eruption 2

Edgewise appliance See Appliance, Edg wise.

dgewise bracket See Appliance, Edgewise.

dwards' procedure See Circumferential supracrestal fibrotomy.

ffective force system See Force system, Effective.

astic cartilage See Cartilage, Elastic.

lastic deformation See Deformation, Elastic.

astic force delivery rate See Stiffness.

astic limit The maximum deformation that a body (e.g. orthodontic wire or appliance part) can undergo before permanent (plastic) deformation occurs. Precise experimental distinction between the proportional limit and the elastic limit is difficult, and for all practical purposes they can be considered indistinguishable.

astic material A material that undergoes no permanent deformation (fully recovers its original shape), after it has been subjected to a certain stress. [Also see Elasticity.]

astic modules See Elastomeric modules.

astic modulus (E) S. Modulus of elasticity.

astic open activator See Appliance, Elastic open activator.

astic range The strain up to which no plastic deformation occurs. [On a stress/strain diagram, the horizontal (strain) coordinate of the elastic limit.]

astic separator See Separator, Elastic.

astic separator pliers See Orthodontic instruments, Elastic separator pliers.

astic strength The load (stress) up to which no plastic deformation occurs. [On a stress/strain diagram, the vertical (stress) coordinate of the elastic limit.]

Elastic thread See Elastomeric modules, Elastomeric thread.

Elasticity The property of a material to exhibit reversible deformation under load (i.e. changing its shape without undergoing permanent deformation). An elastic material regains its original shape when the load is removed. [Also see Modulus of elasticity.]

Elasticity, Modulus of See Modulus of elasticity.

Elastomer (Elastomeric material) A polymer (soft, rubber-like material) containing large molecules with weak interaction among them, cross-linked at certain points to form a three-dimensional structure. Elastomers may be stretched when their chains are pulled apart and uncoiled, but on removal of the stress they snap back to their relaxed state and practically their original dimensions.

Elastomeric chain See Elastomeric modules, Elastomeric chain.

Elastomeric ligature See Elastomeric modules, Elastomeric ligature.

Elastomeric modules Different configurations of elastomeric material in the shape of small circles (ligatures), chains or threads, with various orthodontic applications.

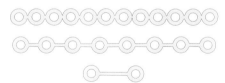

Elastomeric modules

Elastomeric chain A chain of connected elastomeric rings used as a force-producing mechanism for orthodontic tooth movement. Elastomeric chains can be open or closed, depending on whether or not there is a distance between the rings at its passive state.

Elastomeric ligature ("Donut," "O-ring") Small round band of elastomeric material that is stretched around the tie-wings of an orthodontic bracket for the purpose of preventing disengagement of an archwire or auxiliary from a bracket slot.

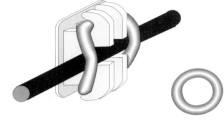

Elastomeric ligature

Elastomeric thread A stretchable thread made of elastomeric material available in various cross-sectional thicknesses. It is used as a force-producing mechanism for tooth movement.

Electromyography (EMG) Detection and recording of changes in the intrinsic electric potentials of skeletal muscles, by means of surface (*surface EMG*) or needle electrodes (*deep EMG*).

Elevation of the mandible See Arthrokinetics of the TMJ.

Elevator masticatory muscles Paired masseter, medial pterygoid and temporalis muscles, the main action of which is to elevate the mandible.

Elgiloy wire See Cobalt-chromium alloy.

Elongation Overall deformation (elastic and plastic) of a material as a result of tensile force application.

Emergence The stage of the eruption process involving the initial penetration of the gingiva by the erupting tooth and its first appearance in the oral cavity. The term sometimes is used to signify breaking through the alveolar bone during eruption.

EMG See Electromyography.

Eminectomy Surgical removal of part of the articular eminence of the temporomandibular joint or recontouring of its surface. Eminectomy occasionally is contemplated as a treatment modality for some types of TMD.

Emission scintigraphy (Planar scintigraphy) Two-dimensional imaging process in which the area of interest is scanned with a gamma camera 2 to 4 hours after the administration of a radio-labeled material. When bone is to be assessed, technetium 99m is the radioisotope of choice due to its tendency to accumulate in areas of osteoblastic activity. Increased uptake of the radioisotope in the tissue scanned is indicative of increased cellular activity (as for instance an active area of growth in children, neoplasia or inflammation).

"En masse" retraction Retraction of a number of teeth (usually the four incisors, or a six anterior teeth) together, as a group.

"End-on" Anteroposterior deviation of an occlusal relationship from the ideal occlusion by one half cusp (half the mesiodistal width of a premolar). The term can be used for either Class II or Class III occlusal relationships.

End-to-end bite See Edge-to-edge bite.

Endochondral bone See Bone, Endochondral.

Endochondral ossification See Ossification, Endochodral.

Endosseous implant See Implant, Endosseous.

Engagement (of the bracket slot) See Bracket slot engagement.

Enucleation Surgical removal of a bone cyst together with its lining, or of a tooth th

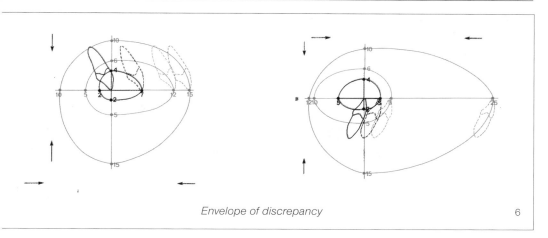

Envelope of discrepancy

6

has not yet emerged into the oral cavity. Enucleation of premolars sometimes is contemplated as part of a serial extraction protocol, but depending on the technique and the situation, it carries a chance of creating a residual bony defect at the site. Enucleation of the mandibular third molars sometimes is advocated as a means to increase the available space in a severely crowded mandibular arch.

Envelope of discrepancy A diagram devised by W.R. Proffit and J.L. Ackerman to illustrate graphically the amount of change that can be produced by orthodontic tooth movement alone (inner envelope), orthodontic tooth movement combined with growth modification (middle envelope), and orthognathic surgery (outer envelope) in the sagittal and vertical planes of space, based on the authors' clinical judgment.

Envelope of motion The three-dimensional space circumscribed by border mandibular movements and by the incisal and occlusal contacts of a given point of the mandible.

Epicanthal folds Excess skin and subcutaneous tissue lateral to the nasal bridge, concealing the medial canthi. Epicanthal folds may be a result of racial phenotype (common in Asians), nasal bridge hypoplasia, orbital hypotelorism, surgery, or trauma.

Epidemiology The science concerned with the frequency and distribution of a disease or state. Its focus is on the total population rather than the individual, and its purpose is disease classification and prevention.

Epithelial attachment See Junctional epithelium.

Epithelialized free soft tissue graft See Graft, Free gingival.

Equilibration, Occlusal See Occlusal equilibration.

Equilibrium The state of a body (i.e. a tooth or dental segment) or a system when the sum of all the forces and the sum of all the moments acting on it is equal to zero. The assumption that a system is in static equilibrium at a given point is the basis for static analysis of all mechanical systems.

    Adult occlusal equilibrium See Occlusal equilibrium, Adult.

    Juvenile occlusal equilibrium See Occlusal equilibrium, Juvenile.

Equivalent force systems See Force system, Equivalent force systems.

105

Erasmus postgraduate program in orthodontics A collaborative effort among 15 European Union (EU) and non-EU countries, initiated by F.P.G.M. van der Linden, with the purpose of developing a 3-year postgraduate orthodontic program curriculum, with a common content of 75%, leaving the remaining 25% for electives. The project, which was funded by a grant through the Erasmus Bureau of the European Cultural Foundation of the EU, was carried out between 1990 and 1992, and stimulated the standardization of postgraduate orthodontic education throughout Europe, as well as in other parts of the world.

Eruption See Tooth eruption.

Eruption, Forced See Forced eruption.

Eruption path The path traversed by a tooth, through surrounding tissues, from the initiation of its eruptive movement until its arrival at its functional position in the mouth.

Eruption theories See Tooth eruption mechanisms.

Eruptive tooth movement See Physiologic tooth movement, Eruptive.

Essix retainer See Retainer, Essix.

Esthetic bracket See Bracket, Esthetic.

Esthetic bends See Bends, Artistic.

Esthetic line of Ricketts (E-line) See Cephalometric lines, E-line.

Esthetic plane of Rees See Cephalometric lines, Rees esthetic plane.

Esthetic plane of Steiner (S-line) See Cephalometric lines, S-line.

Esthetics, Facial See Facial esthetics.

Etching See Acid etching.

Etiologic factors Factors that may be involve in, or cause the development of a diseas or condition.

Etiology The cause of a medical or dental co dition.

Euryprosopic Having a wide and short faci form.

Excursion of the mandible Movement of th mandible away from the median position the intercuspal occlusion position. [Also se Arthrokinetics of the TMJ.]

    Lateral excursion Right or left mov ment of the mandible away from the mi sagittal plane (to the side). [Compare wit Laterotrusion; Mediotrusion.]

    Protrusive excursion Anterior moveme of the mandible from the intercuspal positio

Exfoliation (Shedding) Physiological loss a deciduous tooth prior to the eruption of successor.

Exostosis A hyperplastic osseous overgrow projecting outward from the surface of a bor (e.g. *torus palatinus, torus mandibularis*).

Expansion Enlargement; increase in volum surface or extent. The term often is used refer to the process of widening of the de tal arches.

    Asymmetric expansion At the level the dental arch, asymmetric expansion ca be attempted by pitting the segment teeth that primarily needs to be expande against an anchorage segment of increase size. In practice this is done by incorpora ing more teeth or a larger palatal surface the anchorage segment (anchorage rei forcement) and/or by expanding the tee on the active segment one at a time. In a case, some buccal displacement of th teeth in the anchorage segment will observed as a side effect.

Rapid maxillary (palatal) expansion (RME, RPE) A method of increasing the maxillary arch width by opening the midpalatal suture, thereby achieving some degree of skeletal expansion. The method, which was popularized by A.J. Haas, involves the use of a fixed (cemented or bonded) maxillary appliance of several possible designs, using an expansion screw of the same type as in the Hyrax appliance. The screw typically is activated by at least 0.20 to 0.25 mm (one quarter turn) daily and may produce a force as high as 100 N (10 kg or 20 lb). Expansion usually is continued until the lingual cusps of the maxillary posterior teeth come into contact with the lingual inclines of the buccal cusps of the mandibular posterior teeth. A diastema commonly appears between the central incisors as the midpalatal suture separates, which closes spontaneously in the few weeks following the procedure due to the pull of the supracrestal fibers. When active expansion has been completed, a 3- to 5-month retention period is recommended with the appliance in place. It is advocated that this type of expansion may have more of a skeletal effect and may minimize the amount of dental tipping, which is a common (usually undesirable) side effect of orthodontic arch expansion. [Also see Appliance, Hyrax; Appliance, Haas.]

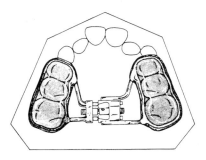

Bonded RME appliance   5

Slow maxillary (palatal) expansion (SME or SPE) A method of increasing the maxillary dental arch width by using a maxillary removable appliance that normally carries an expansion screw in the midline.

The appliance commonly is activated by 0.20 to 0.50 mm (one or two quarter turns) per week and is advocated in patients that require limited expansion, since it produces expansion mainly by dental tipping. [Also see Appliance, Expansion

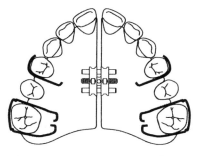

Slow maxillary expansion appliance   11

Surgically assisted rapid maxillary expansion In adult patients in whom the midpalatal suture is fused, the resistance to suture separation can be decreased by bilateral osteotomies of the lateral maxillary buttress, with or without a midpalatal osteotomy. After the lateral osteotomies are performed, the screw is turned a few times in the operating room to achieve separation of the suture and is subsequently turned back. The patient can begin activating the appliance the following day. If correction of a unilateral maxillary palatal crossbite is necessary, the lateral osteotomy can be made only on one side, thus creating a differential anchorage situation.

Expansion appliance See Appliance, Expansion.

Expansion screw (Jackscrew or Glenn Ross screw) A mechanical device incorporated in a removable or fixed appliance used to enlarge the dental arch, usually in the transverse dimension. Expansion screws also can be used as part of a removable appliance for individual tooth movement or for incisor proclination, as well as in a bone distraction device for distraction osteogenesis.

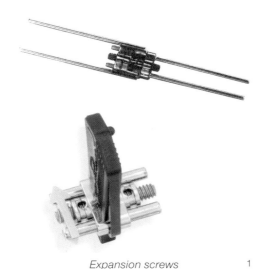

Expansion screws   1

Expansion screw key An instrument used to turn the jackscrew of an expansion appliance.

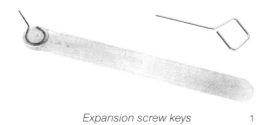

Expansion screw keys   1

Exposure (of a tooth) See Surgical exposure.

External pterygoid muscle See Muscle, Lateral pterygoid.

External resorption See Resorption, External.

External rotation (of the mandible) See Mandibular rotation, Intramatrix.

Extracapsular adhesion See Adhesion, Extracapsular.

Extraction Removal of teeth.

Extraction, Serial See Serial extraction.

Extraction series bracket See Bracket, Extraction series.

Extraoral traction appliance See Appliance, Extraoral traction.

Extraction therapy Orthodontic treatment requiring the extraction of one or more permanent teeth.

Extraction vs. non-extraction debate A long-standing controversial issue in orthodontics, over whether or not extraction of permanent teeth is advisable and necessary as part of orthodontic treatment. This debate started in the early 1900s between E.H. Angle and his former student C.S. Case, and has been continuing, on and off, ever since.

Angle's thesis was that "there shall be a full complement of teeth and each tooth shall be made to occupy its normal position." He believed in the universal applicability of the "normal occlusion theory" in which every tooth must have its ideal position and serve its specific function.

Case, on the other hand, defended the judicious use of extraction as a practical procedure. Following his own precisely set rules, he claimed to extract in only 12% to 15% of his cases.

The climax of this conflict was a fierce debate in 1911 between Case and M. Dewey (who represented Angle's views) at the annual meeting of the National Dental Association (former name of the ADA). It took many years after this episode for the problem to become a matter of calm and objective evaluation and respectful appreciation of various points of view, each of which has made its contribution to orthodontics.

Extraoral anchorage See Anchorage, Extraoral.

Extraoral force See Force, Extraoral.

Extraoral traction The use of extraoral anchorage to apply forces to the dentition or the jaws.

Extraoral traction appliance See Appliance, Extraoral traction.

Extrusion See Orthodontic tooth movement, Extrusion.

Eye-ear plane See Cephalometric lines, Frankfort horizontal plane.

Eyelet A small orthodontic attachment in the shape of a closed helix soldered onto a bonding base or welded directly on an orthodontic band. Eyelets mainly are used as handles for elastic traction. [Also see Attachment, Orthodontic.]

Coil eyelet See "Pigtail" attachment.

F

Face frame See Appliance, Face mask

Face mask See Appliance, Face mask.

Facebow (of an articulator) An instrument used to enable the mounting of dental casts on an articulator. The facebow is used to record the relationship of the patient's maxillary arch with respect to the opening axis of the temporomandibular joint and the Frankfort horizontal plane and subsequently to transfer this relationship to the articulator.

Facebow (of a headgear) The rigid wire component of a headgear used to transfer extraoral forces to the maxilla (or occasionally the mandible) and the teeth. A facebow consists of two coplanar metal bows, brazed or (laser-)welded at the midline. The smaller of the two bows (inner bow) inserts intraorally into specially manufactured tubes that usually are attached to the bands of the maxillary first molars, or incorporated into the acrylic of a removable orthodontic appliance. The hooks at both ends of the larger, outer bow attach to the headgear strap, which produces an extraoral force of variable direction, depending on the type of headgear (cervical, occipital, etc.).

Facebow-adjusting pliers See Orthodontic instruments, Facebow-adjusting pliers.

Facet See Wear facet.

Facial Of or relating to the face. The term also is used to identify the labial surface of an anterior tooth. [Also see Labial.]

Facial angle See Cephalometric measurements (Hard tissue), Facial angle.

Facial asymmetry A term denoting a dissimilarity or disproportionality between the right and left sides of the face, usually meant as an undesirable lack of balance. The asymmetry can be due to the underlying facial skeleton or to the soft tissue drape.

Facial axis angle of Ricketts See Cephalometric measurements (Hard tissue), Facial axis angle of Ricketts.

Facial axis of Ricketts See Cephalometric lines, Facial axis of Ricketts.

Facial concavity A term commonly used in profile analysis. A concave facial profile is one in which an inwardly rounded curve is formed from the forehead to the lips to the chin, as often associated with a Class III malocclusion (Downs' angle of convexity (NAPg) has a negative value). [Modified from the AAO Glossary of Dentofacial Orthopedic Terms, 1993.]

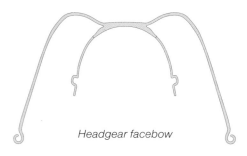

Headgear facebow

cial convexity The opposite of facial concavity, describing an outwardly rounded curve from the forehead to the lips to the chin. Facial convexity indicates a fullness in the lip region relative to the chin and forehead, as is commonly associated with a Class II malocclusion or a bimaxillary protrusion (Downs' angle of convexity (NAPg) has a positive value). [Modified from the AAO Glossary of Dentofacial Orthopedic Terms, 1993.]

cial esthetics A term pertaining to the beauty and appeal of the face. It is an entity which carries a great deal of subjectivity and is impossible to describe and quantify accurately, but it generally is believed that symmetry, balance and proportion play a major role.

cial form The term usually refers to the configuration (shape) of the face from an anterior (frontal) view.

cial growth The physiological process of enlargement and change of the facial skeleton and overlying soft tissues over time.

cial height See Cephalometric measurements (Hard tissue), Facial height.

Facial index See Index, Facial.

Facial line See Cephalometric lines, Facial plane.

Facial mask See Appliance, Face mask.

Facial midline See Midline, Facial.

Facial orthopedics See Orthodontics and dentofacial orthopedics.

Facial pattern A term generally used to describe the facial configuration, or the directional tendency of facial growth, from a lateral (profile) view.

Facial plane (FP) See Cephalometric lines, Facial plane.

Facial type 1. When referring to the lateral (profile) view the facial type can be described as: retrognathic (opisthognathic), mesognathic (orthognathic) or prognathic. **2.** When referring to the frontal view, the three facial type options are: brachycephalic or euryprosopic (wide and short), mesocephalic or mesoprosopic (average) and dolichocephalic or leptoprosopic (long and narrow).

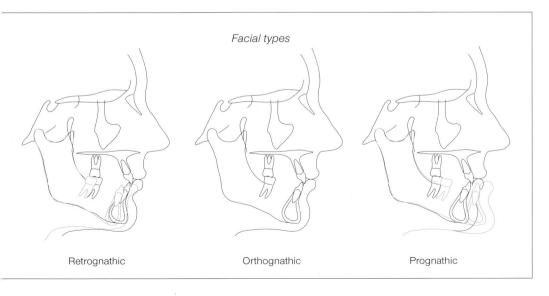

Facial types

Retrognathic   Orthognathic   Prognathic

111

Facies A distinctive facial appearance characteristic of certain disorders (i.e. Down syndrome).

"Adenoid" facies See "Adenoid" facies.

Fatigue Degradation of materials subjected to a number of load changes. Tendency to fracture under cyclic stresses.

Fatigue failure The phenomenon in which stress values well below the ultimate tensile stress of a material can produce a premature fracture because microscopic flaws grow slowly over many cycles of stress. Depending on the type of loading situation, a material can exhibit either static or dynamic fatigue failure.

Dynamic fatigue failure Most prosthetic and restoration fractures develop progressively over many cycles of periodic occlusal loading after initiation of a crack from a critical flaw and subsequently by propagation of the crack until a sudden fracture occurs.

Static fatigue failure Fracture of a material attributed to the interaction of a constantly applied stress with structural flaws over time.

Fee-for-service dentistry A method of paying practitioners on a service-by-service, rather than a salaried or capitated basis. [Taken from the AAO Glossary of Dentofacial Orthopedic Terms, 1993.]

Fenestration Round or oval perforation of the buccal or lingual cortical plate of the alveolar process over the root of a tooth, which does not involve the alveolar crest.

Ferrite One of the three possible lattice structures of iron, on which the different classes of steels also are based. [Also see Austenite; Martensite.] The body-centered cubic (BCC) structure that pure iron has at room temperature. This phase is stable in temperatures as high as 912° C.

FGF See Growth factors.

FH See Cephalometric lines, Frankfort horizontal plane.

FH-NPog See Cephalometric measurement (Hard tissue), Facial angle.

Fibroblast The predominant cell of connective tissue. Because all tissues of the tooth (except enamel) and its supporting apparatus are connective, fibroblasts play an important role in the development, structure and function of a tooth. Fibroblasts function to form the (extracellular) fibers of connective tissue, that is, collagen and elastin. As well, they produce and maintain the ground substance in which they and their fibrous products are enmeshed, and they exhibit contractility and motility, which are utilized in determining the structural organization of connective tissue, especially during embryogenesis. Fibroblasts are the architect, builder and caretaker of connective tissue.

Fibroblast growth factor (FGF) See Growth factors.

Fibrocartilage See Cartilage, Fibrocartilage.

Fibrosis Formation of fibrous connective tissue to replace normal tissue lost through injury or infection.

Fibrotomy See Circumferential supracrestal fibrotomy.

Fibrous ankylosis See Ankylosis.

Fibrous joint See Joint, Fibrous.

Figure-eight ligature A stainless steel ligature tied around two or more brackets or teeth of the same arch, so that its two ends cross over each other at the interproximal spaces, forming a figure of eight. It is used to prevent closed spaces from reopening and to consolidate teeth together, forming a multi-tooth anchorage segment. [Also see Laceback.]

nal splint See Splint, Surgical.

nger spring See Orthodontic springs, Finger spring.

nger-sucking habit See Thumbsucking habit.

nishing The final stage of fixed appliance orthodontic treatment, during which final detailing takes place to idealize individual tooth position.

nishing archwire See Archwire, Finishing.

nishing strips See Abrasive strips.

nite element analysis An engineering technique of stress analysis, the basic concept of which is the visualization of a structure as an assemblage of a finite number of discrete structural elements connected at a finite number of points. The finite elements are formed by figuratively "cutting the original structure into segments." For two-dimensional applications, triangles of various sizes and shapes usually are the finite elements of choice. Each element retains the mechanical characteristics of the original structure. Some characteristics of the material have to be specified (depending on whether it is isotropic or not).
Additionally, a numbering system is required to identify the elements and their connecting points, called "nodes." A coordinate system also must be established to identify uniquely the location of the nodal points. A large number of simultaneous linear equations are computer-generated, which establishes compatibility within each element.
The technique has some very distinct advantages as a research tool, among which is the ability to obtain an estimate of the stresses throughout the structure under consideration. Further, the inclusion of any type of anisotropy and inhomogeneity conceptually is possible by inserting the appropriate distribution of material properties at the nodes of the elements.
However, when it is applied to structures such as a tooth, there are some practical limitations, as relatively little is known about the mechanical properties of dental and especially periodontal tissues.

First branchial arch syndrome See Hemifacial microsomia.

First-order bends See Bends, First-order.

First-order rotation See Rotation (of a tooth), First-order.

First transitional period The period during which the deciduous maxillary and mandibular incisors are replaced by the permanent incisors (starting from the time of exfoliation of the first deciduous incisor, or from the time of emergence of the first permanent molar in the mouth, and ending with the eruption of the last incisor).

Fistula An abnormal passage or communication between two anatomical cavities, or between an anatomical cavity and the external body surface.

   Oronasal fistula A fistula connecting the nasal and oral cavities, a common finding in patients with a history of cleft lip and palate.

Fixation, Surgical Immobilization of bones following a fracture or a surgical procedure to facilitate and accelerate the healing process.

   Intermaxillary fixation (IMF, Maxillomandibular fixation) Traditional method of fixation utilizing stainless steel wires between the maxillary and mandibular teeth to immobilize the mandible. The wires can be ligated on special hooks soldered or crimped on the orthodontic archwires, or on arch bars if no fixed orthodontic appliances are present. Typical duration of IMF is between 6 and 8 weeks, during which the patient is fed liquid diet through the retromolar area. Intermaxillary fixation is sometimes combined with RIF, in which case its duration is shorter.

Rigid internal fixation (RIF) Fixation technique in which bony segments are immobilized by use of small titanium bone plates (fixation plates) and/or screws across the osteotomy or fracture line. Bone plates must be contoured carefully to adapt to the bony surfaces prior to their application. By directly and rigidly fixing bony segments together, the period of intermaxillary fixation can be reduced or completely eliminated after surgery. Rigid internal fixation occasionally is combined with IMF following orthognathic surgery.

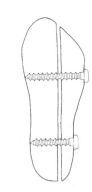

Bicortical screws

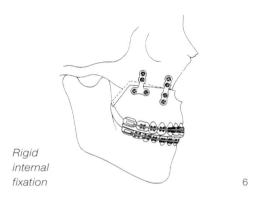

Rigid internal fixation   6

Fixation plate Titanium plates of various configurations that carry holes for placement of osseous screws, used for rigid internal fixation.

Fixation screws Titanium osseous screws (2.0 to 3.5 mm in diameter or larger) used for stabilization of the bone plates in rigid internal fixation.

Bicortical (Position) screw Fully threaded screw that binds in both cortices of the two bony segments to which it is applied. As the screw is tightened, no compression is possible because with the screw threads engaging both segments, the distance between them is maintained.

Lag screw Partially threaded screw (only has threads close to its tip) that is placed so that its threads only bind the cortex of the bony segment that lies farthest away from

the point of entry (i.e. the medial/distal seg ment in the case of a BSSO). [Also se Segment, Distal.] The same size hole drilled in both segments. As the lag scre is tightened, it engages the medial/dist cortex but is free to rotate in the lateral/pro imal cortex, which eventually produces con pression of the segments against eac other.

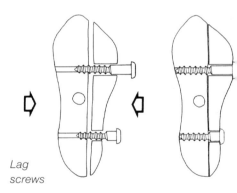

Lag screws

Fixed appliance See Appliance, Fixed.

Fixed/removable appliance See Applianc Fixed/removable.

Fixed retainer See Retainer, Fixed.

Fixture A device that is firmly fastened in plac in a mechanical sense, often used to secu other devices. [In implantology the ter commonly is used to denote the *body* of a osseointegrated dental implant (i.e. the po tion of the implant that is placed into the bone surgically).]

ange A projecting rim of a removable orthodontic appliance, usually consisting of an acrylic extension of its main body. Flanges commonly are used in functional appliances to dictate the desired mandibular position. Vestibular and lingual flanges also serve to remove the pressures from the surrounding soft tissues on the alveolar processes and teeth.

ap A loosened section of tissue, separated from its surrounding tissues except at its base.

Pharyngeal flap See Pharyngeal flap operation.

Repositioned flap A flap that is moved laterally, coronally or apically to a new position.

ared teeth A term used to indicate generalized labial tipping of the maxillary and/or mandibular anterior teeth, or generalized buccal tipping of posterior teeth.

at occlusal splint See Splint, Diagnostic.

exibility The property of certain materials that can undergo a larger strain or deformation under the influence of a relatively small stress. The maximum flexibility is defined as the strain that occurs when the material is stressed to its proportional limit. It is desirable that orthodontic wires and springs have a high flexibility as well as a high value for the elastic limit (the stress above which a wire will not recover its original shape).

exion-extension injury (Whiplash) Sudden, exaggerated traumatic movement of joints through the extremes of their range of motion with hyperflexion and then hyperextension, resulting in ligamentous sprain, muscular strain, inflammation and subsequent reflex muscle splinting.

Flush terminal plane See Terminal plane, Flush.

Flux A substance that promotes the flow of solder over two metal parts by preventing the production of oxides.

FMA See Cephalometric measurements (Hard tissue), Frankfort-mandibular plane angle.

FMIA See Cephalometric measurements (Hard tissue), Frankfort-mandibular incisor angle.

Force The action of one body on another body that tends to change the state of rest or motion of the latter. Orthodontics is based on the application of forces on teeth, under the influence of which tooth movement can be achieved.
Force is a vectorial quantity. This means that to adequately describe a force, its *magnitude, direction* (line of action), *sign* (sense) and *point of application* have to be defined. Forces are depicted in a coordinate system as vectors. The inclination of the vector (or the angle between it and a specified reference line or axis) shows the direction of the force, the length of the vector is proportional to the magnitude of the force, and the arrowhead denotes the sense of the force.
Force, though defined in Newtons, commonly (but, strictly speaking, inaccurately) is reported in mass units (grams or ounces).

Component forces The constituent forces (two or more) of a certain force system.

Concurrent forces Two or more forces that have the same point of application.

Constant force A force whose magnitude remains the same as at the time of activation, for a certain time interval (e.g. from one patient visit to the next). This is a theoretical concept, as in clinical reality a true constant force cannot be generated, but only approximated.

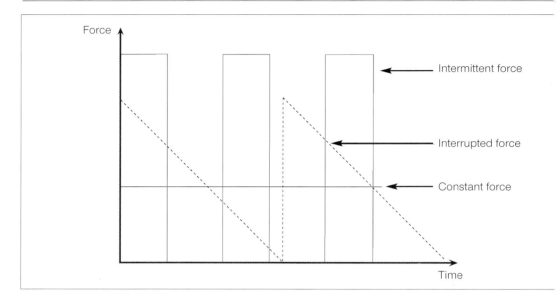

Continuous force A force that is maintained between certain intervals (e.g. does not drop to zero between patient visits).

Coplanar forces Two or more forces whose vectorial direction is on the same plane of space (regardless of their sense).

Extraoral force Force generated by (elastically) deforming an activating element of an orthodontic or orthopedic appliance, located outside the oral cavity. [Also see Anchorage, Extraoral.]

Frictional force See Friction.

Heavy force A force of high magnitude. [Compare with Force, Light.]

Intermittent force A force whose magnitude abruptly drops to zero, as is the case when an orthodontic appliance is removed by the patient and then resumes again, as when the appliance is re-inserted into the mouth. Intermittent forces are produced by all appliances that require patient cooperation, such as removable appliances, headgear, and elastics.

Interrupted force A force whose magnitude declines to zero between activation. Most conventional orthodontic force-producing mechanisms (with the exception of super-elastic wires and coils) generate interrupted forces that sharply or smoothly decline as some tooth movement occurs and require re-activation after a certain time period.

"Jiggling" forces Interrupted force causing the teeth to move in one and then in another direction. Occlusal forces are thought to be of the "jiggling" type, especially in cases of occlusal trauma. No clear cut pressure and tension zones can be identified histologically in affected teeth, but rather there is a combination of pressure and tension. [Also see "Jiggling"; Round-tripping.]

Light force A force of low magnitude. The term is used freely and arbitrarily, as there is neither universal consensus nor sound scientific evidence regarding specific numeric values of magnitude. As well, it is application-dependent: a force that is considered too high for a certain application may be ideal for another.

Normal force (F_N) Any force acting in a direction perpendicular to the plane under consideration. In the case of friction between two bodies, the force acting in a direction perpendicular to the contacting surfaces. The magnitude of the normal force is directly proportional to the magnitude of the frictional force. [Also see Frictional coefficient.]

Optimal force (Optimum force) See Optimal force theory.

Orthodontic force Force applied to teeth for the purpose of effecting tooth movement, generally having a magnitude lower than an orthopedic force. There is no clear distinction between orthodontic and orthopedic forces in terms of magnitude, but rather many widely variable, arbitrary suggestions exist in the literature.

Orthopedic force Force of higher magnitude in relation to an orthodontic force that, when delivered via the teeth for 12 to 16 hours a day, is supposed to produce a skeletal effect on the maxillofacial complex. Little scientific evidence exists regarding the magnitude that a force should have in order to produce a skeletal effect.

Physiologic force A force of such magnitude and temporal characteristics, which is accepted by the biological tissues as equal to a force of a natural process (e.g. the force generating tooth eruption); in other words, a force that has no harmful effects on biological tissues.

Reaction force A force identical in magnitude and direction to the active force that is used for a certain orthodontic application, but of opposite sense. [Also see Newton's laws, Law of action and reaction.]

Resultant force A single force that can substitute two or more individual forces (component forces) acting on a body, and produce the same effect on it. It can be expressed as the vector sum of all compo-

nent forces. The resultant force can be determined by one of two methods: the geometric method or the analytical (trigonometric) method. The analytical method is preferred when the calculation of a resultant of coplanar, non-concurrent forces is to be performed. [Also see Force composition.]

Force composition (Combination of forces) Determination of a resultant force by combination of two or more component forces. When two component forces have a common point of application, the resultant force is determined by considering the two vectors to be sides of a parallelogram (geometric method). The resultant force then is the diagonal of the parallelogram. Its length indicates the magnitude of the resultant force on the same scale as the original forces.

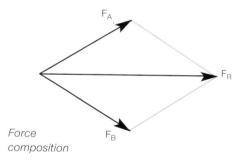

Force composition

It is important to understand that the resultant force will have the identical effect on movement of the tooth as the two separate forces. A tooth or a set of teeth moves in response to the net effect of all forces. If the resultant force is the same, the movement will be the same, regardless of how many individual forces are applied to the tooth and regardless of their direction.

To determine the resultant of more than two forces that have a common point of application, a series of successive parallelograms is constructed. Each time, the resultant from any two forces replaces those forces and is used to construct the next parallelogram. The sequence in which forces are combined is of no consequence.

However, different forces on a tooth usually are not applied at the same point, as was assumed previously. According to the law of transmissibility of force, the point of application of a force may be considered to be anywhere along its line of action. [Also see Law of transmissibility of force.] Consequently, the resultant of two forces with different points of application can be determined by extending their lines of action to construct a common point of application.

Force couple See Couple.

Force decomposition See Force resolution.

Force/deflection rate See Load/deflection rate.

Force delivery A force produced by an orthodontic wire, spring or other auxiliary against a tooth.

Force regime See Mode of force application.

Force resolution (Decomposition of forces) Rather than combining two or more forces into a single resultant, it often is useful to divide a single force into components at right angles to each other (in two or three dimensions). In this instance, the parallelogram procedure for composition of forces is reversed. Every force can be considered as the diagonal of a parallelogram and its components can be drawn along the orthogonal axes. [Also see Global reference frame.]

With more than one force on a tooth, there are two methods for determining the overall component forces. First, the applied forces can be combined into a single resultant [see Force composition], and then this resultant can be resolved into its components. Alternatively, the components for each force can be determined separately, and these components then can be combined to determine the net component vectors.

Force system Combination of all the forces and moments acting on a body. A 3-dimen-

sional force system consists of three forc in the principal dimensions of space (F_x, F_y, F_z) and three moments considered abc the three axes (M_x, M_y, M_z).

Applied force system The force syste acting at the point of application of the forc (usually the bracket of a tooth).

Consistent force system A force syste that only includes forces and moments th are desirable for the intended tooth mov ment.

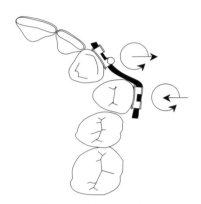

Consistent force system

Effective force system The combinatic of forces and moments considered at t center or resistance (CRes) of a body (toot It can be used to predict the type of mov ment that will occur.

Equivalent force systems Two force sy tems are equivalent if they cause the sar effect on a body. In such a case, the sum all the forces and the sum of all the momer in system A have to be equal to those system B in all three principal dimensio of space.

Inconsistent force system A force sy tem that contains one or more componer (forces or moments) which are not co patible with the intended tooth moveme and thus would lead to unwanted si effects.

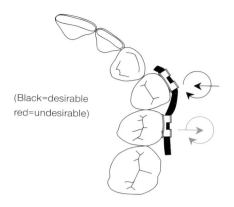

(Black=desirable
red=undesirable)

Inconsistent force system

Statically determinate/indeterminate force system As stated by the first law of Newton, when a body is in static equilibrium then the sum of all the forces and the sum of all the moments acting on it must be equal to zero ($\Sigma F = 0$ and $\Sigma M = 0$). This generates a total of six equations in 3 dimensions. When the number of static equilibrium equations is larger than or equal to the number of unknowns, then the force system is determinate, which allows calculation of the applied forces and moments and prediction (to an extent) of the resulting tooth movement. This is done by considering the system at one specific instant in time and by assuming that it is, at that time, in static equilibrium.

When a wire connects two teeth (or two segments of teeth that have been joined together so that they can be assumed to be rigid bodies and their CRes can be estimated) then specific equilibrium equations may be formulated for them, which allow a description of the force system and an approximate prediction of the tooth movement that will occur (determinate force system).

Conversely, when a continuous wire engages more than two teeth, the forces and moments acting on each tooth will interact with the force systems on the adjacent teeth.

The result is a situation with more unknowns than available equilibrium equations, which does not permit analysis of the resulting forces and moments. The force system then is said to be statically indeterminate.

Forced bite See Mandibular shift.

Anterior forced bite A mandibular shift in an anterior direction from CR to CO. An anterior forced bite may result in an anterior functional crossbite. [Also see Crossbite, Functional.]

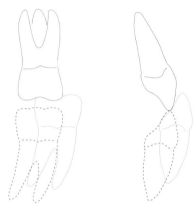

Anterior forced bite

Lateral forced bite A mandibular shift in a lateral direction after an occlusal interference in CR. A lateral forced bite may be the cause a posterior functional crossbite. [Also see Lateroclusion.]

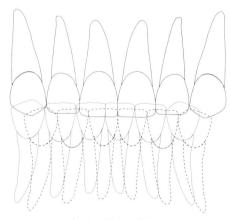

Lateral forced bite

Forced eruption (of a tooth) The application of orthodontic traction to guide an unerupted or impacted tooth into its proper position in the dental arch, usually following its surgical exposure. [Also see Surgical exposure.]

Formability The amount of permanent deformation that a material can withstand before failing. In the case of an orthodontic wire, it represents the amount of permanent bending the wire will tolerate (e.g. while being formed into a clinically useful spring or loop) before it breaks. High formability is a property that an ideal wire alloy for orthodontic purposes should possess.

"Forme fruste" An atypically mild or incomplete manifestation of a disease or anomaly (e.g. *forme fruste* cleft lip).

Forward rotation (of the mandible) See Mandibular rotation, Counter-clockwise.

Fossa Hollow pit, concavity or depression, especially on the surface of a bone or tooth.

Fossa, Glenoid See Glenoid fossa.

FP See Cephalometric lines, Facial plane.

Fracture Break or discontinuity of an entity (pertaining to a fractured bone, tooth, cartilage, but also wire, appliance part, ceramic bracket etc.).

Comminuted fracture A fracture resulting in multiple small segments, fragments or splinters.

Complex fracture A fracture involving vital structures adjacent to the fracture site.

Compound (open) fracture A fracture that has communication with the external surface (e.g. when a bony segment perforates the skin or penetrates the oral mucosa).

Condylar fracture Breakage (discontinuity) of the condyle, which most frequently occurs at the condylar neck. The direction of displacement of the condylar head depends on whether the fracture line above or below the insertion of the lateral pterygoid muscle. A condylar fracture an early age usually is treated conservatively by intermaxillary fixation and/or elastic traction, or sometimes by functional appliances, without an open reduction procedure (provided it is not a comminuted complex fracture).
Following that, there is a good chance regeneration and continued, almost normal growth; however, there typically is an element of an asymmetry that eventually develops, with an associated malocclusion. Usually the growth of the condyle on the affected side is somewhat diminished, and there is a degree of limitation of condylar movement on the affected side. As well, secondary maxillary deformity is not uncommon, with canting of the occlusal plane (up on the affected side).

Displaced fracture A fracture leading to gross discontinuity of the segment involved, as compared with the normal anatomy.

Greenstick fracture An incomplete fracture, in which one side of a bone (one cortical plate) is broken and the other side bent (usually the fracture only involves the convex side of the curve).

Intracapsular fracture A fracture occurring within the capsule of a joint. In the case of the mandibular condyle, an intracapsular fracture involves the portion of the condylar head that is enclosed by the temporomandibular joint capsule.

Open fracture See Fracture, Compound

Pathologic fracture A fracture due to the weakening of bone structure by pathologic processes such as osteomalacia, osteomyelitis, tumors or osteogenesis im perfecta. In instances of severe destruction of bone, fractures of the jaws can occur spontaneously during chewing, yawning or talking.

acture line Linear radiolucency seen on a radiograph indicating a break in a bone or tooth.

anchise dentistry A system for marketing a dental practice, usually under a trade name where permitted by law, in return for a financial investment or other consideration. Participating dental practitioners may also receive the benefits of media advertising, a national referral system, and financial and management consultation. [Taken from the AAO Glossary of Dentofacial Orthopedic Terms, 1993.]

änkel appliance See Appliance, Fränkel.

ankfort horizontal plane (FH) See Cephalometric lines, Frankfort horizontal plane.

ankfort-mandibular incisor angle (FMIA) See Cephalometric measurements (Hard tissue), Frankfort-mandibular incisor angle.

ankfort-mandibular plane angle (FMA) See Cephalometric measurements (Hard tissue), Frankfort-mandibular plane angle.

ee body diagram A depiction of an object (e.g. a tooth) or system as a free body, upon which all the acting forces and moments can be considered, and the Newtonian laws of static equilibrium can be applied, for purposes of mechanical analysis.

ee-end spring See Orthodontic springs, Free-end.

ee gingiva See Gingiva, Free.

ee gingival graft See Graft, Free gingival.

Free graft See Graft, Free.

Free vector A vector whose action is not confined to or associated with a unique line in space. A free vector can produce the same effect on a body regardless of the point on the body where it is applied. The moment of a couple is an example of a free vector commonly encountered in orthodontics.

Freeway space (Interocclusal clearance, Interocclusal separation) The distance between the occlusal surfaces of the maxillary and mandibular teeth when the mandible is in its rest position.

Fremitus Vibration of a tooth due to a premature contact with its antagonist in centric occlusion, which can be clinically detected by palpation.

Frenectomy The surgical repositioning or excision of a (labial) frenum in cases where it is felt that its fibers may interfere with the stability of an orthodontically corrected midline diastema, or with its spontaneous closure during and after eruption of the maxillary canines. Frenectomy also is indicated when a frenum is involved in causing localized gingival recession or in cases of ankyloglossia. [Also see Ankyloglossia.]

Frenum (Frenulum) A fold of mucous membrane and underlying fibrous tissue.

Buccal frenum Smaller attachment of the cheeks on the buccal aspect of the maxillary and mandibular alveolar processes, usually at the level of the premolars.

Labial frenum The band of fibrous tissue connecting the upper or lower lip to the labial aspect of the maxillary and mandibular alveolar process respectively, at the midline.

Lingual frenum A band of fibrous tissue connecting the tongue with the floor of the mouth and the lingual aspect of the mandibular alveolar process at the midline.

When it is short, it may cause a limitation of tongue movements and possible difficulties with speech. [Also see Ankyloglossia.]

Friction A force resisting the relative displacement of two contacting bodies, in a direction tangent to the plane of contact. Because of friction, part of the mechanical energy intended for movement of the two bodies relative to each other is dissipated as thermal energy.

Static friction is the component of frictional force that has to be overcome to initiate motion.

Dynamic (*kinetic*) friction is the component of frictional force that has to be overcome to maintain motion. The static frictional force usually is somewhat higher than the dynamic frictional force.

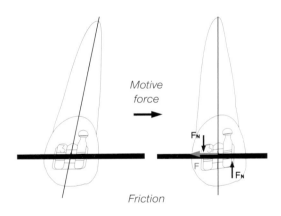

Friction

Frictional coefficient (μ) The law of friction theorized by Coulomb states that the magnitude of the frictional force F is equal to the product of the normal force F_N acting perpendicular to the contact surface, multiplied by the frictional coefficient μ ($F = F_N \times \mu$). The frictional coefficient μ depends on the surface roughness and the combination of the materials involved. It does not depend on the area of the contacting surfaces and varies only slightly with the velocity of movement.

With respect to the type of friction, a static and a dynamic frictional coefficient can be distinguished.

Frictional force See Friction.

Frictionless mechanics See Mechanics Frictionless.

Frontal cephalometric radiograph See Cephalometric radiograph, Posteroanterio

Frontal plane (Coronal plane) Any plane passing longitudinally through the bod from side to side, at right angles to the median plane and dividing the body int front and back parts.

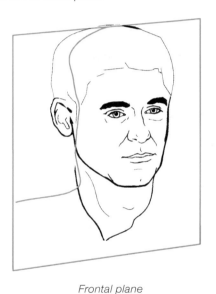

Frontal plane

Frontal resorption (Direct resorption) Se Bone resorption, Frontal.

"Full dimension" archwire See Archwire "Full dimension."

Full thickness periodontal graft See Graf Full thickness periodontal.

"Full" treatment Term commonly used t signify fixed appliance orthodontic trea ment, usually involving both dental arches

Fully programmed bracket See Bracket, Fully programmed.

Function The specialized, normal or proper physiologic activity of an organ or part.

Function regulator See Appliance, Fränkel.

Functional appliance See Appliance, Functional.

Functional crossbite See Crossbite, Functional.

Functional cusps See Cusp, Functional.

Functional jaw orthopedics Treatment with functional appliances, making use of forces created by the musculature of the patient to bring about the desired dentofacial and functional changes.

Functional matrix theory A hypothesis put forth by M.L. Moss to provide a theoretical explanation of the interrelationship between osteogenesis and local functional demands. According to Moss, each function in the head is controlled by a specific functional cranial component. The size, shape and spatial position of the individual cranial components are relatively independent of one another. Each cranial component consists of two parts: a *functional matrix* that actually carries out the function and a *skeletal unit,* whose role is to protect and/or support its specific functional matrix.
Skeletal units may be composed of bone, cartilage or ligaments, but they are not the equivalent of the "bones" of classic osteology. Skeletal units are distinguished as microskeletal or macroskeletal units. The sum of all microskeletal units of a skull component makes up the macroskeletal unit. For example, the mandible is a macroskeletal unit consisting of the condylar, coronoid, angular, alveolar and basal microskeletal units.
The functional matrix includes the functioning spaces and the soft tissue components required for a specific function. Teeth also are a functional matrix. When a functional matrix grows, or changes in size, shape or spatial position, the related skeletal unit will respond accordingly. Movement of teeth with orthodontic treatment induces changes on the alveolar skeletal unit. In a similar fashion, the blood vessels and nerves of the mandibular canal have an effect on the mandibular basal microskeletal unit.
There are two types of functional matrices, the *periosteal* matrix and the *capsular* matrix (their designation indicates the sites of their activity). The periosteal matrices include muscles and teeth, whereas the capsular matrices are conceived of as volumes enclosed and protected by both the neurocranial and the orofacial capsules. In the neural skull the capsular matrix is the neural mass. In the facial skull this matrix consists of the functioning spaces of the oronasopharyngeal and orbital cavities.
The capsular and periosteal matrices have completely different effects on the growth process. Periosteal matrices act upon skeletal units in a direct fashion by the processes of osseous deposition and resorption (or by the processes of cartilaginous and fibrous tissue manipulation). Their net effect is to alter the form (size and shape) of their respective skeletal units. On the other hand, capsular matrices act upon functional cranial components as a whole, in a secondary and indirect manner, by altering the volume of the capsules within which the functional cranial components are embedded. The effect of such growth changes is to cause a passive translation of these cranial components in space.
Cranial growth is a result of combined activity of both types of matrix. Growth is accomplished by both spatial translation and changes in form.

Functional occlusal plane See Cephalometric lines, Occlusal plane.

Functional occlusion See Occlusion, Functional.

Functioning side See Working side.

Furcation The anatomic area of a multi-rooted tooth where the roots diverge.

Fusion Abnormality of dental morphology involving a union of the dentin (and enamel) of two teeth, from two separate tooth buds. [Compare with Gemination and Twinning].

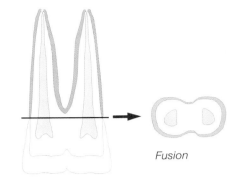

Fusion

G

G See Cephalometric landmarks (Hard tissue), Glabella.

G' See Cephalometric landmarks (Soft tissue), Soft tissue glabella.

Gable bends See Bends, V-bends.

GAGs See Glycosaminoglycans.

Galvanic corrosion See Corrosion, Galvanic.

Gelb splint See Splint, Gelb.

Gemination Abnormality of dental morphology due to incomplete division of a single tooth bud. [Compare with Twinning and Fusion.]

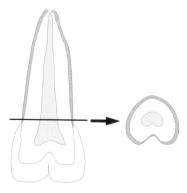

Gemination

Genial Of or pertaining to the chin.

Genioplasty An orthognathic surgical procedure designed to reshape the contour of the

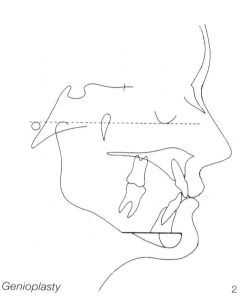

Genioplasty 2

chin, giving it a more esthetic appearance. The procedure is performed intraorally by a vestibular incision and, depending on the situation, can augment or reduce the prominence of the chin in the anteroposterior, vertical or transverse plane of space. This can be performed by various approaches, such as by sliding the distal (genial) segment on the proximal (mandibular) segment and/or by removal of a wedge of bone. Alloplastic grafts to increase the prominence of the chin are no longer widely performed, due to their side effects.

Geometry classes of Burstone See Burstone's geometry classes.

Gigantism A condition of abnormally high growth, resulting from excessive secretion of growth hormone by the pituitary gland, before closure of the epiphyses, brought about by a pituitary adenoma. It is regarded as the childhood form of acromegaly. The growth usually is symmetrical, and patients lack the coarse features seen in acromegaly, but thickening of soft tissue and facial bones may occur after some years' duration. The size of the teeth generally is proportional to the size of the jaws. [Also see Acromegaly.]

Gingiva The fibrous investing tissue, covered by keratinized epithelium, that immediately surrounds a tooth and is contiguous with its periodontal ligament and with the mucosal tissues of the oral cavity. Two types of gingiva can generally be distinguished, attached and free gingiva.

> **Attached gingiva** The portion of the gingiva that is firm, dense, stippled and tightly bound to the underlying tissues, tooth and bone.

> **Free gingiva** The portion of the gingiva that surrounds the tooth but is not directly attached to the tooth surface.

> **Marginal gingiva** The most coronal portion of the free gingiva, which in the healthy situation forms the wall of the gingival crevice.

Gingival col A valley-like depression of the interdental gingiva that connects facial and lingual papillae and conforms to the shape of the interproximal contact area.

Gingival fibers Collagen (predominantly), reticulin and elastic fibers, which together with the different cells (e.g. fibroblasts, macrophages) and the ground substance (proteoglycans and glucoproteins) make up the connective tissue content of the gingiva. Depending on their orientation, they are organized into five principal groupings: the dento-gingival, alveolo-gingival, dento-periosteal, circular and transseptal fibers.

> **Alveolo-gingival fibers** Fibers that radiate coronally from the periosteum of the alveolar crest and extend into the lamina propria of both the free and the attached gingiva.

> **Circular fibers** A small group of fibers that circumscribe the tooth and are present in the free marginal gingiva and in the attached gingiva coronal to the alveolar crest.

> **Dento-gingival fibers** Fibers extending from the cementum laterally into the lamina propria of both the free and the attached gingiva.

> **Dento-periosteal fibers** Fibers which extend from the cementum in the area of the cemento-enamel junction into the periosteum at the alveolar crest.

> **Transseptal fibers** Fibers extending interdentally from the cementum just apical to the base of the junctional epithelium of one tooth over the alveolar crest and inserting into a comparable region of the cementum of the adjacent tooth. Together these fibers constitute the transseptal fiber system, collectively forming an interdental ligament connecting all the teeth of the arch.
> The supracrestal fibers and in particular the transseptal fiber system have been implicated as a major etiologic factor of post retention relapse of an orthodontic correction due to their slow rate of turnover during physiological conditions as well as during orthodontic tooth movement. The reasoning behind advocating a sufficiently prolonged retention period following orthodontic tooth movement is to allow reorganization of the transseptal fiber system, so that clinical stability of the new tooth position is ensured. [Also see Circumferential supracrestal fibrotomy.]

Gingival fibrotomy See Circumferential supracrestal fibrotomy.

Gingival graft See Graft, Free gingival.

Gingival hyperplasia An enlargement of the gingiva owing to an increase in the number of cells.

Gingival papilla See Interdental papilla.

Gingival recession Shift of the gingival margin apical to the cemento-enamel junction, exposing part of the root surface.

Gingival recession, Classification of See Miller classification.

Gingivectomy The excision of a portion of the gingiva, sometimes necessary for continuation of treatment in orthodontic patients with severe gingival hyperplasia due to poor oral hygiene or use of certain medications.

Gingivitis Inflammation of the gingiva.

Gingivoplasty A surgical reshaping of the gingiva to correct a deformity and/or enhance esthetics.

Ginglymoid joint Hinging joint with one convex and one concave surface, with movement in only one plane of space.

Gjessing spring See Orthodontic springs, PG spring.

Glabella (G) See Cephalometric landmarks (Hard tissue), Glabella.

Glass-ionomer cement See Orthodontic cement, Glass-ionomer; Bonding agent.

Glenoid fossa (Mandibular fossa, Temporal fossa, Articular fossa of the temporal bone) A depression on the inferior surface of the squamous portion of the temporal bone at the base of the zygomatic process, in which the mandibular condyle is situated. Posterior to the glenoid fossa is the squamotympanic fissure, which extends mediolaterally. Medially the fossa is limited by the spine of the sphenoid and laterally by the root of the zygomatic process of the temporal bone. Anteriorly, the fossa is bounded by the articular eminence. The middle part of the glenoid fossa is separated from the middle cranial fossa and temporal lobe of the brain by a fairly thin plate of bone.

Global reference frame A coordinate system of three mutually perpendicular, intersecting axes (x = sagittal/anteroposterior, y = vertical/occlusogingival, and z = transverse/mediolateral), used as a reference for various measurements or vector analysis within a dental arch, or in relation to the entire dentofacial complex.
The x-axis is defined as the intersection of the sagittal and occlusal planes, the y-axis

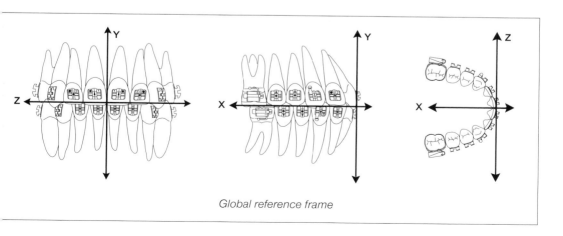

Global reference frame

as the intersection of the sagittal and coronal planes and the z-axis as the intersection of the coronal and occlusal planes.

Glossopexy Any procedure designed to move the tongue anteriorly and attach it to an anterior structure in the mouth. It sometimes is performed on neonates or infants with airway obstruction with or without oropharyngeal or nasopharyngeal intubation, as an alternative to tracheostomy, for airway management.

Glossotomy (Partial glossectomy) A surgical procedure involving excision of part of the tongue. In orthodontics, a glossotomy sometimes is advocated as a modality to alleviate the effects of a large tongue on the dentoskeletal pattern or to help maintain the stability of open bite or Class III corrections. This procedure commonly is performed for similar reasons on patients with severe macroglossia due to specific pathological conditions (e.g. Beckwith-Wiedemann syndrome).

Glycosaminoglycans (GAGs) One of the types of macromolecules that constitute the extracellular matrix. Glycosaminoglycans are long, unbranched polysaccharide chains composed of repeating disaccharide units. Examples of GAGs include *hyaluronic acid*, *dermatan sulfate* and *heparin*.
The major characteristic of GAGs is that they are strongly hydrophilic and have the capacity to withhold water. Thus, GAGs tend to adopt highly extended, so-called random coil conformations, which occupy a large volume relative to their mass (as their polysaccharide chains are too inflexible to fold into more compact structures), and they form gels even at very low concentrations. These gels osmotically absorb large amounts of water into the matrix, enabling the matrix to withstand compressive forces (in contrast to collagen fibrils, which resist stretching forces). Cartilage matrix, for example, resists compression by this mechanism.

Gn See Cephalometric landmarks (Hard tissue), Gnathion.

Gnathion (Gn) See Cephalometric landmarks (Hard tissue), Gnathion.

Gnathology The field of dentistry that deals with static and dynamic aspects of occlusion, the TMJs and the masticatory system as a whole, from an anatomical, histologic, physiological and pathological viewpoint, including the applicable diagnostic, therapeutic and rehabilitative procedures. The term was adopted by B.B. McCollum and his associates, who in the mid-1920s founded the Gnathological Society of California.

Go See Cephalometric landmarks (Hard tissue), Gonion.

Goldenhar syndrome A variant of hemifacial microsomia which additionally may include *epibulbar dermoids* (soft tissue tumors of the cornea of the eyes), lipomas around the orbits and vertebral abnormalities. [See also Hemifacial microsomia.]

Gonial angle See Cephalometric measurements (Hard tissue), Gonial angle.

Gonion (Go) See Cephalometric landmarks (Hard tissue), Gonion.

Goshgarian transpalatal arch See Arch, Transpalatal.

Graft Any material or tissue that is not normally part of an organ or tissue, implanted or transplanted for the purpose of reconstructing or repairing.

Allogenic graft (Allograft, Allogeneic graft) A graft of tissue transplanted from a donor of the same species as the recipient, but having a different genotype. [Compare with Graft, Isologous; see also Graft, Homologous.]

Alloplastic graft (Alloplast) Graft made from inorganic "foreign body" materials, such as inert metals, ceramics or plastics.

Alveolar bone graft A bone graft to the alveolar process, required for orthodontic (moving teeth into a defect of the ridge) or prosthetic (e.g. placement of an implant) reasons, or for reasons of gingival esthetics and health.

An autologous alveolar bone graft commonly is required for the correction of the residual defect of the alveolar process in patients with a history of cleft lip and palate. [Also see Cleft lip and/or palate.] The bone can be taken from various donor sites (most often iliac bone, rib, cranium or chin). In most situations this type of operation is preferably performed when the patient is between approximately 9 and 11 years of age (secondary, or mixed-dentition bone graft), prior to the eruption of the permanent canine on the side of the cleft. The graft stabilizes the segments of the clefted maxilla, aids in closure of any remaining oronasal fistulas, and permits orthodontic closure of the space from the missing lateral incisor(s), or facilitates a prosthetic solution for obliteration of that space.

Autologous (Autogenous) graft A tissue graft transplanted from one site to another in the same individual. [Compare with Graft, Heterologous.]

Costochondral graft An autogenous bone graft used to substitute the mandibular condyle in TMJ reconstruction surgery. The operation involves harvesting the sternal portion of the contralateral fourth, fifth, sixth or seventh rib, together with part of its costal cartilage. The cartilage is trimmed to a size of 2 to 5 mm, as it has been shown that the growth of the grafted side can otherwise exceed that of the essentially normal, contralateral mandibular condyle. The graft is placed at the host site via a pre-auricular or submandibular incision and fixed by means of bone plates and fixation screws. Costochondral grafts are indicated in patients with congenital dysplasia or aplasia of the condyle (e.g. hemifacial microsomia), TMJ ankylosis, osteoarthritis, rheumatoid arthritis, neoplasias or infectious diseases affecting the condyle.

Free graft A tissue graft completely freed from its bed, in contrast to a flap.

Free gingival graft (Epithelialized free soft tissue graft) A keratinized tissue graft transplanted from one area of the mouth (usually the hard palate) to the alveolar area to increase the thickness and width of the keratinized attached gingiva, to achieve root coverage in a tooth with gingival recession and/or to increase the vestibular depth. A common periodontal surgical procedure.

Full thickness periodontal graft (Mucoperiosteal periodontal graft) A free graft consisting of the surface epithelium, connective tissue and the periosteum of the underlying bone.

Heterologous (Xenogenic, Heterogenous) graft A tissue graft transplanted from a donor of a different species than the recipient. [Compare with Graft, Autologous.]

Homologous (Homogenous) graft A tissue graft transplanted from a donor to the same species as the recipient. Homologous grafts are distinguished further into isologous and allogenic.

Isologous (Syngeneic) graft A tissue graft transplanted between genetically identical individuals, such as monozygotic twins or inbred strains. [Compare with Graft, Allogenic; see also Graft, Homologous.]

Split thickness periodontal graft (Partial thickness periodontal graft, Mucosal periodontal graft) A free periodontal tissue graft consisting of epithelium and a thin layer of the underlying connective tissue.

Subepithelial connective tissue graft
A periodontal surgical procedure used to achieve root coverage in teeth with recession. A partial thickness flap is raised at the recipient site and a free connective tissue graft from the palate or the retromolar area is placed. Following that, the primary flap is repositioned coronally to cover the connective tissue graft.

Grating joint sound See Crepitus.

Greater segment See Segment, Greater.

Greenstick fracture See Fracture, Greenstick.

Grinding (of teeth) See Bruxism.

Group function Term used to describe a particular scheme of disclusion of the dental arches during a lateral mandibular excursion. The maxillary and mandibular canines, premolars and, on occasion, molars on the working side come into contact as the mandible moves laterally, causing disarticulation of the remaining teeth.

Growth The age-related increase in size or mass, involving changes in amount of living substance. Growth is the quantitative aspect of biologic development and is measured in units of increase per units of time (e.g. inches per year or grams per day). Enlargement of living matter with growth may be the direct result of cellular division or the indirect product of biologic activity (e.g. bones and teeth). Although growth typically is equated with enlargement, there are instances in which it results in normal decrease in size (e.g. the thymus gland after puberty). [Also see Development.]

Growth axis See Cephalometric lines, Y-axis.

Growth center A location at which independent (genetically controlled) growth occurs, as opposed to a growth site, which is merely a location at which growth occurs.
All growth centers also are growth sites, whereas the reverse is not true. For exam-

ple, as a result mainly of transplantati᠁ studies, it is now known that the sutur᠁ between the membranous bones of the c᠁ nium and the maxilla that previously we᠁ considered as primary growth centers, ac᠁ ally are mere sites of growth. Conversely, t᠁ epiphyseal plates of the long bones are c᠁ sidered to be growth centers, as they c᠁ tinue to grow when transplanted to a n᠁ location or even in culture, which is indi᠁ tive of an innate growth potential.

Growth factors Highly specific serum p᠁ peptides that are directly and specifica᠁ involved in stimulating cell division and/᠁ differentiation. Growth factors act in co᠁ plex manners in regulating a certain fu᠁ tion: most cell types probably depend o᠁ specific combination of growth factors rath᠁ than a single specific growth factor. So᠁ growth factors are present in the circulati᠁ but most act as local chemical mediators᠁ Examples of growth factors include t᠁ *platelet-derived growth factor (PDGF),* whi᠁ stimulates proliferation of connective tiss᠁ cells and is involved in wound-healin᠁ the *insulinlike growth factors I* and *II (IG᠁ and IGF-II),* which stimulate proliferati᠁ of fat cells and connective tissue cel᠁ the *transforming growth factor* β *(TGF-*᠁ which potentates or inhibits the response᠁ most cells to other growth factors and reg᠁ lates differentiation of some cell types; a᠁ the *fibroblast growth factor (FGF),* whi᠁ stimulates proliferation of many cell type᠁ including fibroblasts, endothelial cells a᠁ myoblasts.

Growth potential The amount of growth ᠁ to occur.

Growth prediction In general, an estimati᠁ of the amount of growth to be expected. ᠁ orthodontics, the term refers to the estim᠁ tion of the amount and direction of grow᠁ of the bones of the craniofacial skeleton a᠁ the overlying soft tissues. Due to the larg᠁ inter-individual variation, growth predicti᠁ generally is considered a procedure w᠁ relatively low accuracy.

Growth site A location at which growth occurs. [Compare with Growth center.]

Growth spurt See Pubertal growth spurt.

Growth Study, Bolton-Brush See Bolton-Brush Growth Study.

Growth Study, Burlington See Burlington Growth Study.

Growth Study, Michigan See Michigan Growth Study.

G'Sn-SnPg' See Cephalometric measurements (Soft tissue), Angle of facial convexity.

GTR See Guided tissue regeneration.

Guidance, Anterior See Anterior guidance.

Guidance, Canine See Canine guidance.

Guidance, Condylar See Condylar guidance.

Guidance, Developmental See Developmental guidance.

Guidance, Occlusal See Occlusal guidance.

Guidance of eruption A planned sequence of selective, timed extraction of deciduous teeth with the objective of facilitating the eruption of the permanent successors into improved positions. Guidance of eruption involves no extractions of permanent teeth. [Compare with Serial extraction.]

Guide plane An acrylic surface of a removable or functional appliance that contacts a tooth and transmits the desired intermittent forces to it. A guide plane also may be the part of the functional appliance that serves to induce the desired anterior (or posterior) mandibular position.

Guided tissue regeneration (GTR) Periodontal surgical procedure attempting to regenerate lost periodontal structures through differential tissue responses. Such procedures make use of barrier techniques, where membranes made of materials such

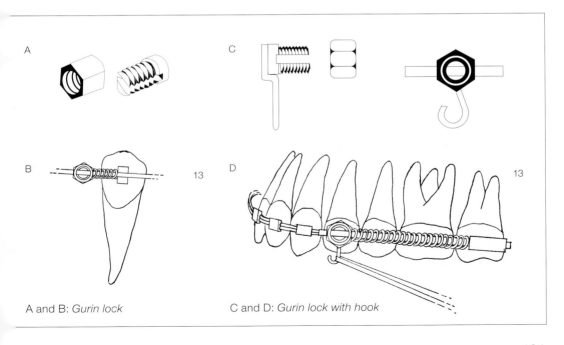

A and B: *Gurin lock*   C and D: *Gurin lock with hook*

as expanded polytetrafluoroethylene, polyglactin, polylactic acid and collagen are employed to exclude the epithelial tissue from the root surface and bone, in the belief that it interferes with regeneration.

"Gummy" smile Excessive amount of gingival exposure upon smiling. [Also see Tooth-to-lip relationship.]

Gurin lock Adjustable archwire attachment that can be locked onto an archwire to serve as a stop, without the need for bending, welding or soldering. A Gurin lock consists of a small screw that is split along its long axis, allowing it to be positioned "riding" the archwire and is secured in place by a hexagon-head lock-nut. Its advantage is that it can be easily removed or repositioned along the archwire at any time, and with no consequences for the archwire. Gurin locks also are available with hooks, used for attachment of elastics directly on the archwire (instead of a Kobayashi hook on a certain tooth). *See illustration previous page.*

H

angle (of Holdaway) See Cephalometric measurements (Soft tissue), H-angle.

line (Harmony line of Holdaway) See Cephalometric lines, H-line.

as appliance See Appliance, Haas.

bit Persistent, repeated action such as sucking of a finger (most commonly the thumb), lip, or other objects. Persistent habits may interfere with the normal development of the teeth or bones as well as with physiologic function. [Also see Thumbsucking habit.]

bit-breaking appliance See Appliance, Habit-breaking.

bit reminder See Appliance, Habit-breaking.

bit therapy Treatment designed to intercept potentially harmful habits, to restore physiologic function and/or to correct a malformation of the teeth or bones caused by a habit. Treatment may consist of counseling or appliance therapy, or both.

bitual occlusion See Occlusion, Centric.

nd and wrist radiograph A radiograph of the carpal, metacarpal and phalangeal bones of the hand and wrist, traditionally used to determine the skeletal maturation status of children, as skeletal or developmental age does not always correspond with chronological age.

The procedure involves the appraisal of the degree of development of various carpal, metacarpal and epiphyseal centers of ossification, in comparison with standards provided from growth studies. The standards are published in an atlas format, based on the average appearance of a hand and wrist radiograph at various chronological ages.

Hard palate See Palate, Hard.

Hard tissue landmarks, Cephalometric See Cephalometric landmarks, Hard tissue.

Hard tissue measurements, Cephalometric See Cephalometric measurements, Hard tissue.

Hard wire cutter See Orthodontic instruments, Hard wire cutter.

Hardening A process used to increase the yield strength and resistance to indentation of a metal.

Work-hardening (Cold-working) Hardening of a wire by repetitive plastic deformation in the cold state. Placing repetitive bends on an orthodontic wire increases its strength and hardness because of work-hardening, but also makes the wire more brittle.

Hardness (of a material) Resistance to indentation on the surface. Depending on the type of indentor used for the hardness test, one can distinguish between *Brinell hardness*, *Rockwell hardness* and *Vickers* *hardness.* Among the properties that are important to the hardness of a material are strength, proportional limit, and ductility.

Harmony line of Holdaway (H-line) See cephalometric lines, H-line.

Harry Barrer retainer See Retainer, Spring.

Harvold cephalometric analysis See Cephalometric analysis, Harvold.

Harvold-Woodside activator See Appliance, Harvold-Woodside activator.

Hawley retainer See Retainer, Hawley.

Hawley wire The labial bow of the Hawley retainer. [Also see Labial bow; Retainer, Hawley.]

Head position, Natural See Natural head position.

Head posture, Natural See Natural head posture.

Headcap See Headstrap.

Headgear Extraoral appliance making use of cervical or cranial anchorage to apply forces to the jaws and teeth, with the purpose of growth modification or tooth movement.
The choice of direction of pull of the headgear usually is based on the patient's facial pattern: the more vertically excessive growth is present, the higher the direction of pull and vice versa. It should be kept in mind, however, that considerable variation in growth response can occur. [Note: To apply Newton's laws for theoretical biomechanical consideration on use of different types of headgears, the facebow is assumed to be completely rigid.]

Asymmetric headgear (Eccentric headgear) A modification in the design of a cervical or straight-pull headgear to achieve differential magnitude of force between the two sides, when attempting

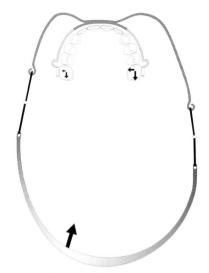

Asymmetric headgear

asymmetric molar distalization. This is usually performed using a facebow with an asymmetric outer bow. One of the arms is kept longer (and/or more laterally offset) on the side that requires the greater distalization to generate a higher force magnitude. The disadvantage of asymmetric headgear traction is the creation of transverse (buccolingual) forces, which are difficult to control and may have detrimental effects on the maxillary arch and the occlusion, especially if an asymmetric headgear is used for a prolonged period.

Cervical headgear (Kloehn-type headgear, Low-pull headgear) A type of headgear consisting of a standard facebow inserting into the headgear tubes of the maxillary first permanent molar attachments and a cervical neckstrap. The cervical headgear, which was made popular by S. Kloehn, is used to restrict anterior growth of the maxilla and to distalize or maintain the sagittal position of the maxillary molars. Because of the cervical anchorage, the direction of the traction with this type of headgear produces an extrusive force on the maxillary first molars, in addition to the distal force. Depending on the orientation and length

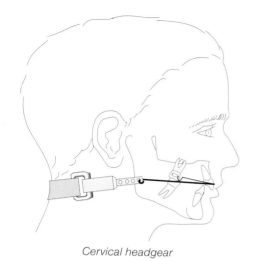

Cervical headgear

the outer bow, as well as the number of teeth included, the vector of the force can be made to pass through, below or above the center of resistance of the unit, resulting in a bodily or tipping movement.

High-pull headgear (Occipital headgear)

This consists of a high-pull headstrap and a standard facebow, the outer arms of which are cut shorter and/or bent upwards slightly, so that the force vector is directed through, below or above the center of resistance of the maxillary first permanent

molars, or that of the entire maxilla. The line of action of the force forms an angle of approximately 45° with the occlusal plane. A high-pull headgear also can be attached to a removable or functional appliance. When a high-pull headgear is used directly on the maxillary first permanent molars without any fixed appliances on the remaining teeth, the insertion of a transpalatal arch on the first molars can serve to prevent undesirable buccal tipping. The objectives of high-pull headgear treatment are restriction of anterior and downward maxillary growth and/ or molar distalization, intrusion, or control of their eruption. The high-pull headgear is commonly used in the treatment of growing patients with Class II malocclusions, increased vertical dimension, minimal overbite and increased gingival exposure on smiling.

J-hook headgear A type of headgear consisting of a high-pull or straight-pull headstrap, attaching to hooks or loops on the archwire by means of a J-hook assembly through the commisures (i.e. without a face-

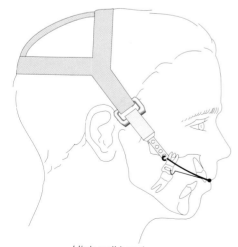

High-pull headgear

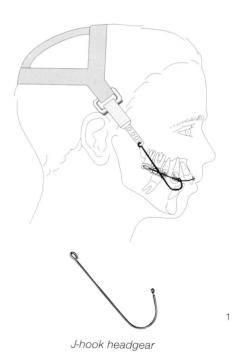

J-hook headgear

bow). A J-hook headgear also may be used to provide the necessary force for distal movement of teeth (such as retraction of canines) with sliding mechanics, by attaching to a sliding jig or directly to the archwire, mesial to the teeth that are to be retracted. Use in conjunction with a removable appliance again is feasible.

Mandibular headgear A headgear directing extraoral forces to the mandibular arch by means of a standard facebow and a cervical neckstrap. Because of the mobility of the mandible, the line of action of the force produced by a mandibular headgear changes depending on the degree of opening.

Reverse-pull headgear (Protraction headgear) See Appliance, Face mask.

Straight-pull headgear (Combination headgear, Horizontal-pull headgear) A headgear with a modified headstrap designed to produce a horizontal force (approximately parallel to the occlusal plane). A similar direction of force can be produced by simultaneously attaching a high-pull headstrap and a cervical neckstrap on the same facebow. Varying the proportions of the total force derived from the

two straps, as well as varying the length a■ inclination of the outer bow, allows the res tant vector to be altered.

Vertical-pull headgear A type of hea gear consisting of a standard facebow a■ a modified headcap, capable of generatin a force vector passing at approximate 65° to the occlusal plane (force vecto passing anteriorly to that would dislod■ the headcap, unless a special custom ma■ headcap is used). This type of headgear used when intrusion of the buccal segmen is attempted. The headcap of a vertical-p■ headgear is usually versatile, in that it h■ multiple notches allowing variation in t■ direction of the traction force.

Headgear facebow See Facebow of a hea■ gear.

Headgear/functional appliance combin■ tion See Appliance, Combined function■ extraoral traction.

Headgear tube See Tube, Headgear.

Headstrap (Headcap) The component ■ an extraoral traction appliance that distr■ utes and transfers reaction forces to t■ cranium. The headstrap allows a posteri■ and upward force vector. It usually carri■ safety-release force modules to reduce t■ chance of accidental injury. Modified hea■ straps also are used with straight-pull (co■ bination) headgears or with vertical-p■ headgears. [Compare with Neckstrap.]

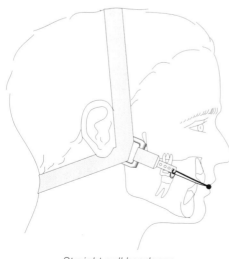

Straight-pull headgear

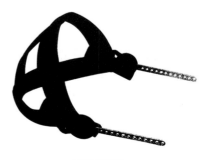

Headstrap

ealth maintenance organization (HMO)
A legal entity that accepts responsibility and financial risk for providing specific services to a defined population during a defined period of time at a fixed price. An organized system of health care delivery that provides comprehensive care to enrollees through designated providers. Enrollees generally are assessed a preset monthly payment for health care services (regardless of the actual treatment costs) and may be required to remain in the program for a specified period of time. Health maintenance organizations usually provide no treatment byalth care practitioners outside the HMO. [Compare with Preferred provider organization.] [Modified from the AAO Glossary of Dentofacial Orthopedic Terms, 1993.]

eat treatment The thermal processing of a material for a certain period of time, above room temperature but below the melting temperature. The effects of heat treatment depend entirely on the temperature, the duration of the process, and the type of material. Heat treating, for example, may harden or soften a metal, or change its grain size or corrosion resistance.

eavy-duty pliers See Orthodontic instruments, Parallel-action pliers with cutter.

eavy force See Force, Heavy.

elix A spiral bend placed in an orthodontic wire in the shape of a closed circle. Used as a stop along the archwire, or for the attach-

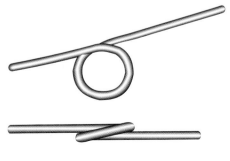

Helix

ment of various modules such as elastics or J-hooks. Additionally, helices can be added in the design of various orthodontic springs to lower their force/deflection rate.

Quad-helix See Appliance, Quad-helix.

Tri-helix See Appliance, Tri-helix.

Hemifacial microsomia (First and second branchial arch syndrome) An umbrella term denoting a family of congenital anomalies characterized by malformation, underdevelopment or absence of certain structures which are derived from the first and second branchial arches during embryological development. Variations of the condition have been named Goldenhar syndrome, oculoauriculovertebral spectrum, necrotic facial dysplasia, otomandibular dysostosis, and craniofacial microsomia.

The disorder can involve the maxilla, mandible, ears, eyes, orbits, nose, frontonasal structures, zygoma, facial soft tissue and musculature, parotid gland and the facial nerve. Unilateral or bilateral cleft lip and/or palate can be co-existing in 7% to 15% of the cases. Cardiac, renal, vertebral and central nervous system abnormalities also have been reported.

The exact mechanism of its etiology remains unknown; however, vascular abnormalities, disturbance of neural crest cell migration, chromosomal abnormalities and certain teratologic agents have been hypothesized. The frequency is approximately 1:5600 live births and there seems to be a male predominance of about 3:2 and a predominance of 3:2 of right-sided versus left-sided involvement in truly unilateral cases.

The disorder is expressed to varying degrees, ranging from a mild facial asymmetry to involvement of many facial structures, unilateral or bilateral, which can be functionally and psychologically debilitating. The clinical appearance most often involves a unilateral hypoplasia of the mandibular condyle and ramus, leading to deviation of the chin to the affected side. Depending on the severity, a number of mandibular posterior teeth may be missing ipsilaterally. Canting of the maxillary occlusal plane (up on the affected side) is a common finding, as are preauricular tags of skin and cartilage.

Treatment of patients with hemifacial microsomia often includes multi-stage procedures such as reconstruction of the mandibular condyle and/or fossa, microvascular free-flap transfer for soft tissue augmentation, auricular reconstruction, facial reanimation, functional appliance treatment, ramus lengthening by distraction osteogenesis or bimaxillary orthognathic surgery.

Hemisection (of a tooth) The surgical separation of an endodontically treated multi-rooted tooth (most commonly a mandibular molar) through the furcation.

Hemostat See Orthodontic instruments, Hemostat.

Herbst appliance See Appliance, Herbst.

Herren activator See Appliance, Herren.

Heterogenous graft See Graft, Heterologous.

Heterologous graft See Graft, Heterologous.

Hickham protraction appliance See Appliance, Hickham.

"High-angle" patient ("Vertical" patient, Long face syndrome, Hyperdivergent face) A general term used to describe a patient with a predominantly vertical growth pattern, a long lower face height and a steep mandibular plane. A Class II malocclusion with an anterior open bite tendency may be associated, typically with excessive gingival exposure on smiling, vertical maxillary excess and lip incompetence. (Referring to the mandibular plane angle.) [Compare with "Low-angle" patient.]

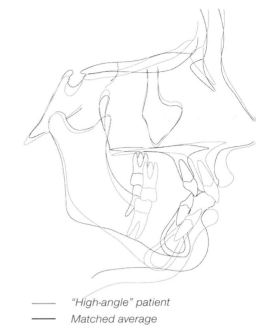

—— *"High-angle" patient*
—— *Matched average*

High labial arch See Arch, E-arch.

High-pull headgear See Headgear, High-pu[

HMO See Health Maintenance Organization.

Hinge axis The theoretical single horizont axis about which the pure rotational mov ment of the mandible occurs, during th initial phase of jaw opening.

Holdaway ratio See Cephalometric measur ments (Hard tissue), Holdaway ratio.

Holdaway's H-angle See Cephalometr measurements (Soft tissue), H-angle.

Holdaway's harmony line (H-line) Se Cephalometric lines, H-line.

Holding arch See Arch, Lingual; Arch, Nanc holding.

Homeostasis of the dentition The sta of equilibrium of the position of the teet as determined by their morphology, th relationship between their supporting bones, the occlusion, the periodontium and forces from muscles and other structures involved.

Homogenous graft See Graft, Homologous.

Homologous graft See Graft, Homologous.

Hooks Attachments soldered, welded or crimped onto an orthodontic archwire, to aid in placement of elastics, headgear (i.e. J-hook), elastic chains, etc., or to facilitate intermaxillary fixation during orthognathic surgery.

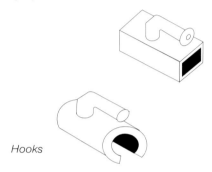

Hooks

"Horizontal" patient See "Low-angle" patient.

Horizontal plane See Transverse plane.

Horizontal-pull headgear See Headgear, Straight-pull.

Horseshoe arch See Arch, Horseshoe.

Host site See Recipient site.

Howes' analysis A plaster cast analysis aimed at evaluating the relationship of the maxillary and mandibular dental arch width to the width of the respective apical bases, taking into account the existing tooth material.
According to A.E. Howes, the ratio of the premolar width (the linear distance between the tips of the buccal cusps of the first premolars bilaterally) over the existing tooth material (the sum of the mesiodistal widths of the first permanent molars, premolars, canines and incisors), in either the maxillary or the mandibular arch, should be approximately 43%. Correspondingly, the ratio of the canine fossa width (the width of the apical base measured on the plaster cast at the level of the apex of the first premolars) over the existing tooth material (the sum of the mesiodistal widths of all the teeth anterior to the second molars, as explained previously) for the same arch should be approximately 44%, whether this concerns the maxillary or the mandibular arch.
When the former ratio is much smaller than the latter, the arch can be expanded to eliminate any existing crowding. If the opposite is true, then according to Howes, extractions are indicated in the presence of crowding.

Howes utility pliers See Orthodontic instruments, Howes utility pliers.

Howship's lacunae Small pits or hollow depressions in bone undergoing resorption, containing osteoclasts. Similar lacunae also can be found in cementum, in which cementoclasts may or may not be located.

Hyaline cartilage See Cartilage, Hyaline.

Hyalinization A term describing the loss of cells from an area of the PDL because of trauma, as seen by light microscopy. Hyalinization occurs often on the compression side of the PDL during tooth movement. When this happens, no remodeling of the alveolar bone can occur because no cells are present; therefore hyalinization causes tooth movement to cease. Only after the hyalinized portion of the ligament is removed by osteoclasts coming from the bone marrow on the endosteal side, does tooth movement start again. [Also see Bone resorption, Frontal and Undermining].

"Hybrid" functional appliance See Appliance, "Hybrid" functional.

Hygienic rapid palatal expander See Appliance, Hyrax.

Hygienist See Dental hygienist.

Hyperdivergent A facial pattern that is characterized by a steep mandibular plane angle, a long anterior lower facial height with an open bite tendency, a retrognathic mandible with an associated Class II malocclusion and lip incompetence. Named so because of the cephalometrically observed excessive divergence of the skeletal planes (mandibular, occlusal and palatal) in relation to each other or to the cranial base. [Compare with Hypodivergent; also see "High-angle" patient.]

Hyperdivergent face See "High-angle" patient.

Hypermobility See Tooth mobility, Increased.

Hypernasality (Rhinolalia aperta) The defective voice quality that is characterized by excessive nasal resonance during speech. It can result from a structural (i.e. hypomobility or shortness of the soft palate in cleft palate patients) or a functional problem of the velopharyngeal mechanism. [Compare with Hyponasality.]

Hyperodontia See Supernumerary teeth.

Hyperplasia Excessive enlargement of a tissue or structure due to increase in the number of cells.

Hypertelorism See Orbital hypertelorism.

Hypertrophic arthritis See Osteoarthritis.

Hypertrophy Excessive enlargement of a organ or structure due to increase in the si but not the number of its individual co stituent cells, as well as increase of interc lular matrix.

Hypodivergent A facial pattern character ed by relative parallelism of the skelet planes (mandibular, occlusal and palat in relation to each other or to the cran base, as observed cephalometrically. Th facial pattern often is associated with Class II, Division 2 malocclusion typica exhibiting a decreased gonial angle, sho anterior lower facial height, deep overbit strong chin and retrusive lips. [Compa with Hyperdivergent; also see "Low-angl patient.]

Hypodivergent face See "Low-angle" patie

Hypodontia Congenital absence of one more, but not all teeth. [Compare wi Supernumerary teeth; Anodontia.]

Hypomobility See Tooth mobility, Reduced

Hyponasality (Rhinolalia clausa) Phonatic with insufficient nasal resonance, usua due to a blockage of the nasal airwa [Compare with Hypernasality.]

Hypoplasia Incomplete or defective develo ment of a tissue or structure. [The ter implies fewer than the usual number cells.]

Hypotelorism See Orbital hypotelorism.

Hyrax appliance See Appliance, Hyrax.

I

Iatrogenic An unfavorable response or condition, caused by medical or dental personnel, diagnostic tests or treatment procedures.

ICP See Occlusion, Centric.

Id See Cephalometric landmarks (Hard tissue), Infradentale.

Ideal occlusion A theoretical concept of an ideal arrangement of the teeth within the dental arches, combined with an ideal interarch relationship, which concentrates optimal esthetics, function, and stability of the dentition and supporting structures. [Also see Six keys of occlusion.]

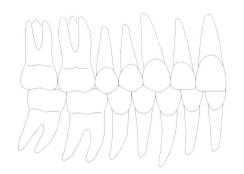

Ideal occlusion

Idiopathic Pain, disease or disorder of unknown etiology.

IGF-I and IGF-II See Growth factors.

Ii See Cephalometric landmarks (Hard tissue), Incision inferius.

Ilizarov technique See Distraction osteogenesis.

Ils See Cephalometric landmarks (Soft tissue), Inferior labial sulcus.

Imaging See Diagnostic imaging.

Imbrication The overlapping of incisors and canines in the same arch, usually due to crowding.

IMF See Fixation (Surgical), Intermaxillary.

Immobilization See Fixation, Surgical; Splinting (of teeth).

IMPA See Cephalometric measurements (Hard tissue), Incisor mandibular plane angle.

Impaction (of food) The forceful wedging of food into the interproximal space during mastication.

Impaction (of the maxilla) An orthognathic surgical procedure involving superior repositioning of the maxilla, usually by means of a Le Fort I osteotomy. A maxillary impaction is used for correction of a high smile line, associated with vertical maxillary excess. In the instance of surgical correction of a skeletal open bite, a *differential* maxillary impaction is performed, whereby the anterior aspect of the maxilla is moved superiorly to a lesser extent than its posterior aspect. *See illustration next page.*

141

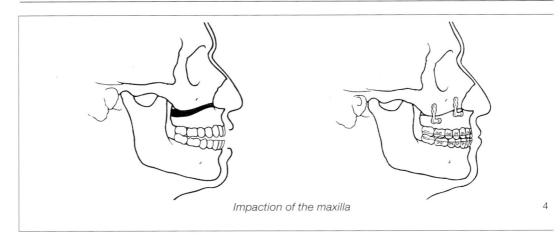

Impaction of the maxilla 4

Impaction (of a tooth) Failure of a tooth to emerge, usually due to insufficient space, or due to the presence of a supernumerary tooth blocking its eruption path. Impaction sometimes occurs with no apparent etiology (idiopathic). Certain conditions (e.g. cleidocranial dysostosis) are accompanied by a high frequency of impacted teeth.

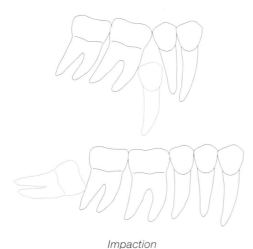

Impaction

Impinging overbite See Overbite, Impinging.

Implant An alloplastic material or device that is surgically placed into the body. In dentistry, implants are placed beneath the mucosal or periosteal layer or within bone for functional, therapeutic or esthetic pu poses. Root-form, endosseous, screw threaded implants are the most common used implants in clinical practice.

Endosseous implant An implant that embedded in mandibular or maxillary bor and projects through the oral mucosa co ering the edentulous ridge.

Orthodontic implant Any implant use during orthodontic treatment as anchorag for orthodontic tooth movement. Orth dontic implants can be placed on the alv olar process, anterior hard palate, retrom lar area, etc. Osseointegrated implants co stitute excellent anchorage for even the mo complicated types of tooth movement, a they do not show any clinically significa reactive movement to orthodontic force (infinite anchorage).

Osseointegrated implant See Osse integration.

Subperiosteal implant An implant th rests on the surface of the bone, benea the periosteum.

Transosteal implant An implant that pe etrates the inferior mandibular border ar also projects through the oral mucosa, co ering the edentulous ridge.

Impression An accurate negative imprint of the maxillary or mandibular dental arch and surrounding structures, from which a positive reproduction (cast, model) can be made. When taking an impression for orthodontic purposes the flanges of the impression tray are extended to allow maximum reproduction of the alveolar process. Alginate is by far the most commonly used impression material in orthodontics. [Also see Orthodontic impression trays; Orthodontic casts.]

Incidence The number of new patients acquiring a disease or condition over a predetermined time period, as generated by an analytic epidemiological investigation of a prospective longitudinal nature. [Compare with Prevalence.]

Incisal Pertaining to, or in the direction of, the incisal edge of the anterior teeth.

Incision inferius (Ii) See Cephalometric landmarks (Hard tissue), Incision inferius.

Incision superius (Is) See Cephalometric landmarks (Hard tissue), Incision superius.

Incisor-mandibular plane angle (IMPA) See Cephalometric measurements (Hard tissue), Incisor-mandibular plane angle.

Inclination (Third order, "Torque") Angular deviation of the long axis of a tooth from a line perpendicular to the occlusal plane, in

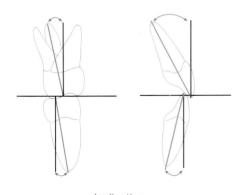

Inclination

the labiolingual, or buccolingual direction. [Compare with Angulation.]

Inclined plane An oblique surface (slope) used to correct a crossbite of one or more incisors. The inclined plane can be part of a removable appliance or it can be fixed on the teeth of the opposing arch. Inclined planes also have been used as part of functional appliances to induce an anterior or posterior mandibular position.

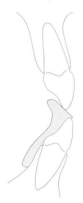

Inclined plane

Incompetent lip seal See Lip incompetence.

Inconsistent force system See Force system, Inconsistent.

Increased tooth mobility See Tooth mobility, Increased.

Index A relative or arbitrary system of measurement used to describe or quantify a condition. The purpose of an index is to reduce the multitude of variables that enter into a diagnosis and influence the assessment of the severity and prognosis of a condition, to a format (numerical or categorical) that permits direct comparison.

Many indices have been advocated in orthodontics; some have been developed to classify malocclusion into types (the Angle classification being a prime example), others to record prevalence of malocclusion in epidemiological studies. In addition, certain occlusal indices (such as the IOTN and PAR index) are meant mainly as methods of determining the need for treatment, or as indicators of the clinical outcome of treatment.

Cephalic index A numerical expression of the ratio between biparietal diameter and fronto-occipital diameter of a living person's head. [Compare with Index, Cranial.] The cephalic index is calculated by the formula "maximum head width x 100/maximum head length." It is used in anthropometry to classify skulls as dolichocephalic (cephalic index up to 75.9), mesocephalic (between 76 and 80.9) or brachycephalic (81 or larger).

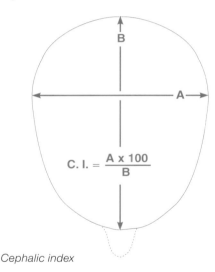

$$C.I. = \frac{A \times 100}{B}$$

Cephalic index

Cranial index The equivalent of the cephalic index in a dry skull; a craniometric measurement.

Facial index A numerical expression of the proportionality of the face. The facial index is calculated by the formula: "facial height x 100/zygomatic width." It is used in anthropometry to classify faces as euryprosopic, mesoprosopic or leptoprosopic.

Index of orthodontic treatment need (IOTN) An index developed by P.H. Brook

and W.C. Shaw in 1989. The IOTN ranks ma occlusions in terms of the significance c their various components for the individual dental health and perceived esthetic impai ment. The intention is to identify thos individuals who would most likely benef from orthodontic treatment. It incorporate a dental health and an esthetic componen The dental health component can b applied either clinically or on study cast: by categorizing each occlusal trait cor tributing to the malocclusion into one c five grades (grade 1 = no need for treatmen grade 5 = great need). The measurement are facilitated by a specially designed rule The esthetic component consists of a 1(point scale illustrated by a series of nun bered photographs to which the patient' situation is compared.

Irregularity index An index introduce by R.M. Little in 1975 for standardize assessment of mandibular anterior crowc ing. It involves measuring the linear dis placement of the anatomic contact point (as distinguished from the clinical contac points) of each mandibular incisor from th respective points of the adjacent teeth. Th sum of these five displacements represent the relative degree of anterior irregularit Perfect alignment from the mesial aspect c the left to the right canine would yield a scor of 0, with increased crowding represente by greater displacement, and thus a highe index score. The measurements are pe formed with a caliper, parallel to the occlusa plane. Vertical discrepancies between adja cent contact points are not taken int account, as it is assumed that correction c such discrepancies would not appreciabl affect anterior arch length. Mesiodistal inte dental spacing also is disregarded, provic ed the teeth in question are in proper arc form. If spacing as well as rotations ar present, only the labiolingual displacemer from the proper arch form is recorded.

Peer assessment rating (PAR) inde An index for recording the severity of malocclusion in the mixed and permaner dentition, developed in 1987 by a group of 10 orthodontists in Great Britain (British Orthodontic Standards Working Party). The index consists of a scoring system of study casts, facilitated by a ruler. Individual scores for the components of alignment and occlusion finally are summed to calculate an overall score. Thus, a score of zero would indicate perfect alignment and occlusion, with scores above zero (but rarely beyond 50) indicating increasing levels of irregularity. The index is applied to both the start and end of treatment study casts, and the change in the total score reflects the success of treatment with regard to the alignment and occlusion.

ndirect bonding See Bonding, Indirect.

ndirect resorption See Bone resorption, Undermining.

ndividual Practice Association (IPA) A partnership, corporation or other legal entity that contracts with an HMO, union, or other provider to provide care to an enrolled group for a fixed monthly amount. In the IPA, the provider can work from his/her office instead of an HMO center or clinic. Fee-for-service patients can be treated alongside those in the IPA plan. Patients in the IPA plan must use a participating provider. The provider must follow IPA practices, accept reimbursement as full payment and comply with IPA peer review and quality assurance procedures. Typically, the IPA pays the provider a percentage of his/her fee, with the remaining percentage held in a reserve pool that may be divided at year's end by the provider if any funds remain. [Taken from the AAO Glossary of Dentofacial Orthopedic Terms, 1993.]

elastic Deviating from a proportional relationship of stress and strain.

elastic deformation See Deformation, Permanent.

Inertia The property of matter that causes it to resist change in motion.

Inertia, Law of See Newton's laws.

Infant maxillary orthopedic treatment See Presurgical infant orthopedics.

Infantile swallow (Visceral swallow) See Swallow, Infantile.

Inferior joint space (Inferior joint compartment) The intra-articular space between the head of the mandibular condyle and the inferior surface of the articular disc of the TMJ. During the early opening stage of mandibular movement, only the inferior joint space is involved (by rotational movement of the condyle). [Also see Joint, Temporomandibular; Superior joint space.]

Inferior labial sulcus (Ils) See Cephalometric landmarks (Soft tissue), Inferior labial sulcus.

Inferior prosthion See Cephalometric landmarks (Hard tissue), Infradentale.

Infinite anchorage See Anchorage, Infinite.

Informed consent The outline by any health professional, including the orthodontist, of the patient's problems along with the possible solutions, in a simplified fashion comprehensible to the reasonable layman, in order to obtain the patient's consent to treatment. The health professional is supposed to establish treatment priorities through discussion with the patient. Reasonable treatment alternatives and the risks and benefits of each alternative should be provided, including that of no treatment. In this way, the patient is able to make an informed decision. Informed consent is a legal requirement prior to treating patients and is encouraged by the American Association of Orthodontists.

Infradentale (Id) See Cephalometric landmarks (Hard tissue), Infradentale.

Infraeruption See Undereruption.

Infraocclusion See Infraposition.

Infraorbital pointer The component of an articulator facebow that records the position of the infraorbital rim to facilitate alignment of the plane of the facebow with the Frankfort horizontal plane.

Infraposition (Infraocclusion) A situation in which a tooth or group of teeth is positioned below the occlusal plane; commonly due to a deleterious habit or to ankylosis. Infraposition is a more general term that contains undereruption. [Compare with Undereruption.]

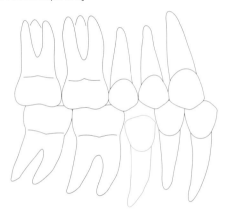

Infraposition

Initiating factors Factors that cause the onset of a disease or disorder.

Inner bow See Facebow (of a headgear).

In-out bends See Bends, First-order.

Insulinlike growth factors I and II (IGF-I and IGF-II) See Growth factors.

Intensifying screen (Rare-earth screen) A screen used to intensify the latent images on an x-ray film. It usually consists of a thin sheet of plastic coated with a fluorescent material, which is mounted in the cassette in close contact with the film. The x-ray cause the screen to produce visible lig which intensifies the generation of the late images on the film, greatly reducing t exposure of the patient to radiation.

Interbracket span (Interbracket distanc The distance between orthodontic bracke (measured between adjacent slot ends) th determines the length of a straight wire co necting them. The smaller the width of t brackets, the longer the interbracket spa the lower the load/deflection rate of the wi and vice versa. [Also see Load/deflectio rate.]

Interceptive orthodontic treatment I tervention in the incipient stages of a pro lem to lessen its severity or possible futu adverse effects and to eliminate its caus Such treatment may take place in the deci uous or transitional dentition and m include redirection of ectopically eruptin teeth, slicing or extraction of deciduo teeth, correction of isolated dental cros bites or recovery of minor space loss.
The presence of complicating factors suc as skeletal disharmonies, overall spac deficiency, or other conditions requirir present or future comprehensive therap are beyond the realm of interceptive ther py. [Modified from the AAO Glossary Dentofacial Orthopedic Terms, 1993.]

Intercuspal position See Occlusion, Centri

Intercuspation See Interdigitation.

Interdental papilla (Gingival papilla) Th portion of the gingiva that occupies the inte proximal spaces. The interdental extensic of the gingiva.

Interdental spacing Spacing between th teeth.

Interdigitation (Intercuspation) The inte locking of the cusps of the posterior tee in the fossae and embrasures of their anta onists.

tergonial line See Cephalometric lines, Intergonial line.

terincisal angle See Cephalometric measurements (Hard tissue), Interincisal angle.

terlabial gap The vertical separation of the lips at rest. A 2- to 3-mm interlabial gap generally is considered to be esthetically pleasing. [See also Cephalometric measurements (Soft tissue), Interlabial gap.]

termaxillary Between the maxilla and the mandible. [Compare with Intramaxillary.]

termaxillary anchorage See Anchorage, Intermaxillary.

termaxillary elastics See Orthodontic elastics, Intermaxillary.

termaxillary fixation (IMF) See Fixation (Surgical), Intermaxillary.

termaxillary mechanics See Mechanics, Intermaxillary.

termaxillary traction See Orthodontic elastics, Intermaxillary.

termediate splint See Splint, Surgical.

termittent force See Force, Intermittent.

ternal derangement Disturbed arrangement of intracapsular joint components that interferes with smooth joint movements. In the TMJ it can be associated with elongation, tear or rupture of the ligaments or capsule, causing altered disc position or morphology. Although this is not always the case, chronic dysfunction of internally deranged TMJs generally is thought to follow a progression to more severe stages of breakdown, eventually leading to degenerative joint disease.

ternal pterygoid muscle See Muscle, Medial pterygoid.

Internal resorption See Resorption, Internal.

Internal rotation (of the mandible) See Mandibular rotation, Total.

International System of Units (SI, Système Internationale d' Unités) Internationally standardized system of physical units consisting of seven basic units from which all others can be derived.

The seven dimensionally independent basic quantities (and their respective units and abbreviations) are: length (meter, m); mass (kilogram, kg); amount of substance (mole, mol); time (second, s); thermodynamic temperature (°Kelvin, °K); electric current (ampere, A); luminous intensity (candela, cd).

Interocclusal clearance See Freeway space.

Interocclusal separation See Freeway space.

Interocclusal splint See Splint.

Interposition of the lip See Lip interposition.

Interposition of the tongue See Tongue interposition.

Interproximal reduction of enamel See Interproximal stripping.

Interproximal stripping (Interproximal reduction of enamel, Reproximation, Slenderizing) Reduction of the mesiodistal width of the teeth by removal of interproximal enamel. This procedure can be achieved by means of handheld or motor-driven abrasive strips, or handpiece-mounted abrasive discs, or by means of a tapered fissure carbide bur. It most commonly is performed in the mandibular or maxillary incisor area in patients with a tooth-size discrepancy. Generalized stripping of the entire arch is advocated by J.J. Sheridan to relieve crowding without extractions. According to him, up to 0.3 or 0.4 mm of enamel can be removed per tooth surface,

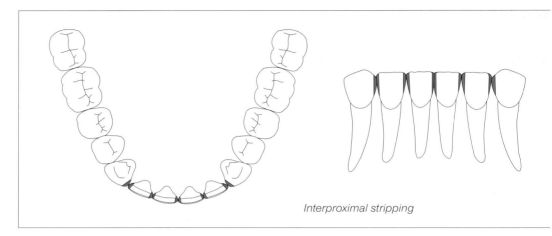

Interproximal stripping

depending on the size and shape of the teeth.

It has been advocated that interproximal stripping, if carried out to an extreme, may cause the mandibular incisor roots to approximate excessively, resulting in thinning of the interradicular alveolar bone, perhaps making it more prone to later periodontal bone loss. Another potential side effect is the resulting enamel roughness that may contribute to increased plaque accumulation.

Interpupillary line   A line connecting the pupils of the eyes, used as a reference in the evaluation of frontal facial asymmetry.

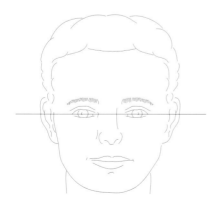

Interpupillary line

Interrupted force   See Force, Interrupted.

Intersegmental   Between segments of tee (usually within the same dental arcl [Compare with Intrasegmental.]

Intersegmental mechanics   See Mechanic Intersegmental.

Interstitial growth   Growth within a tissu Histologically, a characteristic type of grow of soft tissues and cartilage occurring by combination of cellular hyperplasia ar hypertrophy. Interstitial growth does n occur in calcified tissues such as teeth bone.

Intra-articular disc   See Articular disc.

Intracapsular   Located within the capsule a joint.

Intracapsular adhesion   See Adhesio Intracapsular.

Intracapsular fracture   See Fracture, Intr capsular.

Intracoronal retainer   See Retainer, Bond lingual.

Intramatrix rotation (of the mandible)   S Mandibular rotation, Intramatrix.

tramaxillary Within the same dental arch. [Compare with Intermaxillary.]

tramaxillary anchorage See Anchorage, Intramaxillary.

tramaxillary elastics See Orthodontic elastics, Intramaxillary.

tramaxillary tractions See Orthodontic elastics, Intramaxillary.

tramembranous bone See Bone, Intramembranous.

tramembranous ossification See Ossification, Intramembranous.

trasegmental mechanics See Mechanics.

traoral vertical ramus osteotomy (IVRO) See Osteotomy, Transoral vertical ramus.

trasegmental Within the same segment of teeth. [Compare with Intersegmental.]

trasegmental mechanics See Mechanics, Intrasegmental.

trusion See Orthodontic tooth movement, Intrusion.

trusive arch See Arch, Intrusive

visible braces A lay term applied to lingual orthodontic appliances, or to those made of a clear material (ceramic or plastic brackets). [Also see Appliance, Lingual.]

Ion implantation A surface modification technique involving a ballistic process through which an element is imbedded into the surface of a substrate. The main advantage of this process is that the surface properties of the substrate are improved, while the bulk properties and tolerances remain unchanged. Ion implantation is used in orthodontics to optimize the frictional characteristics of β-Ti archwires.

IOTN index See Index, Index of orthodontic treatment need.

IPA See Individual Practice Association.

Ipsilateral Referring to the same side as the one under consideration. [Compare with Contralateral.]

Irregularity index See Index, Irregularity.

Is See Cephalometric landmarks (Hard tissue), Incision superius.

Isologous graft See Graft, Isologous.

Isometric contraction Muscle contraction without change in length.

Isotonic contraction Muscle contraction with shortening of the muscle length, without appreciable change in magnitude of the produced force.

IVRO See Osteotomy, Transoral vertical ramus.

J

J-hook headgear See Headgear, J-hook.

Jackscrew See Expansion screw.

Jasper jumper See Appliance, Jasper jumper.

Jaw Either of the two bony structures (maxilla or mandible) in most vertebrates that border the mouth and bear teeth.

> **Lower jaw** See Mandible.

> **Upper jaw** See Maxilla.

Jaw joint See Joint, Temporomandibular.

Jaw surgery See Orthognathic surgery.

"Jiggling" forces See Force, "Jiggling."

"Jiggling" (of a tooth) Repetitive limited movement of a tooth in one and then in the opposite direction, as is commonly thought to occur under the influence of occlusal forces.
Most types of orthodontic tooth movement in reality take place as a series of minute "jiggling" movements. This translates into continuous reversal of the root surfaces that sustain compression and tension which is, at the histological level, equivalent to round-tripping. [Also see Round-tripping.]

Joint The place of union between two or more bones.

> **Arthrodial joint** A joint that permits gliding movements (translation).

Cartilaginous joint A joint in which cartilage is interposed between the implicated bones and the fibrous tissue (in the sequence: bone-cartilage-fibrous tissue-cartilage-bone). Examples are the costochondral joint and the pubic symphysis. Cartilaginous joints permit little if any movement of the bones involved.

Fibrous joint A joint in which the bones are connected by fibrous tissue. Three types are described:
Suture, a joint that permits little or no movement. Its function also is to permit bone growth. [Also see Suture].
Gomphosis, a joint such as the one that connects a tooth to its surrounding bone by the fibrous periodontal ligament.
Syndesmosis, a joint in which the two bony components are some distance apart, but are connected by a ligament that permits limited movement (e.g. the joint between the fibula and tibia, or that between the radius and ulna).

Ginglymoid joint A joint that permits hinging movement (rotation) in one plane.

Synovial joint A type of joint by which two bones are united and surrounded by a fibrous capsule, thus creating a joint cavity. [Note: The name comes from the latin word *ova* (egg) because the opposing bones of such joints are separated by an enclosed space filled with fluid which, when examined with the naked eye, resembles egg white. The capsule is continuous with periosteum of the bones involved in the joint and lined on its inner surface by a synovial membrane. The synovial membrane secretes synovial fluid that fills the joint cavity. The articulating surfaces of the bones are covered with hyaline cartilage (the temporomandibular, acromioclavicular and sternoclavicular joints are exceptions in that their articulating surfaces are covered by fibrous tissue). The cavity may or may not possess a fibrous articular disc, separating it into two compartments. Various ligaments are associated with synovial joints to strengthen the articulation and limit excess movement.

Synovial joints are classified further by the number of axes in which the bones involved can move (uniaxial or multiaxial) and by the shapes of the articulating surfaces (planar, ginglymoid, pivot, condyloid, saddle, and ball-and-socket). Movements in a synovial joint are initiated and performed by muscles working together in a highly coordinated manner.

Temporomandibular joint (TMJ, Craniomandibular articulation) Paired synovial joint capable of both gliding (translation) and hinge (rotation) movements; thus considered a ginglymoarthrodial joint. The TMJ is formed by the mandibular condyle fitting into the glenoid fossa of the temporal bone. Separating these two bones from direct contact is the articular disc. In the healthy joint, the articular portion of the disc is composed of dense fibrous connective tissue, devoid of any nerves or vessels. Conversely the posterior attachment of the disc is richly vascularized and innervated. The disc also is attached to the condyle both medially and laterally by *collateral (discal) ligaments*. These ligaments permit rotational movement of the disc on the condyle during opening and closing of the mouth. This so-called condyle-disc complex translates out of the fossa during over-extended mouth opening.

Surrounding the joint is a fibrous capsule (*capsular ligament*) that extends from the margins of the glenoid fossa, including the articular eminence anteriorly, to envelop the head of the condyle before fusing inferiorly with the periosteum of the condylar process. Other ligaments reinforcing the joint are the *lateral (temporomandibular) ligament,* which reinforces the lateral wall of the capsule, preventing lateral dislocation of the condyle, as well as the *sphenomandibular* and *stylomandibular* ligaments.

In the healthy joint, rotational movement occurs between the condyle and the inferior surface of the disc (the inferior joint space) during early opening. During later stages of opening, translation takes place in the space between the superior surface of the disc and the fossa (the superior joint space). The synovial fluid serves as a lubricant and also acts as a medium for transporting nutrients to and waste products away from the joint components.

Unlike most synovial joints the articulating surfaces of the TMJs are lined with dense fibrous connective tissue, not hyaline cartilage. This is an important feature because fibrous connective tissue has a greater ability to repair itself than does hyaline cartilage. Movement and stability of the TMJs is achieved by the muscles of mastication. These include the masseter, medial pterygoid and temporal muscles, which predominantly elevate the mandible; the digastric muscles, which assist in mandibular depression; the inferior lateral pterygoid muscles, which assist in protruding the mandible; and the superior lateral pterygoid muscles, which provide stabilization for the condyle and disc during function.

Joint noises See Clicking; Crepitus.

Joint symptoms Symptoms of TMD.

Jones jig See Appliance, Jones jig.

JRA See Arthritis, Juvenile rheumatoid.

"Jumping of the bite" 1. An expression credited to N.W. Kingsley in the late 1800s, referring to the avoidance of the prior intercuspal position by anterior repositioning of the mandible. Such an effect can be brought up by a functional-type appliance for the cor-

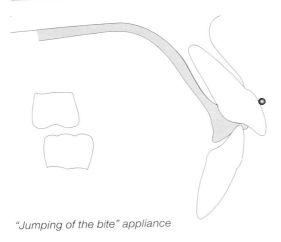

"Jumping of the bite" appliance

rection of mandibular retrognathism. [Also see Appliance, Kingsley.]

2. The same expression also is used to connote correction of an anterior crossbite by movement of the affected tooth over the opposing dental arch.

Junctional epithelium (Epithelial attachment) A single or multiple layer of non-keratinizing cells adhering to the tooth surface at the base of the gingival crevice.

Juvenile occlusal equilibrium See Occlusal equilibrium, Juvenile.

Juvenile rheumatoid arthritis See Arthritis, Juvenile rheumatoid.

K

esling setup See Diagnostic setup.

ey, Torquing See Orthodontic instruments, Torquing key.

ey ridge The radiographic image of the zygomatic process of the maxilla as commonly seen on a lateral cephalometric radiograph.

eys of occlusion See Six keys of occlusion.

Keystoning" The reshaping of the interproximal aspects of the mandibular incisors to provide an interlocking pattern to resist rotational relapse. "Keystoning" is done by oblique interproximal stripping, so that rotational tendency of one tooth would be counteracted by the reverse rotational relapse tendency of its adjacent tooth.

Kinematics See Dynamics, Kinematics.

Kinesiograph Instrument used to record and provide graphic representation of mandibular movements.

Kinetic friction See Friction.

Kinetics See Dynamics, Kinetics.

Kinetor See Appliance, Kinetor.

Kingsley appliance See Appliance, Kingsley.

Kloehn headgear See Headgear, Cervical.

Kobayashi hook (Kobayashi tie, Kobayashi ligature) A ligature fabricated from 0.012-inch (0.30-mm) or 0.014-inch (0.35-mm) annealed stainless steel wire, whose legs are welded onto each other, forming a helical "hook" at its end. It is

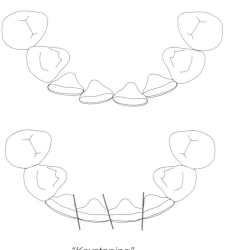

"Keystoning"

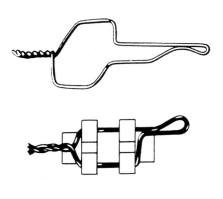

Kobayashi hook   1

placed on a bracket below the archwire or in the same way as a regular stainless steel ligature and it is used for the attachment of orthodontic elastics.

Küfner procedure See Osteotomy, Complete maxillary.

Kyphosis (of the cranial base) See Basilar kyphosis.

L

-loop See Loop, L-.

-point See Cephalometric landmarks (Hard tissue), L-point.

abial Of or pertaining to the lips, or in a direction towards the lips. Also identifies a surface facing the lips. [Compare with Lingual.]

abial bow A part of a removable orthodontic appliance, typically consisting of a stainless steel wire that lies on (or at a distance from) the labial surface of the maxillary or mandibular anterior teeth, usually at the mid-crown level. A labial bow may be embedded in the acrylic of the appliance and cross the occlusal table at the embrasures mesial or distal to the first premolars, or it may be soldered directly onto the molar clasps. It is used to enhance retention of the appliance, to relieve pressure from the lips as well as (when activated) to tip the incisors lingually and close spaces. A labial bow can be covered with clear acrylic in the case of some retainers. [Also see Retainer, Hawley; Retainer, Spring.]

abial crown torque (Lingual root torque)
See Torque, Crown; Torque, Root.

abial frenum See Frenum, Labial.

abial root torque (Lingual crown torque)
See Torque, Root; Torque, Crown.

abiolingual appliance See Appliance, Labiolingual.

Labiolingual tipping Tipping of a tooth in a labiolingual direction. [Also see Inclination.]

Labiolingually In a direction parallel to the sagittal plane (along the x-axis) for anterior teeth. For posterior teeth the term *buccolingually* is appropriate. [Also see Buccolingually; Global reference frame.]

Labiomental sulcus See Mentolabial fold.

Labioversion Labial inclination of one or more teeth.

Labrale inferior (Li) See Cephalometric landmarks (Soft tissue), Labrale inferior.

Labrale superior (Ls) See Cephalometric landmarks (Soft tissue), Labrale superior.

Laceback (Lace) Stainless steel ligature placed passively in a figure-eight mode (usually from the terminal molar to the canine of the same quadrant), as part of the leveling and alignment stage of treatment

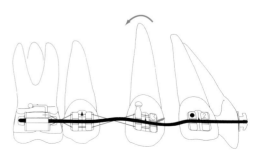

Laceback

155

with the straight-wire appliance. For example, when a canine is slightly upright at the time of insertion of the initial archwire, a laceback serves to maintain the sagittal position of its crown, so that the angulation of the tooth is improved by distal movement of the root. [Also see Figure-eight ligature.]

Lacunae Small pits or hollow cavities. [See also Howship's lacunae.]

Lag screw See Fixation screws, Lag screw.

Lamellar bone See Bone, Lamellar.

Laser An acronym for "Light Amplification by Stimulated Emission of Radiation." A device that transforms light of various frequencies into an intense, small, and nearly nondivergent beam of monochromatic radiation. Dental applications of lasers mainly include various types of soft tissue surgery, offering superior control of bleeding; sealing of blood vessels, lymphatics and nerve endings; and minimal scarring. Lasers also are advocated for curing of composite resins, welding of orthodontic wires and appliances, and debonding of orthodontic brackets. The use of lasers in periodontal scaling, root planing and curettage remains a controversial issue.

Laser welding See Welding, Laser.

Late closing click See Clicking, Late closing.

Late opening click See Clicking, Late opening.

Latent myofascial trigger point See Myofascial trigger point, Latent.

Lateral cephalometric radiograph See Cephalometric radiograph, Lateral.

Lateral excursion of the mandible See Arthrokinetics of the TMJ, Lateral excursion of the mandible.

Lateral forced bite See Forced bite, Lateral.

Lateral pterygoid muscle See Muscle Lateral pterygoid.

Lateroclusion A functional posterior cross bite associated with a lateral shift of the mandible that occurs only in centric occlusion (CO or ICP). In centric relation (CR) the mandible is centered in the midsagittal plane. This type of crossbite is caused by dental interferences and can be treated by maxillary expansion and/or by occlusal equilibration. [Compare with Laterognathia also see Crossbite, Functional; Forced bite Lateral.]

Laterognathia A posterior crossbite in CO associated with a lateral shift of the mandible that does not improve when the mandible is in CR (a true skeletal asymmetry). In severe situations the only treatment option is orthognathic surgery. [Compare with Lateroclusion.]

Laterotrusion The movement away from the median of the ipsilateral (working) half of the mandible and the respective condyle during a lateral mandibular excursion [Compare with Mediotrusion.]

Laterotrusive occlusal contact See Occlusal contact, Working side.

Laterotrusive side See Working side.

Lavage The process of washing out or irrigating a cavity or an organ.

Law of transmissibility of force According to this law, the point of application of any force applied to a rigid body can be considered to lie anywhere along the line of action of the force.

For example, a single retraction force on the crown of a maxillary incisor will have the same effect on the tooth whether it is applied on the labial or on the palatal aspect of the crown, provided the line of action is the same. Similarly, the outer arms of a facebow used with a high-pull headgear can be cut short or bent upwards without changing the force system "felt" by the molars, provided the line of force from the headstrap is the same.

The law of transmissibility of force is applied when combining two or more forces with different points of application to construct their resultant force.

Laws of Newton See Newton's laws.

Leeway space The difference between the combined width of the deciduous canine, first and second molars in each quadrant, and their successors (permanent canine, first and second premolars). The term was introduced by H.N. Nance (1947). The average value is approximately 1.0 mm for each maxillary quadrant and 1.7 mm for each mandibular quadrant, although there are large individual variations. These "spaces" normally are closed by mesial drift of the first permanent molars as the deciduous teeth are replaced.

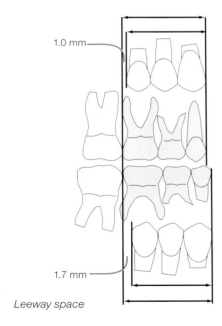

1.0 mm

1.7 mm

Leeway space

Le Fort I, II and III surgical procedures See Osteotomy, Complete maxillary.

Lehman appliance See Appliance, Lehman.

Leong's premolar See Dens evaginatus.

Leptoprosopic Having a narrow and long facial form.

Lesser segment See Segment, Lesser.

Leveling The phase of comprehensive orthodontic treatment aiming at flattening the curve of Spee until the marginal ridges of all the teeth in the arch lie more or less in the same horizontal plane. Thus, leveling refers to correction in the vertical plane.

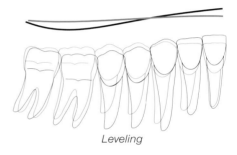

Leveling

Leveling wire Any archwire used for leveling.

Lewis bracket See Bracket, Lewis.

Li See Cephalometric landmarks (Soft tissue), Labrale inferior.

LI-NB/Pg-NB See Cephalometric measurements (Hard tissue), Holdaway ratio.

LI-to-AP distance See Cephalometric measurements (Hard tissue), LI-to-AP distance.

Ligament Flexible band of fibrous tissue composed of parallel collagenous bundles, binding joints together, as well as connecting various bones and cartilages.

Ligament, Periodontal See Periodontal ligament.

Ligaments (of the TMJ) See Joint, Temporomandibular.

Ligamentous position See Centric relation.

Ligature A tie that secures an archwire or other auxiliary in the bracket slot, by being placed under the tie-wings of the bracket. Ligatures are typically made of stainless steel wire, rubber, or elastomeric material.

Elastomeric ligature See Elastomeric modules, Elastomeric ligature.

Stainless steel ligature A ligature made from annealed stainless steel wire (0.008 to 0.012 inch, or 0.20 to 0.30 mm, in diameter) that engages under the bracket tie-wings (usually with the help of a Mathieu-style, Steiner, or Coon ligature-tying plier) and is twisted until it tightens around them, holding the archwire or other orthodontic spring in place. The excess wire is cut and discarded, and the twisted end ("pigtail") is tucked under the archwire for patient comfort. [Also see Stainless steel.]

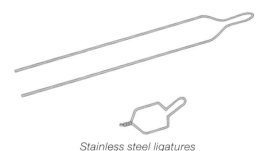

Stainless steel ligatures

Ligature director See Orthodontic instruments, Ligature director.

Light force See Force, Light.

Light-wire appliance See Appliance, Begg.

Light-wire pliers See Orthodontic instruments, Light-wire pliers.

Lightening strips See Abrasive strips.

Limited orthodontic treatment Orthodontic treatment with a limited objective, not involving the entire dentition. It may be directed at the only existing problem, or at only one aspect of a larger problem in which a decision is made to defer or forego more comprehensive therapy. Examples of this type of treatment would be single-arch treatment to improve alignment, partial treatment to close or to open space, or to upright a tooth in preparation for prosthodontic treatment. [Modified from the AAO Glossary of Dentofacial Orthopedic Terms, 1993.]

Line of action See Direction.

Lingual Of or pertaining to the tongue; or in a direction towards the tongue. Also identifies a surface facing the tongue. [Compare with Labial.]

Lingual appliance See Appliance, Lingual.

Lingual arch See Arch, Lingual.

Lingual arch space maintainer See Space maintainer, Lingual arch.

Lingual cleat A low-profile attachment that can be bonded directly to a tooth or welded on a band. Its functions are to accommodate the attachment of elastics, to aid as a seating lug during band fitting, and to facilitate band removal.

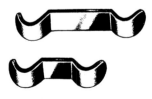

Lingual cleats

Lingual crossbite See Crossbite, Lingual.

Lingual frenum See Frenum, Lingual.

Lingual crown torque See Torque, Crown Torque, Root.

Lingual orthodontics See Appliance, Lingual.

Lingual retainer See Retainer, Bonded lingual.

Lingual root torque (Labial crown torque) See Torque, Root; Torque, Crown.

Lingual sheath See Sheath.

Linguoversion Lingual inclination of one or more teeth.

Lip bumper See Appliance, Lip bumper.

Lip exercises Exercises aiming at stimulating the musculature of the lips, with the objective of achieving a competent lip seal. A key component of functional appliance treatment, stressed by R. Fränkel.

Lip incompetence (Incompetent lip seal) Excessive separation of the lips at rest.

Lip interposition The habit of placing the lower lip between the maxillary and mandibular anterior teeth, or between the mandibular anterior teeth and the palate (often seen in patients with an increased overjet).

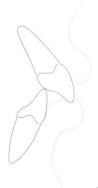

Lip interposition

Lip line See Tooth-to-lip relationship.

Lip protrusion See Protrusion, Lip.

Lip retrusion See Retrusion, Lip.

Lisping Incorrect pronunciation of a sibilant or affricate sound, most commonly heard on /s/ and /z/.

Load/deflection rate (Force/deflection rate) A mechanical characteristic of orthodontic springs or wires, describing the dependence of the magnitude of the generated force on the amount of deflection (deformation, activation). It expresses force per unit displacement of the spring, and is measured in cN/mm (g/mm). A spring with a low load/deflection rate is capable of generating forces that approximate constancy and do not depend very much on the amount of activation. The five major parameters available to the clinician for varying the load/deflection rate are:

1. Wire cross-section The load/deflection rate varies directly with the fourth power of the diameter of a round wire and with the third power of the width (large dimension) of a rectangular wire. Therefore, reducing the cross-section of the wire can reduce the load/deflection characteristics of an orthodontic appliance significantly. [Also see Archwire cross-section.]

2. Wire length The load/deflection rate varies inversely with the third power of the length of a wire segment (or cantilever); thus small increases in wire length can reduce the load/deflection rate dramatically. In continuous archwire multi-attachment appliances, the wire length is, to a great extent, dictated by the interbracket span between adjacent teeth. The addition of loops to the wire can serve in increasing the length, lowering the load/deflection rate. [Also see Interbracket span; Archwire, Multiloop.]

3. Wire material The load/deflection rate is proportional to the modulus of elasticity (E) of the material. For the same size and cross-sectional shape, a wire material with a low E will deliver less force for an equal deflection, than a wire with a high E. [Also see Modulus of elasticity.]

4. Wire configuration Bending loops of various shapes into an archwire reduces its load/deflection rate by increasing the wire length. [Also see Loop; Archwire, Multiloop.]

5. <u>Constraint conditions</u> The load/deflection rate of a wire segment depends on its mode of ligation between two teeth. A wire segment tightly ligated in two edgewise brackets delivers a much higher load, for a standard deflection, than a cantilever of the same material, length and cross-section ligated in only one of the brackets (one fixed end). [Also see Orthodontic spring, Cantilever.]

Lock, Archwire See Gurin lock.

Locking of a joint See Disc displacement without reduction.

Long-axis rotation See Orthodontic tooth movement, Pure rotation.

Long face syndrome See "High-angle" patient.

Loop Orthodontic spring of various shapes and configurations. Loops are used for a number of purposes, such as to lower the load/deflection rate by addition of more wire, to achieve frictionless tooth movement, to avoid the inconsistency of the force system delivered by a straight wire, and to achieve dissociation of forces and moments in the created force system (i.e. changes in forces do not automatically alter the moments). [Also see Load/deflection rate; Archwire, Multiloop.]

Boot loop See Loop, L-.

Box loop A rectangular or square-shaped loop bent into a continuous archwire (the loop has no free end). It is used to increase the flexibility of the wire at a certain localized point where this is necessary (e.g. when there is only one tooth that is not well aligned within the arch), while maintaining rigidity of the archwire in the remainder of the arch for anchorage purposes. A box loop offers flexibility in both the horizontal and vertical plane. [Compare with Loop, Rectangular.]

Closed loop (Reverse loop) A loop be in such a way that the separation betwee its vertical legs is reduced when activate by traction (the base of the loop remain closed–"safety-pin" principle), in contra to an open loop.

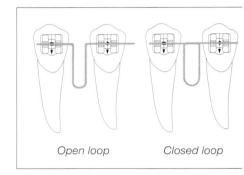

Open loop   *Closed loop*

Closing loop Any loop which, upc mesiodistal-pulling activation, is capab of generating a force in the direction of th activation. A closing loop can be open closed and can have various configuration Closing loops are used for space closur either by movement of an individual too (e.g. canine retraction), or as part of a clc ing loop arch for "en masse" movement teeth.

L-loop (Boot loop) An orthodontic loc in the shape of an "L" (or a "boot"). It cor bines flexibility in both horizontal (mesiodi tal and buccolingual) and vertical dime sion. The L-loop delivers a force system th is different at the two sides of the loop. A a simple rule, the smaller moment is deve oped at the bracket that faces the L-loop. Se *illustration next page.*

Omega loop An Ω-shaped loop use primarily for space closure, or for attachme of intermaxillary elastics.

Open loop A loop whose vertical le separation increases when activated t traction (the base of the loop is open), contrast to a closed loop.

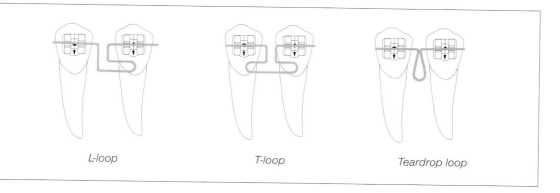

L-loop   T-loop   Teardrop loop

Opening loop A loop used to create space, in a fashion comparable to an open coil spring. The loop is compressed to engage the archwire in the brackets, so deactivation of the loop will tend to increase the arch length. [Also see Orthodontic springs, Coil spring, Open.]

Rectangular loop A rectangular-shaped loop bent into a segmental wire (the posteriorly directed, horizontal end of the loop is free). The rectangular loop is used to overcome problems of inconsistency of force system delivered by a straight wire, where either the forces or the moments are in an undesirable direction. The desired combination of forces and moments can be reached by varying the point of ligation along the horizontal free end of the loop, and by controlling the horizontal dimension of the loop. [Compare with Loop, Box; Loop, Vertical.]

T-loop Orthodontic loop in the shape of a "T." A T-loop is basically a double L-loop, but is more flexible in the vertical plane than an L-loop of the same dimensions that is made from the same orthodontic wire. Used primarily as a force-producing mechanism for space closure or alignment.

Teardrop loop A modified version of a vertical loop with its legs touching each other at its base, giving it the shape of an inverted teardrop. Its advantage is that it required less interbracket space than a regular closed or open loop of the same dimensions.

Vertical loop A simple U-shaped loop that can be bent into a continuous archwire or used as a segmental spring. The greatest degree of flexibility of a vertical loop is in the mesiodistal dimension, somewhat less in the buccolingual, and very little in the ver-

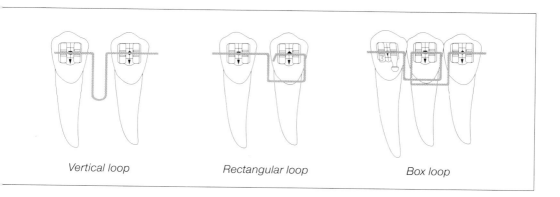

Vertical loop   Rectangular loop   Box loop

tical dimension. When preactivation bends are placed in the wire on either side of a vertical loop, it behaves according to the V-bend principle. Although it does reduce the force/deflection rate, when placed between two misaligned brackets a vertical loop produces a force system corresponding to that of a straight wire. [Compare with Loop, Rectangular.]

Wilson loop A U-shaped loop, similar in shape, but smaller than a Coffin spring, often incorporated in a transpalatal arch (midway between the maxillary first molars), or in a lingual arch (mesial to the mandibular first molars, bilaterally), to facilitate adjustment in the transverse or sagittal direction, respectively.

Louisiana State University activator (L.S.U. activator) See Appliance, Herren activator.

"Low-angle" patient ("Horizontal" patient, Hypodivergent face) A general term used to describe a patient with a pre-

dominantly horizontal growth pattern, short lower face height and a flat mandibular plane. A Class II malocclusion with deep, occasionally impinging overbite may be associated. (Referring to the mandibular plane angle.) [Compare with "High-angle" patient.]

Low-pull headgear See Headgear, Cervical

Lower face-throat angle See Cephalometric measurements (Soft tissue), Lower face throat angle.

Lower facial height See Cephalometric measurements (Hard tissue), Facial height

Lower jaw See Mandible.

Lower lip length See Cephalometric measurements (Soft tissue), Lower lip length.

Ls See Cephalometric landmarks (Soft tissue), Labrale superior.

L.S.U. activator See Appliance, Herren activator.

Lug, Occlusal See Occlusal rest.

Lug, Seating See Seating lug.

Luxation (of the condyle) See Dislocation condyle.

Luxation (of a tooth) Partial or complete detachment of a tooth from its socket. [Also see Subluxation.]

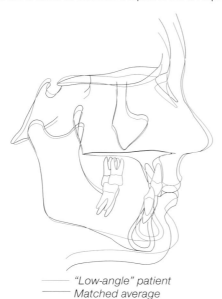

——— "Low-angle" patient
——— Matched average

M

acrodontia A term denoting larger than normal tooth size. Although no standardization is agreed upon, two standard deviations above the mean of the general population can be considered a cut-off point beyond which a diagnosis of macrodontia can be established. [Compare with Microdontia.]

acroglossia Abnormally large tongue, commonly associated with the presence of an open bite and spacing of teeth. Indentations may be evident on the side of the tongue. Macroglossia is a common finding in certain pathologic conditions such as Down syndrome, Beckwith-Wiedemann syndrome, myxedema, cretinism, or hypophyseal gigantism. A partial glossectomy is advocated by some clinicians as a means of treatment in severe situations.

agnetic resonance imaging (MRI) Non-invasive, non-ionizing imaging technique that uses a combination of magnetic fields and radiofrequency waves. As with computerized tomography, the images can be restricted to narrow planes and in this way multisectional views of the body can be obtained.

Human tissues consist of molecules contain hydrogen nuclei (protons). Each proton has an axial spin and because of its charge, behaves like a small magnet. Normally the protons are arranged randomly; however, when the patient is placed in a strong magnetic field the direction of the spin of the protons aligns with that of the field. In addition, the protons precess or wobble with a frequency determined by the strength of the magnetic field, but out of phase with each other. The application of a pulsed, resonant radiofrequency causes the protons to be deflected from their alignment and to precess in phase. With cessation of the radiofrequency, the protons realign with the applied magnetic field by transferring their acquired energy to their surroundings and revert to precessing out of phase. The rate at which the protons realign is referred to as the *T1 relaxation time*; the *T2 relaxation time* is the period in which protons remain in phase before returning to a random pattern. The energy released by the relaxation of the hydrogen nuclei is converted by a computer into a visual image.

Diagnostic MRI allows multiplanar imaging and offers better soft tissue contrast compared with CT. Additionally, it has no known harmful effects to the tissues. On the other hand, it does not display bone as well, since bone has a low signal intensity. Magnetic resonance imaging may be contraindicated in patients with ferromagnetic surgical clips and cardiac pacemakers.

Magnets, Orthodontic See Orthodontic magnets.

Magnification The enlargement of the image of an object on a radiograph in relation to the actual object due to divergence of the x-ray beam (depending on the object-film distance).

Magnitude A characteristic of both scalar and vectorial quantities, denoting size or amount, in physical units of measurement.

Main archwire See Arch, Base.

Main slot See Bracket slot, Main.

Main tube See Tube, Main.

Malar bone See Zygomatic bone.

Malar midfacial augmentation Augmentation of the malar and of the infraorbital and paranasal areas, which may be accomplished by a modified Le Fort I or II osteotomy, or with alloplastic materials or onlay cortical bone grafts placed simultaneously with a Le Fort I osteotomy. [Also see Osteotomy, Küfner.]

Malformation A morphological structural defect of an organ, part of an organ, or a larger area of the body resulting from an intrinsically abnormal developmental process (e.g. cleft lip, or polydactyly). Malformations may be relatively simple or complex. The later the defect is initiated, the simpler the malformation. Malformations initiated earlier during organogenesis tend to have more far-reaching consequences. [Compare with Deformity; Disruption.]

Malformation syndromes Recognized patterns of malformation presumably having the same etiology and currently not interpreted as the consequence of a single localized error in morphogenesis (e.g. Down syndrome).

Malleability The ability of a material to sustain considerable permanent deformation without rupture, under compression (as in hammering, or rolling into a sheet). Malleability is not as dependent on strength of the material as ductility is. Gold is the most ductile and malleable pure metal and silver is second. [Compare with Ductility.]

Malocclusion Any deviation from the normal or ideal occlusion. [Also see Angle classification.]

Mandible The lower jaw, consisting of a curve horizontal portion, the body, and two pe pendicular portions, the rami. Each of th rami carries a coronoid and a condyla process. The condyles articulate with th temporal fossae by means of the tempor mandibular joint. Fifteen pairs of muscle attach on the mandible. Its embryologic development is guided by Meckel's car lage. At birth, the bone consists of two halve united by a synchondrosis (mandibular syr physis), which ossifies during the first pos natal year.

Mandibular advancement See Advance ment of the mandible.

Mandibular autorotation See Autorotatio of the mandible.

Mandibular dental midline See Midlin Mandibular dental.

Mandibular dislocation (Mandibular dis placement) See Dislocation of the co dyle.

Mandibular fossa See Glenoid fossa.

Mandibular headgear See Headgea Mandibular.

Mandibular line See Cephalometric line Mandibular plane.

Mandibular occlusal plane See Cepha lometric lines, Occlusal plane.

Mandibular plane (MP) See Cephalometri lines, Mandibular plane.

Mandibular plane angle See Cephalometri measurements (Hard tissue), Mandibula plane angle.

Mandibular prognathism See Prognathism Mandibular.

Mandibular retrognathism See Retro gnathism, Mandibular.

andibular rotation To visualize the following concepts, one has to imagine the core of the mandible as the bone that surrounds the inferior alveolar nerve. The rest of the mandible consists of its various functional processes. If implants are placed in areas of stable bone away from the functional processes, it can be observed that in most individuals the core of the mandible rotates during growth, in a sense that would tend to decrease the mandibular plane angle (i.e. counterclockwise, with the standard head orientation toward the right side). The concept of mandibular rotation during growth was elucidated mainly by the metallic implant experiments of A. Björk in the 1960s. Following are the most commonly encountered terms on components of mandibular rotation (the terminology varies greatly depending on the source):

Apparent rotation See Mandibular rotation, Matrix.

Backward rotation See Mandibular rotation, Clockwise.

Clockwise rotation (Backward rotation, Posterior rotation) Displacement of the mandible in the direction of mouth opening (clockwise, with the patient facing to the right), due to increased posterior vertical growth. Clockwise mandibular rotation also can occur as a consequence of orthodontic treatment, when posterior teeth are extruded in a non-growing patient. Clockwise rotation of the mandible usually is

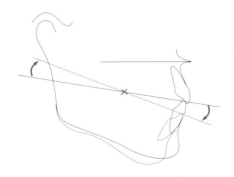

Clockwise mandibular rotation

accompanied by an increase of the anterior lower face height and a reduction of the overbite.

Counterclockwise rotation (Forward rotation, Anterior rotation) Rotation of the mandible in the direction of mouth closing (counterclockwise, with the patient facing to the right), due to increased posterior, compared to anterior growth. Counterclockwise rotation of the mandible would tend to cause a relative reduction in the anterior lower face height and a deepening of the overbite.

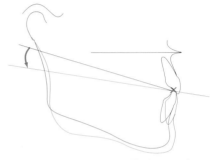

Counterclockwise mandibular rotation

External rotation See Mandibular rotation, Intramatrix.

Forward rotation See Mandibular rotation, Counterclockwise.

Internal rotation See Mandibular rotation, Total.

Intramatrix rotation (External rotation) Rotation within the body of the mandible, due to angular remodeling of the inferior border relative to the core of the mandible (which affects the orientation of the mandibular plane with regard to the cranial base).

Matrix rotation (Apparent rotation) Rotation of the entire mandible around its condylar axis (which affects the orientation of the mandible as a whole relative to the cranial base).

Total rotation (True rotation, Internal rotation) The actual rotation of the core of the mandible (the part of the bone that surrounds the inferior alveolar nerve) relative to the cranial base, which is a combination of the intramatrix and matrix rotation.

True rotation See Mandibular rotation, Total.

Mandibular setback See Setback of the mandible.

Mandibular shift (CR-CO shift, Mandibular slide, Forced bite, Slide in centric) A deflection of the mandible in an anterior, posterior and/or lateral direction, as a result of a premature contact occurring when the mandible is in centric relation. [See also Forced bite; Occlusal interference, Centric.]

Mandibular slide See Mandibular shift.

Mandibular symphysis (Mental symphysis) The line of fusion of the lateral halves of the anterior portion of the mandible at the median plane. It is wide open during fetal life and ossifies by intramembranous ossification in the first year of life, usually before the emergence of the mandibular deciduous central incisors.

Mandibular trismus See Trismus.

Mandibulofacial dysostosis See Treacher Collins syndrome.

Marginal gingiva See Gingiva, Marginal.

Marginal ridge See Ridge, Marginal.

Marking pencil (Arch marker) Wax pencil usually in white or red for marking archwires intraorally to indicate the desired location for adjustment bends or loops.

Martensite A body-centered cubic phase in stainless steels, or a monoclinic, triclinic or hexagonal crystalline structure of nickel-titanium alloys. The martensitic phase of nick-el-titanium exists at lower temperatures an is characterized by high ductility. It is forme as a result of quenching (rapid cooling) cold working the austenite phase. [See als Austenite; Martensitic transformation.]

Martensitic transformation The transitic into a crystalline structure called *martens* by displacement of the atoms, during co ing down from a higher temperatu phase called *austenite*, as occurs in allo such as steel or nickel-titanium. In nickel-ti nium alloys martensitic transformatic involves only a shearing movement of th atoms, without sliding of crystals past ea other. Thus, the transformation can t reversed when increasing the temperatur The temperature at which the phase chang occurs is termed *transition temperatur* This temperature depends on the compo tion and mode of fabrication of the alloy. the martensitic phase (below the transitic temperature), the wire has higher ductili whereas in the austenite phase (above th transition temperature) it is more resista to permanent deformation. A wire that deformed while in the martensitic phas recovers its original shape at the return the austenite phase (*shape memory* effe A martensitic transformation also can t induced by mechanical loading in shap memory alloys while in the austenite phas just above their transition temperature. such a case the wire exhibits *superelast* behavior. [Also see Nickel-titanium allo Superelasticity; Transition temperature.]

Maryland bridge See Resin-bonded prosth sis.

Mass, Center of See Center of mass.

Masseter muscle See Muscle, Masseter.

Mastication The process of chewing th food, in preparation for deglutition.

Masticatory mucosa See Mucosa, Mas catory.

asticatory muscles A group of skeletal muscles providing movement of the mandible and safeguarding the stability of the TMJs. The masticatory muscles involve the masseter, medial pterygoid and temporal muscles, which predominantly elevate the mandible (mouth closing); the digastric muscles, which assist in mandibular depression (mouth opening); the inferior lateral pterygoid muscles, which assist in protrusion and in contralateral movements of the mandible; and the superior lateral pterygoid muscles, which provide stability for the condyle and disc during function. The masticatory muscles are recruited during talking, swallowing and masticating, as well as during nonfunctional (parafunctional) actions such as grinding and clenching. Motor innervation of the muscles of mastication is supplied by the trigeminal nerve (CV). [Also see Muscle.]

ateria alba White accumulation or aggregation of microorganisms, desquamated epithelial cells, blood cells and food debris, loosely adhered to surfaces of teeth, soft tissues, dental restorations and orthodontic appliances.

athieu-style ligature-tying pliers See Orthodontic instruments, Mathieu-style ligature-tying pliers.

atrix rotation (of the mandible) See Mandibular rotation, Matrix.

aturation The qualitative changes that occur with ripening or aging. Rapid maturation as well as accelerated physical growth occurs during puberty.

ature swallow See Swallow, Somatic.

axian separator See Separator, Maxian elastic.

axilla (Upper jaw) An irregularly shaped paired bone that makes up a major part of the bony framework of the facial skeleton. It consists of the body of the maxilla and the zygomatic, nasal, palatine and alveolar processes. The suture between the right and left portions of the maxilla persists into adulthood.

Maxillary Of or pertaining to the upper jaw.

Maxillary dental midline See Midline, Maxillary dental.

Maxillary impaction See Impaction of the maxilla.

Maxillary incisor-lip line relationship See Tooth-to-lip relationship.

Maxillary inferior repositioning See Downgrafting of the maxilla.

Maxillary occlusal plane See Cephalometric lines, Occlusal plane.

Maxillary osteotomy See Osteotomy, Complete Maxillary.

Maxillary prognathism See Prognathism, Maxillary.

Maxillary retrognathism See Retrognathism, Maxillary.

Maxillary superior repositioning See Impaction of the maxilla.

Maxillomandibular fixation See Fixation, (Surgical), Intermaxillary.

Maximum anchorage See Anchorage, Maximum.

Maximum elastic strain (of a material) See Working range.

Maximum intercuspal position See Occlusion, Centric.

McNamara cephalometric analysis See Cephalometric analysis, McNamara.

Mechanical moment (of a force) See Moment of a force.

Me See Cephalometric landmarks (Hard tissue), Menton.

Me' See Cephalometric landmarks (Soft tissue), Soft tissue menton.

Mechanics The physical science that deals with the state of rest or motion of bodies under the action of forces. Mechanics includes two sub-disciplines, statics and dynamics, and is also associated very closely with materials science. In orthodontics the term often is used as a synonym for mechanotherapy.

Cantilever mechanics Orthodontic mechanotherapy using cantilever springs to generate the appropriate force systems for specific types of tooth movement. Because full bracket engagement is allowed only at the fixed end of the cantilever with one-point contact at the other end, a statically determinate force system is achieved. This allows determination of the produced forces and moments at both ends of the cantilever by simple measurements and calculations. Moreover, the cantilever offers the possibility of a low load/deflection rate and a relatively long range of deactivation, generating an almost continuous force that generally is considered desirable for tooth movement. [Also see Orthodontic springs, Cantilever.]

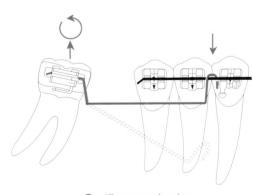

Cantilever mechanics

Class I mechanics Orthodontic mechanotherapy utilizing intramaxillary anchorage for tooth movement.

Class II mechanics Orthodontic mechanotherapy making use of intermaxillary anchorage (e.g. elastics) between the anterior aspect of the maxillary and the posterior aspect of the mandibular arch.

Class III mechanics Orthodontic mechanotherapy utilizing intermaxillary anchorage (e.g. elastics) between the anterior aspect of the mandibular and the posterior aspect of the maxillary arch.

Continuous archwire mechanics Orthodontic mechanotherapy utilizing continuous archwires in the entire dental arch (as opposed to segments of archwire encompassing segments of teeth).

Frictionless mechanics The use of strategies or appliances that do not involve friction between archwire and bracket during tooth movement (e.g. retraction of a tooth by means of a segmental spring).

Intermaxillary mechanics The application of forces and/or moments from one arch to the other.

Intersegmental mechanics The application of forces and/or moments from one segment of teeth to another.

Intrasegmental mechanics The application of forces and moments between teeth that belong to the same segment of an arch.

Segmental arch mechanics (Sectional mechanics) Orthodontic mechanotherapy in which not all teeth within an arch are included in the same archwire, but rather anchorage and active segments are created by consolidating teeth together using wire segments. Various orthodontic loops and springs (e.g. cantilever springs) and different types of arches (e.g. intrusion arches) are used to generate the force systems required for movement of the active segments. Advantages of segmental arch mechanics include the avoidance of friction and the ability to design statically determinate force systems.

Sliding mechanics Mechanotherapy involving sliding of brackets along the archwire during tooth movement (i.e. the classic "pearls on a chain" example). The archwire generates the counter-moment necessary for bodily movement of the teeth. Frictional forces are present when tooth movement is performed by sliding mechanics.

Mechanotherapy Collective term encompassing all procedures, appliances, and strategies adopted in specific phases of orthodontic treatment. [Also see Mechanics.]

Meckel's cartilage A curved cylindrical rod of cartilage derived from the first branchial arch that embryologically has a close positional relationship and guides the development of the mandible. The greater part of Meckel's cartilage disappears without contributing directly to the formation of the bone of the mandible. Only a small part of the cartilage between the future mental foramen and the midline contributes to the mandible by endochondral ossification. The cartilage at the mandibular symphysis is not derived from Meckel's cartilage but differentiates from the connective tissue in the midline.
After the 10th embryonic week, by which time the rudimentary mandible is formed (almost entirely by intramembranous ossification), Meckel's cartilage forms the malleus and incus of the inner ear, the anterior ligament of the malleus, and the sphenomandibular ligament. [Compare with Reichert's cartilage.]

Medial pterygoid muscle See Muscle, Medial pterygoid.

Median plane (Midsagittal plane) The imaginary plane passing longitudinally

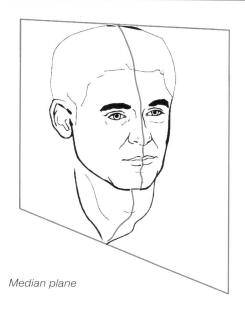

Median plane

through the middle of the body, dividing it into left and right halves. [See also Sagittal plane.]

Mediolaterally In a direction perpendicular to the sagittal plane of the dentofacial complex (along the z-axis). For incisor teeth this coincides with the mesiodistal direction. For all other teeth, it signifies a buccolingual direction. [Also see Global reference frame.]

Mediotrusion Movement in a medial direction of the contralateral (non-working) half of the mandible and the respective condyle during a lateral mandibular excursion. [Compare with Laterotrusion.]

Mediotrusive occlusal contact See Occlusal contact, Non-working side.

Mediotrusive side See Non-working side.

Mediotrusive side interference See Occlusal interference, Non-working side.

Membranous bone See Bone, Intramembranous.

Meniscectomy See Discectomy.

Meniscus See Articular disc.

Mental symphysis See Mandibular symphysis.

Mentolabial fold (Labiomental sulcus) The shallow groove created where the curvature of the lower lip merges with that of the chin.

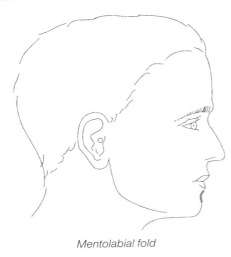

Mentolabial fold

Menton (Me) See Cephalometric landmarks (Hard tissue), Menton.

Merrifield's profile line See Cephalometric lines, Z-line.

Merrifield's Z-angle See Cephalometric measurements (Soft tissue), Z-angle.

Mershon band pusher See Orthodontic instruments, Band pusher.

Mesial Toward the midline, following the dental arch. The term is used to describe surfaces of teeth as well as direction. [Compare with Distal.]

Mesial drift (Mesial migration) See Drift (of teeth), Mesial.

Mesial step See Terminal plane, Mesial step.

Mesial tipping Tipping of the crown of a tooth in the mesial direction.

Mesioclusion See Angle classification, Class III malocclusion.

Mesiodens A supernumerary tooth in the midline of the maxillary alveolar process. A mesiodens often is unerupted, and it may interfere with the eruption and position of the maxillary permanent central incisors.

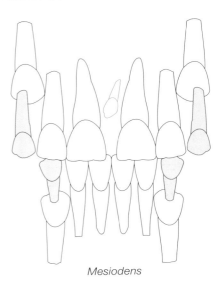

Mesiodens

Mesiodistal tipping See Rotation, Second order.

Mesiodistally In a direction along the dental arch. For incisor teeth this term signifies a direction approximately perpendicular to the sagittal plane (along the z-axis), whereas for all other teeth it actually indicates a direction approximately parallel to the sagittal plane (along the x-axis). [Also see Global reference frame.]

Mesocephalic Anthropometric term used to denote a cranial form of average proportions (cephalic index between 76.0 and 80.9).

Mesognathic See Orthognathic.

Metal bracket See Bracket, Metal.

Methyl methacrylate See Acrylic.

MGJ See Mucogingival junction.

Michigan Growth Study (University of Michigan Growth Study) The University of Michigan Elementary and Secondary School Growth Study was founded by Dean W. Olsen in 1935. It consists of 714 subjects, primarily of Northern European ancestry, on whom anthropometric, psychometric and craniofacial growth data were obtained on an annual basis while they were enrolled as students in the University School, a laboratory school located within the School of Education on the Ann Arbor campus. Collection of cephalometric and other data of orthodontic interest started in 1953 under the direction of R.E. Moyers. The number of annual records was variable among subjects and depended on the number of years that each student attended the University School. Major data collection ended in 1970, but several long-term recall studies have been conducted since that time. The Michigan Growth Study material is currently housed at the Schools of Education and Dentistry, University of Michigan in Ann Arbor.

Microdontia A term denoting smaller than normal tooth size. [Compare with Macrodontia.]

Micrognathia Abnormally small jaw size.

Mid-closing click See Clicking, Mid-closing.

Mid-opening click See Clicking, Mid-opening.

Midline A central reference line of a structure about which symmetry between the right and left halves can be evaluated.

Facial midline An imaginary line splitting the face in two approximately equal right and left halves. In the ideal situation of absolute symmetry, the facial midline can be considered as a perpendicular to the interpupillary line from glabella, passing through the tip of the nose, the midpoint of the philtrum of the upper lip and the midline of the chin.

Mandibular dental midline A line perpendicular to the mandibular occlusal plane, passing through the interproximal contact point between the mandibular central incisors (or, in absence of contact, the midpoint of the diastema between them).

Maxillary dental midline A line perpendicular to the maxillary occlusal plane, passing through the interproximal contact point between the maxillary central incisors (or, in absence of contact, the midpoint of the diastema between them).

Midline of the chin A line drawn perpendicular to the mandibular plane, dividing the chin in two (right and left) halves.

Midline deviation See Midline discrepancy.

Midline diastema A space between the central incisors of the maxillary (common) or mandibular arch (relatively rare), which may be associated with the presence of a hyperplastic labial frenum, or tongue frenum in the case of a mandibular diastema.

Midline discrepancy (Midline shift, Midline deviation) Incongruency between the midlines of the maxillary and mandibular dental arch and/or between them and the facial midline.

Midline of the chin See Midline, Midline of the chin.

Midline shift See Midline discrepancy.

Midsagittal plane See Median plane.

Migraine headache Periodic, recurrent, intense throbbing headache, frequently unilateral and often accompanied by photophobia, exaggerated sensitivity to sound, and nausea or vomiting, aggravated by routine physical activity. The classification of migraine is based on descriptive characteristics rather than known physiologic mechanisms. Migraine headaches should be differentiated from TMD-related symptoms.

Migration, Pathologic Spontaneous movement of a tooth out of its natural position, usually as a result of periodontal disease.

Migration, Physiologic See Drift (of teeth).

Miller classification A classification of gingival recession, widely used in periodontology, introduced by P.D. Miller (1985) as follows:

Class I Gingival recession in which the marginal tissues have not receded beyond the mucogingival junction and there is no loss of interproximal soft tissue or bone. In such recessions 100% root coverage is possible.

Class II Gingival recession in which the marginal tissues have receded beyond the mucogingival junction, still with no loss of the interproximal soft tissue or bone. Again, 100% root coverage is possible in such recessions.

Class III Class I or Class II gingival recession, combined with loss of interproximal bone, such that the soft tissue now is apical to the cementoenamel interproximal junction but coronal to the marginal tissue. 100% root coverage is not possible.

Class IV Gingival recession combined with loss of interproximal bone that is such that one or both of the adjacent interdental areas is level with the marginal gingiva. No root coverage is possible in Class IV recessions.

Minimum anchorage See Anchorage, Minimum.

Mixed dentition See Dentition, Mixed.

Mixed dentition analysis The analysis of space available for alignment of the permanent teeth, when the patient is in the mixed dentition (which involves estimation of the size of the unerupted permanent teeth).

There are three basic approaches to this:

1. Measurement of the size of the unerupted teeth on radiographs. This method is best performed with individual periapical films, but the accuracy is still limited by the inevitable presence of distortion, especially in the case of the canines. In addition appropriate compensation for enlargement is required, which dictates the use of a proportionality ratio (e.g. true width of deciduous molar/radiographically measured width of deciduous molar = true width of unerupted premolar/radiographically measured width of unerupted premolar).

2. Estimation from proportionality tables without the use of radiographs. These data have been tabulated for white American children by R.E. Moyers based on the combined mesiodistal width of the mandibular permanent incisors, which is used to predict the size of both the mandibular and maxillary unerupted canines and premolars. The size of the mandibular incisors correlates better with the size of the maxillary canine and premolars than does the size of the maxillary incisors, because maxillary lateral incisors show great variability in size and shape. This method shows a tendency to overestimate the size of unerupted teeth.

An alternative method for predicting the size of the unerupted canines and premolars by using the width of the mandibular incisors is the method developed by M.M. Tanaka and L.E. Johnston, Jr. According to that, the width of the mandibular canine and premolars in one quadrant can be calculated by adding 10.5 mm to half of the measured mesiodistal width of the four mandibular incisors. Similarly, the width of the maxillary canine and premolars in one quadrant can be determined by adding 11.0 mm to half of the measured mesiodistal width of the four mandibular incisors. The method shows a small tendency toward overestimating the unerupted tooth sizes. Its advantage is that it does not require radiographs or reference tables.

3. Combination of the radiographic and prediction table methods. Since the major problem with using radiographic images comes in evaluating the canine teeth, another option is to use the size of the permanent incisors measured from the dental casts and the size of the permanent premolars measured from the films to predict the size of the unerupted canines. Graphs are available (such as that by R.N. Staley and R.E. Kerber) that allow determination of the mandibular canine from the sum of incisor and premolar widths. The technique is limited to the mandibular arch and requires periapical radiographs.

ML See Cephalometric lines, Mandibular plane.

Mobility (of the teeth) See Tooth mobility.

Mode of force application (Force regime) The time-related aspect of orthodontic force application: the magnitude of a *continuous* force is more or less maintained between activations, that of an *intermittent* force declines with time until a reactivation is performed, whereas that of an *interrupted* force drops to zero between activations (the force is removed temporarily). [See also Force.]

Model surgery A simulation of the actual surgical procedure using the patient's presurgical casts, which are mounted on an articulator. The purposes of this simulation are to verify that the movements planned by the surgical prediction tracing actually can be performed and to relate the casts in the position where the surgical splints will be fabricated. If both jaws are to be repositioned, the maxillary cast is moved first and fixed on the articulator. In this position, the first surgical splint (intermediate splint) is made. Then the mandibular cast is repositioned to simulate the occlusion at the completion of surgery. The final surgical splint is made with the casts in this position. The model surgery is based on a combination of the surgical prediction and the presurgical clinical diagnostic information. [Also see Splint, Surgical.]

Model trimmer A device used for trimming plaster and stone casts. Its main component

is a large rotating grinding wheel, which is kept wet by a stream of water to reduce dust and keep the cutting wheel clean.

Modeling (of bone) A process involving independent sites of resorption and formation that change the intrinsic form (shape and/or size) of a bone, in contrast to the term *remodeling,* which signifies a specific coupled sequence of resorption and formation events to replace previously existing bone. Bone modeling is the dominant process in growth as well as in adaptation to applied loads such as those produced with headgear, rapid palatal expansion, functional appliances, etc. Traumatic or surgical wounding usually results in intense but localized modeling and remodeling responses. Following fractures, osteotomies or placement of endosseous implants, the processes of callus formation and resorption of necrotic osseous margins are modeling processes. In contrast, replacement of the devitalized cortical bone surrounding these sites is a remodeling activity. [Also see Remodeling (of bone).]

Models, Plaster See Orthodontic casts.

Moderate anchorage See Anchorage, Moderate.

Modified arrowhead clasp See Clasp, Adams.

Modulus of elasticity E (Young's modulus of elasticity, E-modulus) The slope of the stress/strain curve in its linear portion (below the elastic limit) ($E = \sigma/\varepsilon$). It is an inherent property of the material, which measures its stiffness. A material with a high modulus of elasticity deforms less than a material with a low modulus, when subjected to identical loads. The modulus of elasticity of a certain material is not influenced by its geometrical shape (length and cross-sectional area) and it cannot be altered appreciably by heat treatment, work-hardening, or any other type of conditioning. The modulus of elasticity of an orthodontic wire determines its load/deflection rate, and it can be changed only by changing the wire material. [Also see Load/ deflection rate; Stress/strain diagram.]

Moiré diffraction Technique with many applications in medicine, used mainly to map three-dimensional contour. In orthodontics it has been used for evaluation of facial asymmetry. The technique uses a series of lines produced by a transparent grid. The grid is placed in front of the object that is to be contour-mapped. A light source is offset from the viewing angle. The light passes through the diffraction grading twice: firstly on its way from the source to the object and secondly after it has been reflected off the object. It then is recorded by a film or viewed by an investigator. An interference pattern of light and dark lines or fringes is created; each fringe represents a set of equidistant points from the grid. The fringes appear superimposed on the object as a series of contour plots of similar elevation. The method is limited by the viewing angle of the system to the object. Areas of rapid elevation change on the object are difficult to characterize because of inability to distinguish the line separation. This requires evaluation of the object from different viewing angles.

Molar derotation See Derotation of molars.

Molar distalization See Distalization, Molar.

Molar tube See Tube.

Molar uprighting See Uprighting, Molar.

Moment Rotational tendency.

Counter-moment When a single force is applied at the bracket of a tooth, uncontrolled tipping probably will result, due to generation of a moment (since the force is applied at a distance from the center of resistance of the tooth). This will tend to move the crown in the direction of the force and the apex in the opposite direction. If bodily movement of the tooth is desired, a reverse

moment *(counter-moment)* must be applied simultaneously to prevent the unwanted movement of the apex.

This counter-moment can be generated either by a second force or, more commonly, by a couple. When sliding mechanics is used for retraction of a canine, the counter moment is generated by a couple, formed by contact of the archwire with the mesial gingival and distal-occlusal wings of the canine bracket, following a small initial unopposed distal tipping movement. When segmental spring (loop) is used for canine retraction, the counter-moment is generated by the spring itself. [Also see Moment-to-force ratio; Canine retraction.]

Moment of a couple Unlike the curvilinear motion produced by a moment of force, the moment of a couple produces tendency to pure rotation around the center of mass (when applied on a free body), or around the center of resistance (when partially constrained body, e.g. a tooth, is involved).

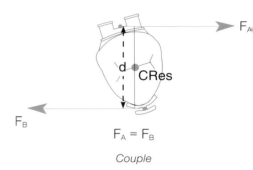

$$F_A = F_B$$

Couple

The moment produced by a couple is a vectorial quantity. It has a magnitude equal to the product of the magnitude of one of the two forces F, times the perpendicular distance d between the two forces ($M_{couple} = F$ x d); thus it is measured in units of force x distance (i.e. N mm, or g mm). Its direction is perpendicular to the plane of the pair of the forces, and its sense is either clockwise or counterclockwise, as viewed looking into the plane of the couple.

A couple can be applied anywhere on a rigid object, creating the same rotational effect. This is why the moment of a couple is said to be a *free vector*. [Also see Couple.]

Moment of a force The moment of a force about a specified point or line is a measure of the potential of that force to rotate the body, upon which the force acts, about the particular point or line.

The moment M of a force F about a point is also a vectorial quantity. Its magnitude is given by the formula $M = F \times d$ (where d is the *moment arm*). A moment of a force is also measured in units of force x distance (i.e. N mm, or g mm). The direction of the moment vector is perpendicular to the plane defined by the force vector and the point about which the moment is considered. The sense of the vector is determined by a rule associated with the rotational tendency, as viewed from above the plane of the force vector and the point about which the moment is considered. By convention, counter-clockwise moments (out of the plane) are said to be positive, whereas clockwise moments (into the plane) are considered negative.

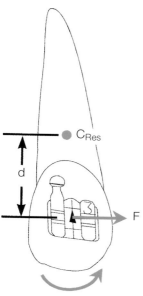

Moment of a force

The shorter the moment arm, the smaller the moment of a force. A moment of a force acting on a body can be considered about any specific point on the body; in orthodontics the center of resistance is commonly used. A force passing through an arbitrary point obviously produces no moment about it.

Moment arm The perpendicular distance (d) of the point about which the moment is determined to the line of action of the force producing the moment.

Moment-to-force ratio The ratio of magnitudes of the uprighting (counter-)moment applied at the bracket of a tooth to control the location of the center of rotation, to the tooth-moving force that is applied at the same point (the bracket).

The counter-moment usually is the moment of a couple. In terms of sense, the counter-moment always is opposite to that of the moment of the force, relative to the center of resistance. Since moments are measured in gram millimeters and forces in grams, the ratio of the two has units of millimeters; this represents the distance away from the bracket that a single force will produce the same effect. [However, it has become conventional in orthodontics to ignore these units and just speak of the moment-to-force ratio as a pure number.]

The moment-to-force ratio is used in two-dimensional analysis as an indicator of the type of tooth movement that will occur.

C.J. Burstone and R.J. Pryputniewicz estimated the different moment-to-force ratios required for various types of tooth movement for a 3-D model of an ideal maxillary central incisor with intact periodontium. When only a force is applied at the bracket of a tooth (M/F ratio of zero), the center of rotation is at, or just apical to, its center of resistance. The resulting tooth movement is uncontrolled tipping. The more the counter-moment increases, the more the center of rotation moves in an apical direction. With a distance from the bracket to the center of resistance of 10 mm, the center of rotation approaches infinity as the M/F ratio approaches 10:1. As soon as the M/F ratio exceeds 10:1, the net moment at the center of resistance changes direction, since the magnitude of the counter-moment is now greater than that of the moment produced by the applied force. The center of rotation is slightly incisal to the center of resistance. When the M/F ratio becomes 12:1 or 13:1, the center of rotation is displaced at the incisal edge, resulting in pure root movement. Further increase of the M/F ratio up to about 20:1 causes the center of rotation to gradually move to a location just incisal to the center of resistance. It is obvious that small changes in the M/F ratio have major effects on the clinically observed tooth movement.

As mentioned previously, it is the ratio between the applied counter-moment and force (and not their absolute magnitudes) that determines the type of tooth movement. However, this mechanical principle does not take into account the fact that the magnitudes of forces and couples are important in determining the biologic response to an orthodontic force system. [Also see Orthodontic tooth movement.]

Monobloc See Appliance, Activator.

Monson, Curve of See Curve of Monson.

Mosquito pliers See Orthodontic instruments, Hemostat.

Mouth breathing The habit of breathing primarily through the oral cavity, which traditionally has been associated with some detrimental dentofacial changes and associated malocclusion. Specifically, the theory is that breathing through the mouth, rather than the nose, could bring about some postural changes, namely tipping of the head back and lowering of the mandible and tongue, in order to facilitate respiration. If these postural changes are maintained, face height may increase and the posterior teeth may overerupt, with resulting downward and backward rotation of the mandible,

steep mandibular plane and open bite tendency. As well, the change in equilibrium between the soft tissues and the jaws and teeth could result in compensatory dental changes, such as a constricted maxillary arch, tendency to a crossbite and upright mandibular incisors. In addition, mouth breathing creates xerostomia, which can predispose to gingival hyperplasia and inflammation, as well as caries, at least in the anterior aspect of the dental arches.

The possible association of mouth breathing and the above described craniofacial pattern, as well as its relationship to nasal airway obstruction, is yet another controversial issue, which has led to many referrals of orthodontic patients for adenoidectomy over the years. [Also see "Adenoid" facies

Mouthguard See Appliance, Mouthguard.

MP See Cephalometric lines, Mandibular plane

MPDS (Myofascial pain dysfunction syndrome) See Myofascial pain.

MRI See Magnetic resonance imaging.

Mucogingival junction (MGJ) The junction between the keratinized gingiva and the non-keratinized oral mucosa.

Mucogingival surgery Periodontal surgical procedures used to correct defects in the morphology, position and/or amount of gingiva.

Mucoperiosteal periodontal graft See Graft, Full thickness periodontal.

Mucosa The epithelial lining of body cavities opening to the outside, consisting of mucous membrane.

Alveolar mucosa Mucosa covering the basal part of the alveolar process, continuing without demarcation into the vestibular fornix and the floor of the mouth. It is loosely attached to the periosteum by means of connective tissue, and thus is mobile.

Masticatory mucosa The gingiva and the mucosal covering of the hard palate.

Oral mucosa The tissue lining the oral cavity.

ucosal periodontal graft See Graft, Split thickness periodontal.

ühlemann appliance See Appliance, Propulsor.

ultidisciplinary treatment Coordinated collaboration of multiple specialties in the treatment of a single individual.

ultifactorial Resulting from the combined action of several factors.

ultiloop archwire See Archwire, Multiloop.

ultiple piece maxillary surgery See Osteotomy, Multiple piece maxillary.

ultistrand wire See Orthodontic wire, Multistrand.

uscle Tissue composed of contractile fibers that effect movements of an organ or body part. Muscle types include striated (skeletal and cardiac) muscles and non-striated, smooth (visceral) muscles.

Buccinator muscle A broad, thin muscle, quadrilateral in form, that occupies the space between the jaws at the side of the face. It originates from the outer surface of the maxillary and mandibular alveolar processes corresponding to the three molars and from the anterior surface of the pterygomaxillary ligament. Its fibers converge toward the angle of the mouth where they become continuous with the fibers of the orbicularis oris. The buccinator muscles compress the cheeks so that during mastication food is kept between the occlusal surfaces of the teeth. As well, when the cheeks have been previously distended with air, the buccinator muscles expel it from the mouth, as in blowing a trumpet.

Digastric muscle Muscle consisting of an anterior and a posterior belly, united by an intermediate rounded tendon. The origin of the posterior belly is at the digastric notch of the mastoid process and the insertion of the anterior belly is at a depression on the inner side of the lower border of the mandible near the symphysis. The central tendon of the digastric muscle perforates the stylohyoid muscle. The function of the digastric muscle is to raise the hyoid bone and base of the tongue and depress the mandible.

Lateral (External) pterygoid muscle A short thick muscle originating from the lateral pterygoid plate (inferior head) and the greater wing of the sphenoid (superior head), extending posterolaterally toward the mandibular condyle. It inserts into a depression in front of the neck of the condyle, into the capsule of the TMJ and sometimes into the articular disc. The lateral pterygoid functions to translate the mandible and is active on mouth opening and near final mouth closure.

Masseter muscle A short, thick muscle, somewhat quadrilateral in form, consisting of two portions, superficial and deep. The superficial masseter (which is larger) originates from the zygomatic process and arch and inserts on the angle and the lower half of the outer surface of the ramus of the mandible. The deep masseter originates from the zygomatic arch and inserts on the upper half of the ramus and the coronoid process of the mandible. The fibers of the two portions are united at their insertion. The masseter is the most powerful muscle of mastication, that functions to elevate the mandible.

Medial (Internal) pterygoid muscle A thick quadrilateral muscle resembling the masseter in form. It originates from the maxillary tuberosity and medial surface of the lateral pterygoid plate and extends in a posterior inferior and lateral direction to insert on the medial surface of the ramus and angle of the mandible. It functions to elevate and protrude the mandible.

Orbicularis oris A muscle consisting of numerous strata of muscular fibers, having different directions, that surround the orifice of the mouth. Some of these fibers are derived partially from the other facial muscles that are inserting into the lips, and some are proper to the lips themselves. The orbicularis oris produces the direct closure of the lips, can apply pressure with the lips on the alveolar arches, or can cause the lips to protrude forward.

Scalene muscles Three muscles situated at the side of the neck. They originate from the transverse process of the cervical vertebrae and insert on the first and second rib. They act to stabilize the cervical vertebrae or incline the neck to the side. They also are accessory muscles to respiration.

Sternocleidomastoid muscle A large thick muscle that passes obliquely across the side of the neck, arising with two heads from the sternum and clavicle. It inserts into the outer surface of the mastoid process and the superior nuchal line of the occipital bone. The sternocleidomastoid rotates and extends the head and flexes the vertebral column.

Suprahyoid muscles A group of muscles comprising the digastric, geniohyoid, mylohyoid and stylohyoid. All these muscles attach to the superior aspect of the hyoid bone and act to stabilize and elevate the hyoid bone and depress the mandible. Part of the relapse of orthognathic corrections by mandibular advancement has been attributed to the pull of the suprahyoid musculature.

Temporalis muscle A broad, fan-shaped muscle situated at the side of the head. It originates from the temporal fossa and inserts into the coronoid process and the anterior aspect of the ramus of the mandible. The anterior portion of the muscle consists of fibers that are directed almost verticall' whereas the posterior portion contain fibers with a more oblique or almost hor zontal orientation. Contraction of the anter or portion of the temporalis functions to ele vate the mandible, whereas the posterio portion mainly assists in retruding it.

Trapezius muscle A broad, flat, triangu lar muscle covering the upper and poster or aspect of the neck and shoulders. It orig nates from the superior nuchal line of th occipital bone and from the spinous proces of the seventh cervical and all the thoraci vertebrae, inserting on the clavicle an scapula. The trapezius elevates the shou der and rotates the scapula.

Muscle contraction The development of ter sion or shortening of a muscle.

Muscle cramp See Muscle spasm.

Muscle exercises See Myofunctional therap

Muscle relaxation appliance See Splin Relaxation.

Muscle spasm (Myospasm, Muscl cramp) Spasmodic continuous involuntar contraction of a muscle or group of muscle typically associated with acute pain and dy function. [Compare with Protective muscl splinting.]

Muscle splinting See Protective muscl splinting.

Myalgia Muscle pain.

Myofascial Pertaining to the muscle and i attaching fascia.

Myofascial pain (Myofascial pain dys function syndrome, MPDS) Region pain referred from or emanating aroun active myofascial trigger points.

Myofascial trigger point Hyperirritable spot, usually within a taut band of skeletal muscle or in the muscle fascia that is painful on compression and can give rise to characteristic referred pain, tenderness and autonomic phenomena. Myofascial trigger points are subdivided into active and latent.

Active myofascial trigger point Myofascial trigger point responsible for local or referred current pain, or symptoms without stimulation through palpation.

Latent myofascial trigger point Myofascial trigger point with all the characteristics of an active myofascial trigger point, including referred pain with palpation, but not currently causing spontaneous clinical pain or symptoms.

Myofunctional therapy (Muscle exercises) Therapy aiming at improvement of muscle function and the habitual position of soft tissues (e.g. therapy for correction of a tongue-thrust habit) to prevent or maintain the correction of any occlusal or dental abnormalities associated with them. The concept was introduced to orthodontics by A. Rogers in 1918.

Myositis Inflammation of muscle tissue.

Myospasm See Muscle spasm.

N

N (Na) See Cephalometric landmarks (Hard tissue), Nasion.

N' (Na') See Cephalometric landmarks (Soft tissue), Soft tissue nasion.

Nance appliance See Arch, Nance holding.

NAPog See Cephalometric measurements (Hard tissue), Angle of convexity.

Nasal floor See Cephalometric lines, Palatal plane.

Nasal obstruction Inhibition of normal nasal breathing due to a mechanical impediment of the nasopharyngeal airway. Nasal obstruction generally induces mouth breathing, but the reverse is not always true (i.e. the presence of mouth breathing does not necessarily suggest nasal obstruction), as mouth breathing could be habitual. [Also see "Adenoid facies."]

Nasion (N, Na) See Cephalometric landmarks (Hard tissue), Nasion.

Nasion-perpendicular See Cephalometric lines, Nasion-prependicular.

Nasion-Sella line (NSL) See Cephalometric lines, Sella-Nasion line.

Nasolabial angle (NLA) See Cephalometric measurements (Soft tissue), Nasolabial angle.

Natural head position A standardized orientation of the head that is reproducible for each individual and is used as a mean of standardization during analysis of dentofacial morphology. The concept of natural head position was introduced by C.F.A. Moorrees and M.R Kean in 1958 and now is a common method of head orientation for cephalometric radiography.
To accomplish natural head position, the patient is asked to look into a mirror placed in front of him/her at eye level (as if he/she were looking at the horizon), with the inter pupillary line parallel to the floor. Advocates of this method maintain that registration of the head in its natural position while obtaining a cephalogram has the advantage that an extracranial line (the true vertical or a line perpendicular to that) can be used as a reference line for cephalometric analysis, thus bypassing the difficulties imposed by the biologic variation of intracranial reference lines. [Compare with Natural head posture.]

Natural head posture An individually characteristic physiologic posture of the head during functional activities (e.g. breathing, walking), used to study the relationship between posture and morphologic characteristics. Natural head posture is a dynamic physiologic posture of the head, as opposed to natural head position, a static head orientation. [Compare with Natural head position.]

Natural undercuts See Undercuts, Natural

eckstrap The component of an extraoral appliance (e.g. cervical headgear) that distributes and transfers reaction forces to the cervical area.

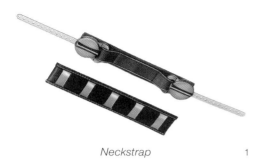

Neckstrap   1

egative overbite See Open bite.

egative overjet See Overjet, Negative.

eonatal maxillary orthopedic treatment See Presurgical infant orthopedics.

euralgia Paroxysmal or constant pain, typically with sharp, stabbing, itching or burning character, in the distribution of a nerve.

euromuscular Concerning both nerves and muscles.

eurotrophism The hypothesis that skeletal growth is under control of the nervous system, assumedly by transmission of substances through the axons of the nerves, much like neural activity controls muscle growth and activity.

eutral position During the activation process of an orthodontic spring, the position of the spring with only the activation moments placed on it (but with zero force).

eutroclusion See Angle classification, Class I malocclusion.

ewton (N) The unit of force in SI, defined as the force required to give a mass of 1 kilogram an acceleration of 1 meter per second squared. [Also see International System of Units.]

Newton's laws All principles of mechanics are based on three physical laws presented in 1686 by Sir I. Newton in his "Philosophea Naturalis Mathematica." The laws of Newton are:

I. Law of inertia When the sum of all the external forces acting on a body is zero, the motion of the body is unchanged (the body either remains at rest, or continues its motion at a straight line with a constant velocity).

II. Law of acceleration If the sum of all the forces acting on a body is not equal to zero, the motion of the body is accelerated along the line of action of the resultant force. The acceleration is proportional to the resultant force and inversely proportional to the mass of the body.

III. Law of action and reaction To every force (action) in a given system, there is an equal and opposite reaction force, so that the sum of all the forces (ΣF) and the sum of all the moments (ΣM) in the system always is equal to zero.

Nickel-titanium alloy (Ni-Ti) Family of alloys primarily consisting of nickel (approximately 55%), titanium (approximately 45%) and optionally of third elements such as cobalt or copper. Nickel-titanium alloys were first reported in the orthodontic literature by G.F. Andreasen in 1971. The name of the first commercially available product was *Nitinol*. Nitinol was developed originally for the U.S. Navy, in the early 1960s, by W.F. Buehler, a research metallurgist at the Naval Ordnance Laboratory in Maryland. [The name *nitinol* is an acronym derived from *ni*ckel and *ti*tanium composition, along with the suffix *-nol* which stands for Naval Ordnance Laboratory.]

Although the original nitinol wire (Unitek/3M) did not exhibit superelastic behavior, it possessed two features of considerable importance for clinical orthodontics:

1. A very low elastic modulus (E), corresponding to about one-fifth of the force delivery of stainless steel wires, and half the force delivery of beta-titanium archwires of the same length and cross-sectional dimensions.

2. An extremely wide working range.

A "second generation" superelastic Chinese nickel-titanium alloy (marketed as "Ni-Ti" by Ormco/Sybron) exhibits non-linear loading and unloading characteristics more pronounced than those of the original nitinol wire.

A "third generation" Japanese nickel-titanium alloy (marketed as "Sentalloy" by GAC International) was subsequently introduced, which also exhibits superelastic behavior. [The name *Sentalloy* is an acronym of the words *superelastic nickel titanium alloy*.] The unloading characteristics of this type of Ni-Ti alloys exhibit initial and final regions of relatively steep slope, along with an extensive intermediate region where there is little or no change in stress.

The superelastic behavior and shape memory characteristics of nickel-titanium alloys are based on a reversible transformation between the austenitic and martensitic Ni-Ti phases. [Also see Martensitic transformation; Shape memory.]

Some of the available nickel-titanium wires are termed *thermally activated* wires due to the fact that their transition temperature is close to the level of body temperature.

Nickel-titanium alloys have characteristic properties that are very useful in orthodontics, namely superelasticity, excellent springback, large working range and low stiffness. However, Ni-Ti wires cannot be soldered or welded without losing their properties, and their friction coefficient is higher than that of stainless steel (although still lower than that of beta-titanium). Ion-implantation may aid in reducing the frictional resistance of nickel-titanium wires. [Also see Martensitic transformation.]

Nickel-titanium wire See Nickel-titanium alloy.

Nightguard (Bruxism appliance) A removable acrylic interocclusal appliance worn at night to prevent or reduce dental wear resulting from bruxism.

Ni-Ti See Nickel-titanium alloy.

Nitinol See Nickel-titanium alloy.

NLA See Cephalometric measurements (Soft tissue), Nasolabial angle.

No. 139 pliers See Orthodontic instrument, Bird-beak pliers.

No. 142 pliers See Orthodontic instrument, Tweed arch-adjusting pliers.

Nociception Stimulation of specialized nerve endings designed to transmit information to the central nervous system concerning potential or actual tissue damage (painful sensation).

Non-arcon articulator See Articulator, Non-arcon.

Non-extraction therapy Orthodontic treatment without any extractions of permanent teeth (wisdom teeth generally excluded).

Non-functional cusps See Cusp, Non-functional.

Non-functioning side See Non-working side.

Non-invasive Denoting any diagnostic or therapeutic procedure that does not require penetration of the skin or entrance into a cavity or organ of the body.

Non-occlusion Any situation in which teeth do not have maximal contact with their antagonists in habitual occlusion. Non-occlusion may be caused by disturbances in tooth eruption (e.g. ankylosis) or by factors that inhibit further eruption, such as digit-sucking or tongue interposition.

According to its localization, non-occlusion can be classified as anterior, posterior or

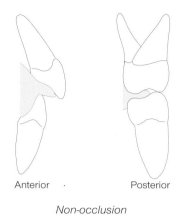

Anterior   ·   Posterior

Non-occlusion   2

total non-occlusion. [Compare with Open bite.]

Anterior non-occlusion   Non-occlusion in the incisor area, which may be combined with some degree of vertical overlap of the incisors, as frequently seen in Class II, Division 1 malocclusions.

Posterior non-occlusion   Non-occlusion in the premolar or molar area, with great variation in the number of teeth and in the occlusal surfaces involved.

Total non-occlusion   A situation characterized by absence of maximal occlusal contact of all posterior teeth, combined with an anterior non-occlusion. In total non-occlusions the tongue usually is positioned between all opposing teeth most of the time.

on-reducing disc   See Disc displacement without reduction.

Non-steroidal anti-inflammatory drug (NSAID)   Class of anti-inflammatory medications that also provide analgesia, but lack the detrimental side effects associated with steroid use.

Non-supporting cusp   See Cusp, Non-functional.

Non-working side (Mediotrusive side, Non-functioning side, Balancing side)   The side opposite to the functioning (working) side on a lateral excursion of the mandible. The side the mandible is moving away from, during a lateral excursion.

Non-working side contact   See Occlusal contact, Non-working side.

Non-working side interference   See Occlusal interference, Non-working side.

Normal force   See Force, Normal.

Normal mobility   See Tooth mobility, Physiologic.

Normal occlusion theory of Angle   See Extraction vs. non-extraction debate.

NSAID   See Non-steroidal anti-inflammatory drug.

NSBa   See Cephalometric measurements (Hard tissue), Cranial base angle.

NSL   See Cephalometric lines, Sella-Nasion.

Nuclear magnetic resonance imaging   See Magnetic resonance imaging.

O

"O-ring"   See Elastomeric modules, Elastomeric ligature.

Oblique cephalometric radiograph   See Cephalometric radiograph, Oblique.

Obstructive sleep apnea (OSA, Obstructive sleep apnea syndrome, OSAS)   Breathing abnormality occurring during sleep, characterized by repeated collapse of the upper airway, producing hypopnea, apnea and, ultimately, desaturation of hemoglobin. The hypopneic and apneic episodes produce frequent arousal from sleep patterns. The effects of repeated desaturation significantly alter normal cardiovascular and pulmonary function, resulting in pulmonary and systemic hypertension as well as arrhythmias, which if untreated can lead to death.

The etiology of OSA appears to be neurogenic failure to preserve the patency of the pharyngeal airway during sleep. The condition often is combined with airway obstruction at various anatomic locations, such as the nasal cavity, adenoids, soft palate, tonsils or base of the tongue. Obesity is considered a predisposing factor in the etiology. In the adult OSA population, males are affected 10 to 20 times more often than females. Almost all apneic patients snore loudly at night. The diagnosis of OSA is made by polysomnography (multiphysiologic sleep recording).

Various treatment modalities advocated include weight loss (if patient is obese), nasal continuous positive air pressure (nasal CPAP), or surgical uvulo-palato-pharyngoplasty (UPPP). Removable intraoral appliances that advance the mandible sometimes are used to re-establish the patency of the airway, as well as to determine whether an orthognathic surgical correction is indicated.

Obturator   A dental prosthesis or appliance used to close a congenital or acquired opening. Sometimes used to cover a remaining oronasal fistula or to facilitate the velopharyngeal mechanism in a patient with a history of cleft lip and palate.

Occipital anchorage   See Anchorage, Occipital.

Occipital headgear   See Headgear, High-pull.

Occlusal   Pertaining to the masticatory surfaces of the posterior teeth. (Also may be used to identify a coronal direction.)

Occlusal adjustment   See Occlusal equilibration.

Occlusal contact   A contact between maxillary and mandibular teeth during occlusion.

   Non-working side contact (Mediotrusive contact, Balancing contact) A contact between maxillary and mandibular teeth on the side opposite to the working side during a lateral mandibular excursion. [Note: The term *non-working contact* is used when there is at least one simultaneous contact on the working side. If the occlusal contact on the non-working side causes disclsion of the teeth on the working side, the term *non-working interference* is used.] [Also see Occlusal interference, Non-working side.]

Working side contact (Laterotrusive occlusal contact) A contact between maxillary and mandibular teeth on the ipsilateral side during guided lateral excursive movement of the mandible.

Occlusal dysfunction A malocclusion with impaired function.

Occlusal equilibration (Occlusal adjustment) Selective grinding of occlusal surfaces of the teeth in an effort to eliminate premature contacts and occlusal interferences, to achieve balancing of the functional occlusal load on the teeth, to eliminate occlusal trauma, to address muscle tension and associated pain, to improve functional relations or to aid in the stabilization of orthodontic results.

Occlusal equilibrium The stage of eruptive tooth movement starting at the point that a tooth reaches the occlusal level and is in complete function. Occlusal equilibrium is divided into juvenile and adult phases.

Adult occlusal equilibrium The final phase of tooth eruption after the end of the pubertal growth spurt. During this phase the rate of tooth eruption is extremely slow. [Compare with Post-emergent spurt; also see Physiologic tooth movement.]

Juvenile occlusal equilibrium The phase of tooth eruption after the post-emergent spurt and during the period of the pubertal growth spurt. During the juvenile equilibrium, teeth that are in function erupt at a rate that parallels the rate of vertical growth of the mandibular ramus. The rate of tooth eruption during this stage is much slower than during the post-emergent spurt, but faster than during the adult equilibrium. [Compare with Post-emergent spurt; also see Physiologic tooth movement.]

Occlusal guidance The contact pattern between teeth during dentally guided mandibular movement away from or toward maximum intercuspation.

Occlusal interference (Premature occlusal contact, Supracontact, Deflective occlusal contact, "Prematurity") Undesirable occlusal contact that may produce mandibular deviation during closure to maximum intercuspation or may hinder smooth passage to and from the intercuspal position.

Centric interference A premature contact occurring when the mandible closes with the condyles in their optimum position in the glenoid fossae (centric relation), which causes a deflection (shift) of the mandible in an anterior, posterior and/or lateral direction.

Non-working side interference (Mediotrusive side interference, Balancing interference) A contact between maxillary and mandibular teeth on the non-working side that causes disclusion of the teeth on the working side during a lateral mandibular excursion. [Compare with Occlusal contact, Non-working side.]

Protrusive interference An occlusal contact between maxillary and mandibular posterior teeth discluding the incisors during a protrusive mandibular excursion.

Occlusal lug See Occlusal rest.

Occlusal plane (OP) An imaginary surface that passes through the occlusion of the teeth. This surface usually is curved and is, strictly speaking, not a plane, but commonly is approximated by one (straight line in the lateral view), based on specific reference points within the dental arches. The maxillary occlusal plane passes through the occlusal cusps of the posterior teeth and the incisal edges of the maxillary incisors. The mandibular occlusal plane is tangent to the occlusal cusps of the posterior teeth and the incial edges of the mandibular incisors. [Also see Cephalometric lines, Occlusal plane.]

Occlusal prematurity See Occlusal interference.

Occlusal rest (Occlusal lug, Occlusal stop) The part of a removable appliance that rests on the occlusal surface of a tooth and prevents movement of the appliance toward the soft tissue. Occlusal rests sometimes are soldered on fixed appliances, such as a "band and loop" space maintainer, to resist dislodgment of the appliance as a result of the forces of mastication.

Occlusal splint See Splint.

Occlusal stop See Occlusal rest.

Occlusal trauma (Traumatic occlusion, Trauma from occlusion, Periodontal trauma) **1.** Injury to the periodontium resulting from occlusal forces in excess of the reparative capacity of the periodontal attachment. The affected teeth usually exhibit widening of the PDL space, wear facets and some degree of hypermobility. [Also see Tooth mobility, Increased.] **2.** The same term sometimes is used to denote a palatally impinging overbite. [Also see Overbite, Impinging.]

Primary occlusal trauma Injury to the periodontium from occlusal loading of excessive magnitude or non-physiologic direction or duration in teeth with normal periodontal structures.

Secondary occlusal trauma Injury to the periodontium from occlusal loading of excessive magnitude or non-physiologic direction or duration in teeth already affected with periodontal disease.

Occlusal wear See Attrition.

Occlusion The relationship of the maxillary and mandibular teeth, as they are brought into functional contact.

Centric occlusion (CO, Intercuspa position, ICP, Habitual occlusion Mandibular position dictated by maximun and habitual intercuspation of the maxillary and mandibular teeth. It is a dentally deter mined position, independent of condyla position.

Functional occlusion (Physiologica occlusion) A static and dynamic relation ship of the teeth combining minimum stres on the temporomandibular joint, optima function of the orofacial complex, stabilit and esthetics of the dentition and protectior and health of the periodontium.

Habitual occlusion See Occlusion Centric.

Optimal occlusion (Ideal occlusion An ideal relationship of maxillary anc mandibular teeth combining a functiona occlusion (as described above) with the absence of malocclusion (as described b the six keys of occlusion).

Physiological occlusion See Occlusior Functional.

Traumatic occlusion See Occlusal trau ma.

Occlusion, Six keys of See Six keys of occlu sion.

Occlusogingivally (Occlusoapically) In direction perpendicular to the occlusa plane, along the y-axis. [Also see Global re erence frame.]

Occlusogram A graphic representation c the arches from the occlusal view. Oc clusograms are mainly used as treatmer planning aids to assist in defining the spe cific tooth movements required within an between arches (in the sagittal and trans verse planes) to achieve treatment goals. A occlusogram is essentially a two-dimer sional diagnostic setup and is directly co related with the Visual Treatment Objectiv

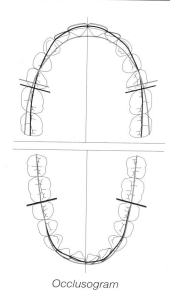

Occlusogram

(VTO). It can be constructed from tracings of photographic or photostatic copies of the occlusal aspects of the maxillary and mandibular study casts. The tracings of the teeth of both arches are superimposed on each other to reproduce the existing occlusal relationship, using index points that are marked on the models and subsequently transferred to the tracings. Anticipated movements of individual teeth as well as the need for extractions then can be determined, to simulate the desired treatment goal. [Also see Visual treatment objective; Diagnostic setup.]

Occult cleft See Submucous cleft palate.

Oculoauriculovertebral spectrum See Hemifacial microsomia.

Offsets See Bends, First-order.

Oligodontia The congenital absence of multiple teeth (a severe form of hypodontia). In many such patients, the existing teeth are smaller than normal and can be shaped atypically. [Compare with Anodontia.]

Omega loop See Loop, Omega.

Omega pliers See Orthodontic instruments, Tweed loop-forming pliers.

One-jaw surgery See Orthognathic surgery, Single-jaw.

One-piece maxillary osteotomy See Osteotomy, One-piece maxillary.

OP See Occlusal plane.

Op See Cephalometric landmarks (Hard tissue), Opisthion.

Open activator See Appliance, Open activator.

Open bite (Negative overbite) Inherited, developmental or acquired malocclusion whereby no vertical overlap exists between

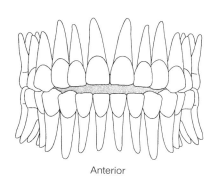

Anterior

Open bite

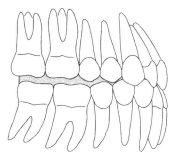

Posterior

maxillary and mandibular anterior teeth (*anterior* open bite), or no vertical contact is exhibited between maxillary and mandibular posterior teeth (*posterior* open bite). An open bite may be localized and thus involve only a few teeth due to a digit-sucking habit or other local factors (*dental* open bite), or it may be caused by divergence of the skeletal planes (*skeletal* open bite or *apertognathia*). [Compare with Non-occlusion.]

Open coil spring See Orthodontic springs, Coil spring, Open.

Open curettage See Curettage, Open.

Open fracture See Fracture, Compound.

Open lock See Dislocation of the condyle.

Open loop See Loop, Open.

Open spring See Orthodontic springs, Open.

Opening loop See Loop, Opening.

Opening of the bite The correction of a deep bite. This can be performed by extrusion of posterior teeth, often resulting in clockwise rotation of the mandible (increased separation between the mandibular and palatal planes); by intrusion of the anterior teeth; or by a combination of the two methods (*relative intrusion* of the anterior teeth). [Also see Bite raising.]

Opisthion (Op) See Cephalometric landmarks (Hard tissue), Opisthion.

OPT See Panoramic radiograph.

Optical pliers See Orthodontic instruments, Tweed loop-forming pliers.

Optimal force theory The hypothesis that there exists a force of certain magnitude and temporal characteristics (continuous vs. intermittent, constant vs. declining, etc.) that is capable of producing a maximum rate of tooth movement with no tissue damage and maximum patient comfort. The optim force for tooth movement may differ for eac tooth, or for each individual patient.

Optimal occlusion See Occlusion, Optimal

Optimum force See Optimal force theory.

Or See Cephalometric landmarks (Hard tissue Orbitale.

Oral mucosa See Mucosa, Oral.

Oral screen See Appliance, Oral screen.

Orbicularis oris See Muscle, Orbicularis or

Orbital hypertelorism The increased di tance between the medial orbital wall reflecting an increased distance betwee the orbits (greater than 2 standard devi tions from the norm). The anatomic lan marks used commonly for the measur ment of interorbital distance are the *dacr on* points (bilaterally). Hypertelorism described on the basis of skeletal measur ments, because the presence of epicanth folds or strabismus (exotropia), or other so tissue variations such as increased distanc between the medial canthi (telecanthu clinically may give a false impression hypertelorism.
Orbital hypertelorism is common in a nur ber of craniofacial malformations such Crouzon syndrome and frontonasal dyspl sia. [Compare with Telecanthus; Orbit hypotelorism.]

Orbital hypotelorism The decreased di tance between the medial orbital walls, common finding in patients born with ma formations such as a median cleft. A patie with orbital hypotelorism has a much great chance of severe brain abnormality tha does one with hypertelorism. [Compare wi Orbital hypertelorism.]

Orbitale (Or) See Cephalometric landmar (Hard tissue), Orbitale.

Orofacial Pertaining to the mouth and face.

Oronasal communication See Fistula, Oronasal.

Oronasal fistula See Fistula, Oronasal.

Ortho- A prefix meaning straight or correct.

Orthodontic appliance See Appliance, Orthodontic.

Orthodontic attachment See Attachment, Orthodontic.

Orthodontic band A ring, usually made of a thin strip of stainless steel, that serves to secure orthodontic attachments to a tooth. Bands are prefabricated in varying shapes to fit closely around the crowns of specific teeth. Each shape comes in different sizes to accommodate individual tooth size variation. Most bands have an occluso-gingival taper to fit the tooth, with the incisal edge straight and the cervical edge contoured, similar to the cementoenamel junction. Orthodontic bands can be plain or have buccal (brackets or tubes) or lingual (buttons, sheaths, cleats, seating lugs) attachments welded or brazed on them. The inner surface of the band can be conditioned by various methods such as pattern rolling, sandblasting, photo- or laser-etching to increase retention.

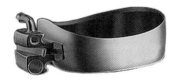

Orthodontic band 1

Orthodontic board See Board, Orthodontic.

Orthodontic casts (Orthodontic models) Positive reproductions of the maxillary and mandibular dental arches and alveolar processes, including the hard palate, mucobuccal, mucolabial and sublingual folds and associated muscle and frenum attachments. Orthodontic casts usually are constructed from an alginate impression and poured in plaster.

Study casts (Diagnostic casts, Study models) Casts poured in white plaster and used for diagnosis and treatment planning. Study casts are important parts of the patient's permanent record. They usually are obtained prior to and at the end of active treatment as well as between distinct treatment phases (e.g. immediately prior to orthognathic surgery).

Working casts Casts poured commonly in hard plaster and used for appliance fabrication, or as a means for detailed evaluation of the interdigitation during orthodontic treatment (e.g. to assess whether the arches are ready for orthognathic surgery).

Orthodontic cement Dental cement used for fixation of orthodontic bands to the teeth.

Glass-ionomer cement A polyelectrolyte dental cement produced by mixing a fluoride-containing aluminum silicate glass powder and a solution of polyacrylic acid. Due to ion transfer between the calcium of the tooth and the polyacrylic acid of the glass-ionomer cement, a high bonding strength can be achieved, especially when there is good moisture control. This inherent adhesion to tooth structure, as well as their long-term release of fluoride ions (with cariostatic potential) are the two main advantages of glass-ionomer cements.

Resin-modified glass-ionomer cement (Dual-cured glass-ionomer cement) The combination of conventional glass-ionomer chemistry with methacrylate resin technology has led to the creation of resin-modified glass-ionomer cements. [Note: Such cements are often incorrectly referred to as *light-cured* glass-ionomer cements; the term *dual-cured* is more appropriate because the original acid-base reaction is supplemented by light-activated polymerization.]

Resin-modified glass-ionomer cements are easier to use than conventional glass-ionomer cements. The supplementary light polymerization allows a longer working time, a rapid hardening on command, and a more rapid early development of strength and resistance against aqueous attack.

Enamel bonding strength is reported to be improved over that of conventional glass-ionomer cements, although it is still inferior to that of resin composites.

Zinc oxide-eugenol (ZOE) cement A dental cement produced by mixing an active form of zinc oxide powder and eugenol. Zinc oxide-eugenol chelate is formed, which causes the cement to set and harden. Zinc oxide-eugenol cement exhibits a relatively low strength and poor resistance to abrasion and disintegration. It can be reinforced by the inclusion of a polymeric and/or inorganic filler in the powder or by the solution of a polymer in the eugenol liquid.

Zinc phosphate cement An opaque dental cement produced by mixing a deactivated zinc oxide powder (that also contains minor amounts of other oxides, such as magnesium oxide) and a liquid consisting of phosphoric acid, water and metallic salts (such as aluminum and zinc phosphates). Phosphate salts are formed, which cause the cement to set and harden. Some zinc phosphate cements also contain copper for its antibacterial properties (i.e. *black* or *red copper cement*).

Orthodontic displacement See Orthodontic tooth movement.

Orthodontic elastics (Rubber bands) Flexible bands, usually made of elastomeric material, used to produce forces for tooth movement. Depending on their purpose, location and orientation, they are categorized as follows:

Anterior diagonal elastics (Anterior oblique elastics) Anterior intermaxillary elastics crossing the midline (e.g. extending from the maxillary right canine to the mandibular left lateral incisor), often used to facilitate the correction of non-coinciding maxillary and mandibular dental midlines.

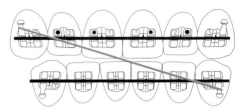

Anterior diagonal elastics

Asymmetric elastics Various combinations of intermaxillary elastics (e.g. Class I elastics on one side and Class II elastics on the other) used to correct an asymmetry in the buccal segment occlusion, with or without an associated midline discrepancy.

Box elastics See Orthodontic elastics, Vertical.

Class I elastics See Orthodontic elastics, Intramaxillary.

Class II elastics Intermaxillary elastics extending unilaterally or bilaterally from the anterior aspect of the maxillary dental arch to the posterior aspect of the mandibular one (e.g. from the maxillary canines to the

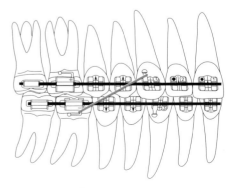

Class II elastics

mandibular first molars). They are used to aid in Class II correction, to reduce the overjet, to minimize anchorage loss during maxillary incisor retraction by taking advantage of intermaxillary anchorage, etc. In addition to the desired sagittal force, Class II elastics create vertical forces (especially when the patient opens their mouth) as well as certain transverse forces, both of which often are undesirable.

Class III elastics Intermaxillary elastics with the opposite orientation to Class II elastics (from the anterior aspect of the mandibular dental arch to the posterior aspect of the maxillary one). As in the instance of Class II elastics, Class III elastics can be used unilaterally or bilaterally. They have various applications: to facilitate protraction of maxillary posterior teeth, to improve the incisor relationship in an edge-to-edge or anterior crossbite situation, or to

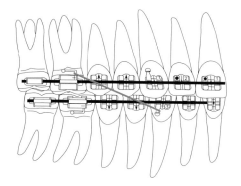

Class III elastics

make use of intermaxillary anchorage during mandibular incisor retraction. In addition to the desired sagittal force, Class III elastics create vertical forces (especially when the patient opens their mouth), as well as certain transverse forces, both of which often are undesirable.

Crossbite elastics (Criss-cross elastics, Through-the-bite elastics) Elastics extending from the palatal (lingual) aspect of one or more maxillary teeth, to the buccal

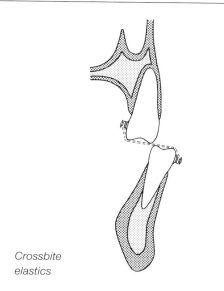

Crossbite elastics

2

aspect of one or more mandibular teeth (or the reverse), to aid in correction of a crossbite. Crossbite elastics create vertical forces in addition to the desirable transverse or anteroposterior forces; they therefore should be used with caution, especially in patients with minimal overbite and long anterior lower facial height.

Intermaxillary elastics (Intermaxillary traction) Elastics running between maxillary and mandibular teeth for sagittal, transverse or vertical coordination of the arches, or a combination of the above. Class II, Class III and crossbite elastics are all examples of intermaxillary traction. Intermaxillary elastics generate forces in all three planes of space, only some of which are usually desirable. They therefore should be used with caution, especially in patients with minimal overbite and long anterior lower facial height.

Intramaxillary elastics (Class I elastics, Intramaxillary traction) Elastic traction between teeth or groups of teeth of the same arch. For example, patients sometimes are requested to wear such elastics during canine retraction using sliding mechanics. *See illustration next page.*

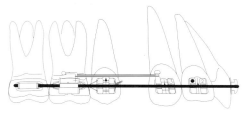

Intramaxillary elastics

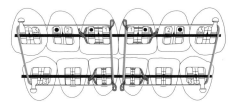

Anterior box elastics

Separating elastic See Separator.

Through-the-bite elastics See Orthodontic elastics, Crossbite.

Transpalatal elastics Intramaxillary form of elastic traction extending across the palatal vault (e.g. between two lingual cleats on the second molar bands) in an attempt to constrict the maxillary arch form, or to reciprocally move buccally displaced teeth into the arch.

Vertical elastics (Up-down elastics, Box elastics, Triangular elastics, Zig-zag elastics, "Spaghetti" elastics) Intermaxillary elastics in various configurations, aiming at extrusion of teeth. They are used to aid in settling (improve the interdigitation) in the final stages of active treatment, to achieve closure of a localized open bite, or to aid in postsurgical leveling of the mandibular curve of Spee by premolar extrusion (e.g. in Class II, Division 2 patients with short lower facial height).

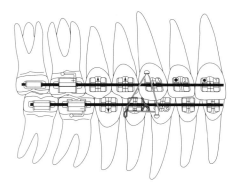

Triangular elastics

Orthodontic force See Force, Orthodontic.

Orthodontic implant See Implant, Orthodontic.

Orthodontic impression trays Stainless steel, aluminum or plastic trays used to receive the impression material (usually alginate) during orthodontic impression taking. An orthodontic impression tray consists of a main body and a handle, which is either welded or riveted to the body. The maxillary tray allows for coverage of the maxillary alveolar process and the palate, whereas the mandibular tray allows for coverage of the mandibular alveolar process. Some tray bodies are perforated to increase retention of the impression material. Trays are available in various sizes and shapes. The flanges of the tray are usually extended with rope wax to achieve representation of the full depth of the vestibule during taking of impressions for orthodontic study models.

Orthodontic instruments Orthodontic procedures demand the use of many specialized instruments, along with several also used in other areas of dentistry. The most commonly used orthodontic instruments are:

Adams pliers (Universal pliers) Heavy wire pliers with sharply tapered beaks forming a four-sided pyramid when closed. Used for bending heavy-gauge wires and adjusting removable appliances.

Arch-forming pliers (Arch-contouring pliers, De la Rossa pliers) Pliers with straight, thick, parallel beaks; the concave

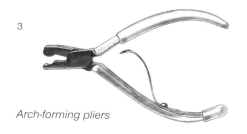

Arch-forming pliers

beak fits around the opposing cylindrical one. The cylindrical beak may have grooves of varying sizes or may be non-grooved. Used to form and contour archwires, either round or rectangular, as well as to incorporate (reverse) curve of Spee into an archwire.

Band burnisher (Beaver-tail burnisher) Stainless steel instrument with a heavy, hollow handle for palm grip, similar to a Mershon band pusher. The shank ends in an angled beaver-tail-shaped tip that can be smooth or serrated and flattened for easier access to band margins under buccal tubes or bracket wings. Used for burnishing and adapting margins of bands to the tooth contour.

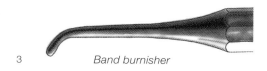

Band burnisher

Band-contouring pliers Pliers with two long, tapering and slightly bowed beaks. The convex tip at the end of the one beak fits into the opposing concave tip in a ball- and-socket manner. The diameter and shape of the tips vary with the manufacturer. Used for adaptation and contouring of stainless steel orthodontic bands.

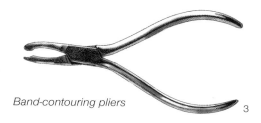

Band-contouring pliers

Band pusher (Mershon band pusher) Stainless steel instrument with a large, tapering handle for palm grip and a long shank with an angled tip. The tip is rectangular and serrated to prevent slippage of the instrument during use. Used for positioning and seating the band properly, as well as for burnishing or adapting the edges of the band around the tooth.

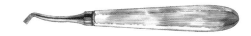

Band pusher

Band-removing (Debanding) pliers, Anterior Pliers with a longer, flat-sided curved beak placed on the incisal edge of teeth, opposing a shorter, sharper beak positioned under the gingival aspect of the band or attachment. The longer incisal beak may have a replaceable plastic or rubber tip to prevent fractures of the incisal edge of the teeth. The beaks generally do not make contact when the handles are closed fully. Used to remove bands from anterior teeth.

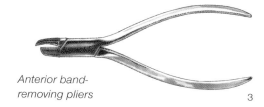

Anterior band-removing pliers

Band-removing (Debanding) pliers, Posterior Pliers with two beaks, one longer than the other. The longer beak, which carries a replaceable plastic cap, is placed on the occlusal surface of a tooth, while the

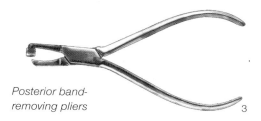

Posterior band-removing pliers

193

shorter, sharpened beak engages and lifts the gingival margin of the band. Anterior and posterior band removing pliers can be combined in a "Universal" design.

Band seater (Band biter) Plastic or metal instrument consisting of a handle and a bite stick that makes use of the patient's biting force to aid the clinician in seating a band. The tip of the bite stick has two sides. The one that is placed on the occlusal margin of the band is made of stainless steel and is available in several sizes and shapes. As well, it usually is serrated to minimize slippage of the instrument during use. The opposite side of the tip, which comes in contact with the patient's teeth during biting, usually consists of a plastic bite shelf.

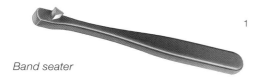

1

Band seater

Bird-beak (no. 139) pliers Pliers with two short beaks (one of which is conical and the other pyramidal in shape) used for bending small wires and springs.

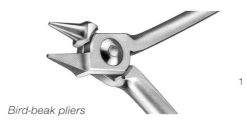

1

Bird-beak pliers

Bracket-positioning instrument (Bracket-height gauge) Device of various designs used to facilitate the placement of brackets at standard distances from the incisal edges or occlusal surfaces of specific teeth. It usually has a ledge that rests on the incisal edge (occlusal surface) of the tooth, while a shorter arm is inserted into the bracket slot.

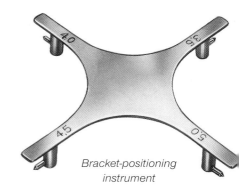

Bracket-positioning
instrument

Bracket-removing pliers (Debondin pliers) Pliers used to remove bracket bonded to teeth. There are various design depending on the type of bracket (e.g. stai less steel, ceramic, plastic). The standar design for stainless steel brackets has tw mirror-image jaws with the sharp cutting tip formed around a cylindrical opening. Th cutting tips generally do not make conta when the handles are closed fully. Th bracket is removed by peel and shear force by placing the cutting tips at the bracke adhesive junction and squeezing.

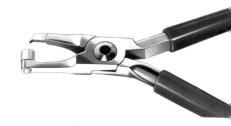

Bracket-removing pliers

Conversion instrument An orthodonti instrument that is inserted into the mesi opening of a convertible tube and function in a "can-opener" fashion to remove its co vertible cap and thus turn it into a bracke [Also see Conversion of a tube into a brac et; Tube, Convertible.]

Coon ligature-tying pliers Revers action pliers (squeezing the handles i creases the separation of the tips), consis

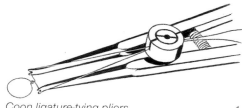

Coon ligature-tying pliers 1

ing of two opposing mirror-image parts (handle, shank and tip, all one piece) joined just below the shank by a round metal cylinder with a channel. The opposing handles are attached by a spring that holds them apart, causing the tips to touch when the instrument is passive. It is used for tying metal ligatures. The opposing tips are blunted and forked to facilitate retention of the ligature wire. As the handles are compressed, spreading the tips, the channel locks the ligature wire automatically. Because of the reverse action, the initial twist and the pressure are exerted at the bracket-archwire junction and then twisted away from the bracket. This gives the ligature a tighter fit around the bracket, forcing the archwire further into the slot.

Distal-end cutter A special wire cutter with the juxtaposed cutting edges set at right angles to the long axis of the instrument to facilitate cutting of the distal end of the archwire, intraorally. May have a safety hold mechanism provided either by a thick wire running parallel to the cutting edges, or by a rectangular shoulder immediately below

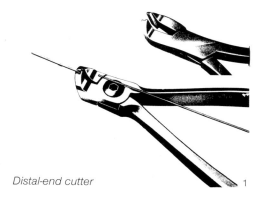

Distal-end cutter 1

the cutting edges. This mechanism serves to grip the loose end of the cut archwire and prevent it from being lost in the mouth, so that it can be discarded easily. It can be used to cut round wires up to 0.020 inch or 0.51 mm in diameter and rectangular wires up to 0.022 x 0.028 inch or 0.56 x 0.70 mm.

Elastic separator pliers (Separator pliers) Reverse-action pliers (squeezing the handles increases the separation of the beaks) with two long beaks that are angled for better access. The beaks are connected with a circular hinge and carry tapered, grooved, blunted tips, which can retain elastic separators (modules). They are used to stretch, hold and place elastic separators.

Facebow-adjusting pliers Heavy-duty pliers with a box-jointed pivot construction, having two parallel beaks and an opposing one that fits between the former when the pliers are closed. Each beak has a rounded notch at a right angle to the beak near the tip on the opposing surfaces. Used for adjusting the inner and outer arches of facebows, or for contouring wires of large diameter (up to 0.062 inch or 1.55 mm).

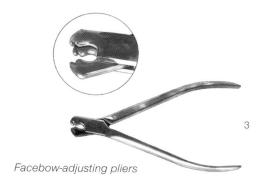

Facebow-adjusting pliers

Hard wire cutter Cutter of design similar to a pin and ligature wire cutter, only larger, and capable of cutting full-dimension archwires.

Hemostat (Mosquito pliers) Small and light pliers with scissor-like design, provided with a mechanical locking mechanism locat-

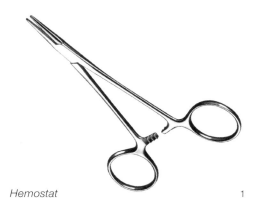

Hemostat 1

Used to tuck and direct stainless ste ligatures under the archwire or brack wings, or to push archwires or auxiliaries in position.

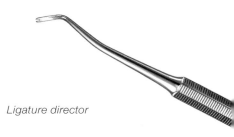

Ligature director

ed between the handles. The handles are available in various lengths. The serrated beaks can be either straight or curved and they may be notched to aid in retention of elastomeric ligatures. Used for placement of elastomeric ligatures (donuts).

Howes utility pliers Pliers with two long, round beaks tapered to a pyramid shape and bowed, terminating in juxta-posed flat round serrated pads. The pads are positioned at right angles to the long axis of the beaks; their diameter varies with the manufacturer. The beaks may be straight or offset at a 45° angle. Used mainly for gripping and handling archwires and stain-less steel ligatures during placement in the mouth.

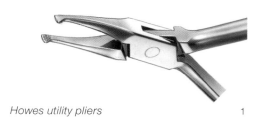

Howes utility pliers 1

Ligature director (Pitchfork instru-ment) Stainless steel instrument carrying a straight or angled tip with a notch capable of engaging wires. Available in double-ended versions or in combination with amalgam-pluggers, scalers or other tips.

Light-wire pliers Essentially identical bird-beak pliers, only with longer and mo slender beaks. Some designs have one more grooves at the tip of the pyramid beak to aid in making reproducible loop and helices. Used mainly to form variou loop designs in orthodontic wires (genera ly light, round wires), to make minor adjus ment bends in archwires or to place met spring separators. [Also see Orthodont wire, Australian.]

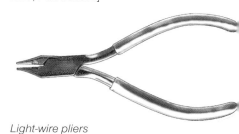

Light-wire pliers

Mathieu-style ligature-tying plier Pliers with long, thin handles equipped wit a positive-locking ratchet and spring fc

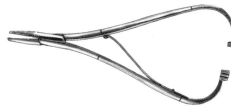

Mathieu-style ligature-tying pliers

instant opening and closing. The opposing tips are serrated and may have tungsten carbide inserts for longer instrument life. The tips vary in length and taper by the manufacturer. The pliers are available in various sizes. Used mainly for tying stainless steel ligatures as well as for placing elastomeric ligatures (donuts).

Parallel-action pliers with cutter (Sargent heavy-duty pliers) Heavy-duty pliers with parallel, flat, serrated opposing beaks. One of the beaks carries a wire cutter on its non-serrated side. Used mainly for bending, cutting or holding large-diameter wires in laboratory procedures.

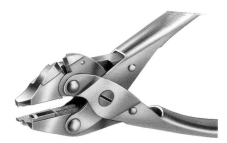

Parallel-action pliers with cutter   1

Pin and ligature wire cutter Cutter with two tapered and pointed opposing beaks, terminating in delicate and sharp cutting edges. The cutting edges may have carbide inserts that can be sharpened or replaced when dull or damaged, without replacing the entire instrument. It is available in various angles, the straight and 15° to the long axis being the most common. The tape and

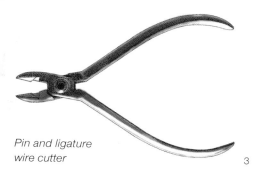

Pin and ligature wire cutter   3

size of the tips vary with the manufacturer. Used to cut soft ligature wires (generally up to 0.016 inch or 0.41 mm) and arch-retaining pins.

Separator pliers See Orthodontic instruments, Elastic separator pliers.

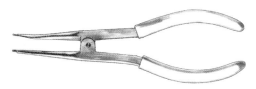

Separator pliers   3

Serrated amalgam-plugger A single-ended or double-ended (in combination with a ligature director or other tip) stainless steel instrument, sometimes used to seat and position bands or to tuck steel ligatures. The tip is available in various lengths, angles and diameters and usually is serrated for better control in pushing motion.

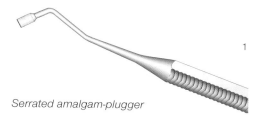

Serrated amalgam-plugger

Steiner ligature-tying pliers Identical to the Coon ligature-tying pliers, differing only in that the round metal cylinder at the shank of the instrument does not carry the special channel to engage the end of the ligature wire. The ligature wire is retained on

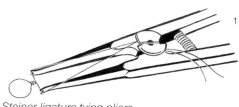

Steiner ligature-tying pliers

the instrument by manually wrapping its free ends around the round metal cylinder.

Torquing key Usually a cross-shaped stainless steel instrument, each of the four ends of which carries a milled slot to engage the wire for placement of torque. Each slot is a different size to accommodate various gauge wires. Used to place torque in an archwire or to assist full engagement of a wire into a bracket slot. Various other kinds of torquing keys are used in combination with special pliers to place torque for an individual tooth.

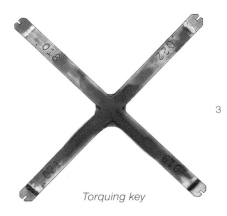

3

Torquing key

Triple-beaked pliers (Three-jaw pliers, Clasp-adjusting pliers) Pliers similar to but smaller than the facebow-adjusting pliers, with a box-jointed pivot construction. The double-sectioned beak is opposed by a single beak, so that a squeezing motion can produce a sharp bend in the wire. Used for adjusting wires, particularly labial bows

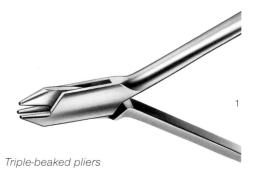

1

Triple-beaked pliers

or clasps on retainers, as well as for placir a curve on flexible or heavier wires, or stai less steel tubing.

Turret Tubular metal device of variou circumferences carrying grooves of variou calibrated sizes, used to shape straig lengths of orthodontic wire into an arch forr Some turrets are equipped with angulate grooves to place torque into rectangular wi during shaping of the arch form.

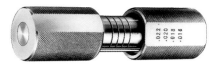

Turret

Tweed arch-adjusting (no. 142) plie Pliers used exclusively for handling adjusting square or rectangular wires. Th beaks are symmetrically flattened blade that are parallel at a separation of 0.020 inc (0.51 mm).

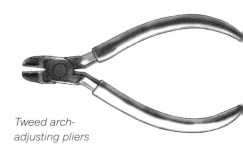

Tweed arch-adjusting pliers

Tweed loop-forming pliers (Omeg pliers, Optical pliers) Pliers with tw opposed parallel beaks, one with concav and one with round cross-section. Th round beak generally is stepped, havin three sections of different diameters (mo commonly 0.045, 0.060, and 0.075 inc or 1.12, 1.50 and 1.90 mm). The tip of th round beak may be replaceable. Used t form various loops or short curved sectior in orthodontic wire. *See illustration ne page.*

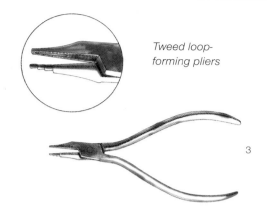

Tweed loop-forming pliers

3

Weingart utility pliers Pliers with two long, slender beaks with opposing, serrated tips. The tips are oblong and pointed and can be straight or curved from the long axis of the pliers to provide a better working angle for intraoral adjustments. Used for holding or gripping the archwire to place it and remove it from the mouth, or to make adjustment bends.

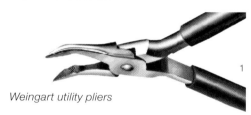

Weingart utility pliers

1

rthodontic magnets Magnets have had various applications in medicine (mainly to aid in fracture healing) and in dentistry (mainly for retention of prostheses). The miniaturization of magnets as a result of the introduction of rare-earth or lanthanide elements facilitated their intraoral applications. In orthodontics, magnetic forces from repelling or attracting poles have been utilized to achieve palatal expansion, intrusion of posterior teeth, molar distalization, forced eruption of unerupted teeth, anterior repositioning of the mandible during treatment with some functional appliances, retraction or alignment of teeth, as well as retention of diastema closure. Neodymium-iron-boron ($Nd_2Fe_{14}B$) and samarium-cobalt ($SmCo_5$) are the types of rare-earth

magnets most commonly used. The greatest disadvantage of magnets is their low corrosion resistance in the presence of saliva. Corrosion products are toxic to the tissues, for which reason magnets must be coated with appropriate materials (usually parylene or acrylic), or be enclosed in a stainless steel casing, when intended for intraoral use. The possibility of adverse effects of magnetic fields on cells and tissues is an issue of controversy.

Orthodontic models See Orthodontic casts.

Orthodontic pliers See Orthodontic instruments.

Orthodontic retainer See Retainer.

Orthodontic specialist See Orthodontist.

Orthodontic springs Force-producing modules or appliance components, made of metal.

Cantilever spring In principle, any piece of wire, one end of which is inserted fully into a bracket or tube, while the other end is ligated to another unit with only a one-point contact. The advantage of using cantilever mechanics is that the created force system can be estimated easily at both units (statically determinate force system) by knowing the length of the cantilever and by measuring the force exerted at its ligated end with a force gauge. Moreover, the relatively long range of deactivation of the spring results in a low magnitude continuous force (low load/deflection ratio) that generally is considered desirable for tooth movement. [Also see Mechanics, Cantilever.]

Closed spring A spring (usually part of a removable appliance) having both ends attached.

Coffin spring An omega-shaped (Ω) spring made of heavy-gauge wire, spanning across the palate as part of some removable orthodontic appliances (e.g. the Bimler or

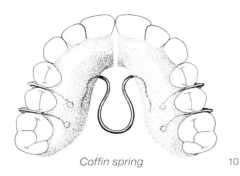

Coffin spring 10

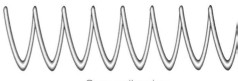

Open coil spring

the Crozat appliance). The function of a Coffin spring is to offer the possibility of expansion or constriction of the maxillary dental arch.

Coil spring, Closed Spring made of fine (typically 0.010 to 0.012 inch, or 0.25 to 0.30 mm) orthodontic wire wound into a coil whose helices tightly contact each other; thus it cannot be compressed. A closed coil spring usually comes in a spool and is cut to the appropriate length according to the intended application. It most commonly is used to maintain a space during fixed appliance orthodontic treatment (e.g. the space of a missing tooth that eventually will be replaced prosthetically).

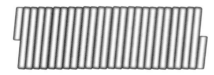

Closed coil spring

Coil spring, Open Spring made of fine (typically 0.010 to 0.012 inch, or 0.25 to 0.30 mm) orthodontic wire wound into a coil whose helices are spaced, so it can be compressed along its long axis. An open coil spring comes in a spool and usually is cut to a length larger than the interbracket distance between the teeth that are intended to be moved away from each other. It is compressed prior to insertion, generating equal and opposite forces on either end.

Coil spring, Retraction (Pletche spring, Closing coil spring) Sprin made of fine (typically 0.010 to 0.012 inch or 0.25 to 0.30 mm) orthodontic wire woun into a coil with tightly contacting helices. Th coils are prefabricated from superelastic c stainless steel wire and come in predete mined lengths with two eyelets on eithe end. Retraction coil springs are used to ger erate forces for retraction of teeth or spac closure by extending them beyond their in tial length.

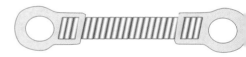

Retraction coil spring

Crefcoeur spring See Appliance, Cre coeur.

Finger spring A free-end spring usual incorporated in removable orthodonti appliances to produce various tipping mov

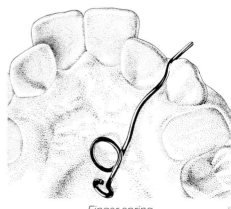

Finger spring

ments of teeth. Finger springs can contain helices to increase the effective wire length for added flexibility.

Free-end spring (Open spring) A broad category of springs (usually part of a removable appliance) having only one end embedded in acrylic.

Gjessing spring See Orthodontic springs, PG spring.

Open spring See Orthodontic springs, Free-end spring.

PG spring (Gjessing spring) A universal retraction spring made of 0.016 x 0.022-inch stainless steel wire, introduced by P. Gjessing. The spring consists of a 10 mm-long, double, ovoid-shaped, closed loop extending gingivally, continuing with a small (2 mm in diameter) occlusal helix. This configuration was designed to reduce the load/deflection rate to approximately 45 g per millimeter of activation. The spring also has an anti-tip moment-to-force ratio of approximately 11:1 and an anti-rotation moment-to-force ratio of approximately 7:1. It is meant to be used as a segmental spring for frictionless segmental canine retraction by translation, or for "en masse" retraction of the maxillary incisors without undesirable lingual tipping. The spring is supposed to be activated every 4 to 6 weeks, to the point where the double loop is separated, which is calibrated to produce approximately 100 g of force.

Root spring An orthodontic spring that can cause movement of the root of a tooth with relatively little movement of the crown. Uprighting springs and torquing springs both are subcategories of root springs.

Rotation spring Auxiliary orthodontic spring, commonly used with single brackets (usually inserted into the vertical slot) to generate the moment required for rotation of a tooth around its long axis.

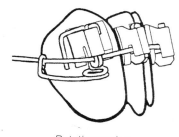

Rotation spring   9

Separating spring See Separator.

Side-winder spring See Appliance, Tip-Edge.

Torquing spring Auxiliary orthodontic spring used to move the root of a tooth in the labiolingual or buccolingual direction.

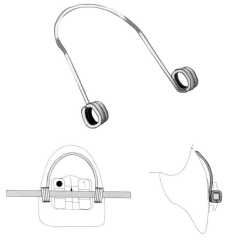

Torquing spring

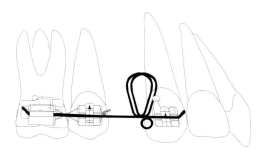

PG retraction spring

Uprighting spring Auxiliary orthodontic spring used to move the root of a tooth in the mesiodistal direction. Uprighting springs commonly are used in the bracket vertical slot with the Begg technique and its modifications (e.g. the side-winder springs of the Tip-Edge appliance).

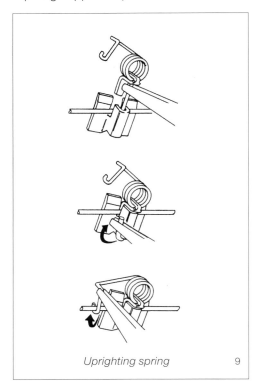

Uprighting spring   9

Z-spring (Recurved spring) A spring bent in the form of a "Z," commonly incor-

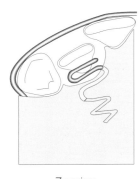

Z-spring

porated into a removable appliance to ti an individual tooth or groups of teeth buc cally or labially.

Orthodontic technique See Technique.

Orthodontic tooth movement Movement (a tooth under the influence of a mechanica force. Orthodontic tooth movement is po sible because of the regenerative an remodeling capacity of the alveolar bon and the periodontal ligament. The mecha nism regulating the transduction of mechanical stimulus into specific cellula activity is not yet entirely understood. Th types of orthodontic tooth movement gen erally are classified as follows:

Extrusion A translational type of toot movement parallel to the long axis of th tooth in the direction of the occlusal plane

Intrusion A translational type of toot movement parallel to the long axis of th tooth in an apical direction.

Pure crown movement The type (tooth movement for which the center (rotation is at the apex of a tooth. [Note: th term is somewhat misleading, as this type (movement also affects part of the root.]

Pure root movement The type of toot movement for which the center of rotatic is at the incisal edge (or for all practical pu poses, at the bracket) of a tooth. For a average maxillary central incisor with intac periodontium the M/F ratio for this type (movement is estimated to be 12:1 to 13: Pure root movement is the intended typ of movement when "torquing" incisc teeth, when uprighting canine roots follov ing extraction space closure, or whe uprighting mesially tipped molars. [Note the term is somewhat misleading, as th type of movement also affects part of th crown.]

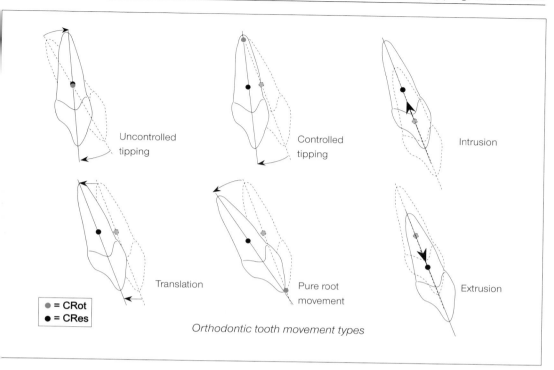

Orthodontic tooth movement types

Pure rotation Rotation of a tooth about its long axis, most evident when viewing the tooth from an occlusal perspective. To achieve this type of tooth movement, the application of a couple is required.

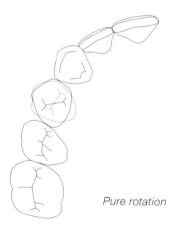

Pure rotation

Tipping, Controlled A type of tooth movement consisting of rotation about the apex of the tooth. It is achieved clinically by the application of a force at the level of the bracket (as in uncontrolled tipping) as well as a counter-moment to prevent movement of the root apex in the opposite direction. For an average maxillary central incisor with no periodontal loss, the M/F ratio for controlled tipping is estimated to be between 7:1 and 8:1.

Tipping, Uncontrolled (Simple) A single horizontal force applied to the crown of the tooth at the level of the bracket will cause movement of the crown and the apex of a tooth in opposite directions. The center of rotation for this movement is approximately at (or slightly apical to) the center of resistance of the tooth. This is the simplest type of tooth movement, but it often is undesirable. The moment-to-force ratio for uncontrolled tipping is 0:1 (no counter-moment is applied, but only a single force).

Translation (Bodily movement) The type of tooth movement during which all points on a tooth move in the same direction by the same amount. During bodily movement, the center of rotation can be assumed to lie at infinity. A single force passing through the center of resistance can produce translation of a tooth along its line of action. Alternatively, a force and a (counter-)moment have to be applied at the bracket of a tooth. For an average maxillary central incisor tooth with intact periodontium, a moment-to-force ratio of approximately 10:1 at the level of the bracket is typical of translation.

Orthodontic tooth movement rate See Rate of orthodontic tooth movement.

Orthodontic wire In orthodontics, wires of various alloys having various cross-sectional shapes and dimensions are used. Some characteristic ones are described below:

Australian wire A round austenitic stainless steel wire, introduced by the A.J. Wilcock Co. in Australia, and selected by P.R. Begg as the main material from which archwires were made for his light-wire technique. The wire is heat-treated and cold-drawn down to its proper diameter from round wire of larger diameter. It exhibits high toughness and tensile strength, combined with increased resilience, but low corrosion resistance because of the presence of copper as an alloying element of the steel. There are various grades of Australian wire, but Begg mainly used the 0.016-inch (0.41-mm), so-called "Special Plus" wire. Another characteristic of the wire is its brittleness. It is recommended that when bending Australian wire, the flat rather than the round beak of the pliers be used and that the bend be placed very slowly, to avoid breakage. Following bending, the archwire can be heat-treated, which makes it harder and more resistant to permanent deformation.

Braided wire See Orthodontic wire, Multistrand.

Coaxial wire See Orthodontic wire, Multistrand.

Elgiloy wire See Cobalt-chromium alloy.

Finishing wire See Archwire, Finishing.

Multiloop wire See Archwire, Multiloop.

Multistrand wire (Braided wire, Coaxial wire) Orthodontic wire fabricated by braiding multiple strands of wire of the same material and usually of the same diameter. This method of combining a number of strands of wire that individually would not be strong enough for a particular application is used to achieve a wire with high flexibility and adequate strength. Multistrand archwires can be round or rectangular and commonly are used for initial alignment.

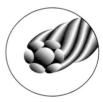

Multistrand wire

Nickel-titanium wire See Nickel-titanium alloy.

Rectangular wire An orthodontic wire with rectangular cross-section. [Also see Archwire cross-section.]

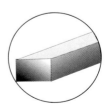

Rectangular wire

Round wire An orthodontic wire with round cross-section. [Also see Archwire cross-section.] *See illustration next page.*

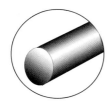

Round wire

Square wire An orthodontic wire with square cross-section. [Also see Archwire cross-section.]

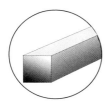

Square wire

Stabilizing wire See Archwire, Stabilizing.

Stainless steel wire See Stainless steel.

TMA wire See Beta-titanium alloy.

Orthodontic wire cross-section See Archwire cross-section.

Orthodontics, American Board of See Board, Orthodontic, American Board of Orthodontics.

Orthodontics and dentofacial orthopedics The area and specialty of dentistry concerned with the supervision, guidance and correction of the growing or mature dentofacial structures, including those conditions that require movement of teeth or correction of malrelationships and malformations of their related structures and the adjustment of relationships between and among teeth and facial bones by the application of forces and/or the stimulation and redirection of functional forces within the craniofacial complex. Major responsibilities of orthodontic practice include the diagno-

sis, prevention, interception and treatment of all forms of malocclusion of the teeth and associated alterations of their surrounding structures; the design, application and control of functional and corrective appliances; and the guidance of the dentition and its supporting structures to attain and maintain optimal occlusal relations, physiologic function and esthetic harmony of facial structures. [Modified from the AAO Glossary of Dentofacial Orthopedic Terms, 1993.]

Orthodontist (Orthodontic specialist) A graduate of an accredited dental school who additionally has followed a postgraduate full-time academic program in orthodontics, in accordance with the requirements of his/her national, state, or provincial law. The duration of the postgraduate orthodontic training varies in different countries or areas of the world. For example, in the USA a two-year full-time academic training beyond general dental school is required to obtain the title of orthodontist, whereas in the European Union the minimum requirement is three years.

Orthodontists, World Federation of See World Federation of Orthodontists.

Orthognathic (Mesognathic) A facial type with normal anteroposterior relationship of the maxilla and mandible in relation to each other and to the cranial base. [See also Facial type.]

Orthognathic surgery Surgical repositioning of all or parts of the maxilla and/or mandible to correct malpositions or deformities. Usually accomplished in conjunction with orthodontic treatment. [Also see Osteotomy.]

Bimaxillary surgery (Two-jaw surgery)
Orthognathic surgical procedure involving repositioning of both the maxilla and the mandible.

Single-jaw surgery (One-jaw surgery)
Orthognathic surgical procedure during

which either the mandible or the maxilla are surgically repositioned.

Orthopantomogram (OPT)   See Panoramic radiograph.

Orthopedic   Attempting to correct abnormal form or relationship of bone structures.

Orthopedic appliance   See Appliance, Orthopedic.

Orthopedic force   See Force, Orthopedic.

Orthopedics, Dentofacial   See Orthodontics and dentofacial orthopedics.

Orthopedics, Presurgical infant   See Presurgical infant orthopedics.

OSA   See Obstructive sleep apnea.

Osseointegrated implant   See Osseointegration.

Osseointegration   A direct structural connection between bone and the surface of an implant. The host bone responds in a safe, predictable and versatile manner to the placement of an implant, with a healing cascade leading to interfacial osteogenesis and immobility of the implant.

Osseous   Bony.

Ossification   Formation and development of bone. Histologically two types of ossification are distinguished: endochondral and intramembranous.

   Endochondral ossification   Bone formation taking place on a cartilage matrix; the cartilage immediately preceding bone in development. This type of ossification occurs embryologically as the chondrocranium ossifies at the epiphyses of all long bones, vertebrae and ribs, at the head of the mandibular condyle, and at the synchondroses of the base of the skull.

Intramembranous ossification   Bone formation directly within a connective tissue membrane, without any intermediate formation of cartilage. This type of ossification occurs embryonically at many sites, such as the cranial vault, the maxilla, the body of the mandible, and at the diaphyses (mid shaft) of long bones, initially by proliferation and condensation of mesenchymal cells. As vascularity increases at these sites of condensed mesenchyme, osteoblasts differentiate and begin to produce bone matrix de novo.

Ostectomy   Surgical removal of a bone, or part of a bone.

Osteoarthritis (Degenerative joint disease, DJD, Degenerative arthritis)   Chronic disease resulting in joint deformity caused by degenerative changes in the articular cartilage, fibrous connective tissue and/or disc. In its late stage it is accompanied by proliferation of new bony tissue at the margins of the joint surface, known as marginal osteophytes, lipping, spurs, or ridges. The fibrillation and breakdown of cartilage is not an inflammatory process, but the breakdown is accompanied by inflammation. The most common etiologic factor that either causes or contributes to osteoarthritis is overloading of the joint structures. In the case of the TMJ it often is painful, and symptoms are accentuated by jaw movement. Crepitation is a common finding.

Osteoarthrosis   Chronic non-inflammatory joint disorder characterized by progressive deterioration and loss of articular cartilage and subchondral bone.

Osteoblast   Uninucleated cell that synthesizes both collagenous and noncollagenous bone proteins (the organic matrix, osteoid). Osteoblasts are responsible for mineralization and are thought to derive from multipotent mesenchymal cells or, alternatively, from perivascular cells. The osteoblast generally is considered to differentiate through a precursor cell, the preosteoblast.

Osteoblasts secrete, in addition to Type I and Type V collagen, small amounts of several noncollagenous proteins and a variety of cytokines. Under physiologic conditions supporting resorption rather than formation of bone, osteoblasts can be stimulated by lymphokines and by prostaglandins to produce interleukin 6, a factor that increases the resorbing activity of the osteoclast.

steoclast Large multinucleated type of cell involved in the degradation and removal of hard tissue. Osteoclasts are derived from monocytes and typically are found against the bone surface, occupying shallow depressions called *Howship's lacunae.* To break down hard tissue, osteoclasts attach to mineralized tissue and create a sealed environment that is first acidified to cause demineralization. Following that, the organic matrix is broken down through the secretion of proteolytic enzymes.

steoconductive material A material that acts as a scaffold for new bone formation. [Compare with Osteoinductive material.]

steocyte As osteoblasts secrete bone matrix, some of them become entrapped in bone and are then called osteocytes. The number of osteoblasts that become osteocytes depends on the rate of bone formation: the more rapid the formation, the more osteocytes are present per unit volume. As a general rule, embryonic (woven) bone has more osteocytes than does lamellar bone.

steogenesis imperfecta As a diagnostic term, osteogenesis imperfecta represents a heterogeneous group of inherited disorders characterized by defects in both mineralized and non-mineralized connective tissues, resulting from mutations in Type I collagen. Males and females are affected equally, and the incidence is between 1 in 5,000 and 1 in 14,000 live births. The classification of the clinical features of the various types of osteogenesis imperfecta according to D.O. Sillence is as follows:

Type I: Normal stature, increased frequency of fractures prior to puberty and after menopause, little or no deformity following fracture repair, hearing loss in about 50% of families, blue sclerae, dentinogenesis imperfecta is uncommon.

Type II: Death in the perinatal period due to extreme bone fragility, poor mineralization of the calvarium, intrauterine fractures of endochondral and membranous bones, blue/black sclerae in virtually all affected individuals, long bone and rib deformities.

Type III: Short stature, characteristic facies, long bone deformity following fracture repair, scoliosis, dentinogenesis imperfecta common, hearing loss common, scleral discoloration variable, reduced lifespan.

Type IV: Mild to moderate short stature, mild to moderate long bone deformity following fracture repair, normal scleral hue, dentinogenesis imperfecta is common, hearing loss occurs in some families.

Osteoinductive material A material that causes the conversion of mesenchymal cells into bone progenitor cells. [Compare with Osteoconductive material.]

Osteomyelitis Inflammation of bone, especially of the marrow, caused by pathogenic organisms.

Osteophyte Bony outgrowth. Marginal adaptation of a joint, formed by bony tissue. In the case of the TMJ, the anterior aspect of the mandibular condyle (in the region of the attachment of the lateral pterygoid muscle) is a relatively common location where osteophytes can be found.

Osteotomy Surgical procedure involving the cutting of bone. Some commonly encountered types of osteotomies in orthognathic procedures are:

Anterior maxillary segmental (subapical) osteotomy Osteotomy of the anterior maxillary segment, usually from canine to canine, with displacement in a posterior, inferior, superior or rotational manner. Most commonly a combination of posterior and

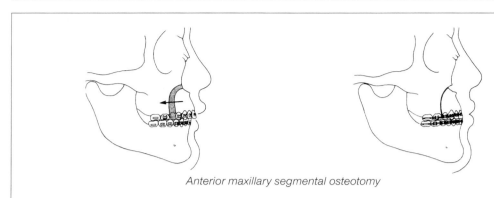

Anterior maxillary segmental osteotomy   4

inferior repositioning of the anterior segment is performed, into the space created by simultaneous extraction of the maxillary first premolars. Anterior repositioning of the segment is almost impossible because of difficulties in stabilization and fixation, even with bone grafting, and because the soft tissue pedicles often are insufficient to cover the surgical defects. The most popular techniques for this type of osteotomy are the Wassmund and Wunderer technique:

Wassmund technique An approach t anterior maxillary segmental osteotom described by M. Wassmund (1927), whic relies on maintaining both the labial an palatal pedicles for vascular supply to th anterior maxillary segment. The osteo tomies are carried out through mucosal tu nels created on the vestibular side by ver cal incisions at the midline and at the lev

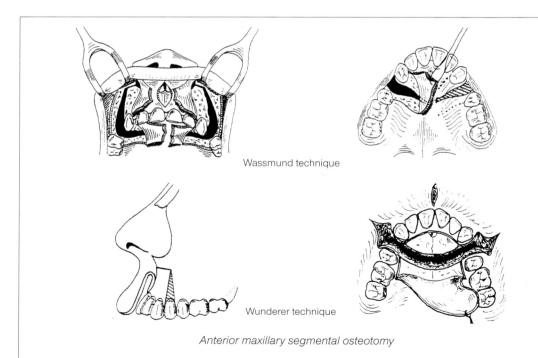

Wassmund technique

Wunderer technique

Anterior maxillary segmental osteotomy   14

of the first premolar and through palatal tunnels created by connecting the extraction sockets of the first premolars to a midpalatal incision.

Wunderer technique An alternative approach to anterior maxillary segmental osteotomy described by S. Wunderer (1963). The technique relies on the vestibular pedicle for vascular supply to the anterior maxillary segment, together with some blood supply from the incisive canal. Bilateral vertical incisions are performed on the vestibular side at the level of the first premolars. These are connected by a transpalatal horizontal incision, allowing reflection of the palatal flap posteriorly.

Bilateral sagittal split osteotomy (BSSO)
A mandibular orthognathic surgical procedure first reported in the English literature by R. Trauner and H.L. Obwegeser (1957), and subsequently modified by others. In this procedure the rami of the mandible are split parallel with the sagittal plane to allow repositioning of the mandibular body into a more favorable relationship with the maxilla and the face. The procedure currently is routinely performed through an intraoral approach and can be used for advancement, setback and rotation of the distal (mandibular) segment. [Also see Segment, Distal; Segment, Proximal.]

When the distal segment is advanced, a gap is created in the buccal plate. When it is set back, a section of the buccal plate is

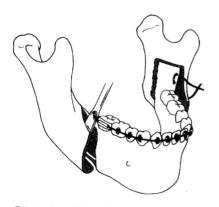

Bilateral sagittal split osteotomy   6

removed to allow good approximation of the buccal cortex of the proximal segment against the lingual cortex of the distal segment on each side. The osteotomy design spares the mandibular nerve and provides a broad interface of the bony segments to aid with fixation and healing. Fixation is achieved by bone screws or bone plates, or through circumosseous fixation wires in combination with IMF.

Complete maxillary osteotomy
Maxillary osteotomies traditionally are described in comparison with the common fracture patterns of the midfacial skeleton, named after the work of R. Le Fort (1900). The Le Fort I, II and III fractures indicate the general levels at which the maxilla may be sectioned selectively from the rest of the skull, although the osteotomies are tailored to the individual patients and may deviate from the known fracture patterns.

Le Fort I osteotomy The most frequently performed of all midfacial osteotomies. It sections the midface through the walls of the maxillary sinuses, the lateral nasal walls and the nasal septum, at a level just superior to the apices of the maxillary teeth. Starting at the inferior-lateral margin of the pyriform aperture of the nose, the osteotomy line traverses the lateral walls of the maxillary sinus approximately 3 to 4 mm above the apices of the canine, premolars and molars. It passes across the canine fossa to the base of the zygomatic buttress and curves around and above the maxillary tuberosity to the lowest part of the pterygomaxillary fissure, where it crosses the posterior wall of the sinus at the same level. It then turns anteriorly through the lateral wall of the nose below the inferior turbinate to join the point of origin. The cut is made bilaterally. Following this, the pterygomaxillary plates are separated from the posterior aspects of the maxillary tuberosities, and the nasal septum is detached from the superior aspect of the hard palate by dividing it along its length with a chisel, so that the maxillary segment is freed. The Le Fort I osteotomy offers a great number of options as the freed maxilla can

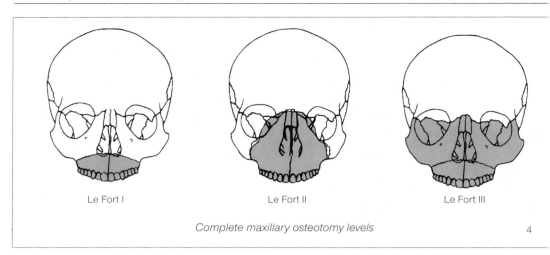

Le Fort I   Le Fort II   Le Fort III

Complete maxillary osteotomy levels

4

be reoriented in all spatial planes. Further segmentation of the maxilla can be performed to correct transverse, anteroposterior and vertical discrepancies between the maxilla and the mandible.

Le Fort II osteotomy A pyramid-shaped osteotomy that is identical to the Le Fort I procedure from the pterygoid column to the zygomatic buttress. From that point, instead of continuing anteriorly to the pyriform aperture of the nose, the cut is directed superiorly, towards the orbit. The cut is kept anteromedial to the infraorbital foramen and crosses the inferior orbital margin at a point halfway between the lacrimal duct medially and the infraorbital canal laterally. It then is continued posteriorly along the floor of the orbit and at right angles to the orbital rim until past the lacrimal groove and its contained lacrimal sac. The cut then is turned medially and anteriorly across the apex of the lacrimal groove and emerges medially to the orbit, just below the midpoint of the medial canthal attachment. The frontal process of the maxilla then is crossed and the cut becomes continuous with the osteotomy of the other side across the nasal bones. The nasal septum is divided at a higher level than during the Le Fort I osteotomy, passing from the nasal bones anteriorly in a downward and backward direction to the posterior part of the septum just above the

posterior nasal spine. The lateral nasal wall are fractured during mobilization of the maxilla at levels corresponding to the septal cut

Le Fort III osteotomy The basic Le Fort I osteotomy, as originally described by F Tessier (1971), was designed to achiev anteroposterior movement of the whol facial mass, establishing normal denta occlusion and increasing orbital capacit enlarging both the height and the depth c the orbits. The aim is to separate the facia mass from the cranial base along the inte frontofacial and the inter-pterygomaxillar planes. To do this, the osteotomy traverses on each side, the medial orbital wall, th orbital floor and the lateral orbital wall t reach the region of the frontozygomati suture. The frontal process of the zygoma ic bone then is split sagittally (effectivel splitting the lateral wall of the orbit) an the cut is continued inferiorly to complet division of the zygoma. The two sides ar connected centrally through the frontona sal area, as in the Le Fort II osteotomy Pterygomaxillary and septal separation the are completed as in the Le Fort II operatio and the central facial block is mobilized.

Many variants of Le Fort III procedures exis that can be applied in the treatment of a var ety of craniofacial problems and can b combined with surgery of the cranial vault

Küfner osteotomy A modification of th

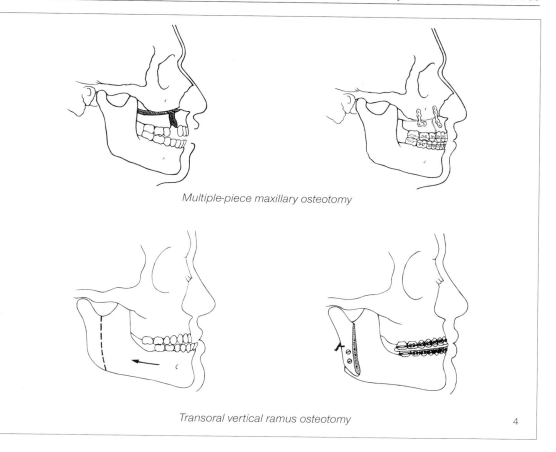

Multiple-piece maxillary osteotomy

Transoral vertical ramus osteotomy

4

Le Fort II osteotomy originally described by J. Küfner (1971). It is intended for patients with good nasal bridge and projection, but exhibiting retrusion of the infraorbital region and maxillary dentoalveolar area, with zygomatic flatness. The difference is that the osteotomy does not involve the nasal bridge, but is extended laterally to include the infraorbital rim and zygomatic process.

Cortical osteotomy See Corticotomy.

Multiple-piece maxillary osteotomy
When a severe transverse discrepancy between the maxillary and mandibular arches exists, a two- or a three- and sometimes even a four-piece maxillary procedure is performed, following a Le Fort I osteotomy, to reposition each segment separately

to an ideal relationship with the mandibular arch. Due to the increased risks entailed in the segmental procedures, most clinicians prefer to limit the number of segments into which they divide the maxilla. [Compare with Osteotomy, One-piece maxillary.]

One-piece maxillary osteotomy (Single-piece maxillary osteotomy, Total maxillary osteotomy) Any osteotomy that mobilizes the maxilla as a whole. [Compare with Osteotomy, Multiple-piecemaxillary.]

Transoral vertical ramus osteotomy (TOVRO, Intraoral vertical ramus Osteotomy, IVRO) A vertical osteotomy of the mandibular ramus performed via a transoral approach for correction of mandibular prognathism. It commonly is carried out in conjunction with a coronoidectomy. The coronoid fragment with attached temporalis tendon is allowed to retract. The line of the osteotomy extends from an area in front of the condyle to a point at or near the angle of the mandible.

This osteotomy is reserved for patients who require a mandibular setback, as it necessitates full-thickness overlap between the mandibular segments. After the setback the condylar segment lies laterally to the distal mandibular segment. Stabilization can be provided by a circumramus suture or wire, by rigid fixation screws, or alternatively no stabilization is used. In the latter case, patients are left in intermaxillary fixation for 4 to 6 weeks. The TOVRO is advocated to be less likely than the BSSO to produce neurosensory changes.

Outer bow See Facebow (of a headgear).

Overbite (Vertical overbite) The degree of vertical overlap of the mandibular incisors by their maxillary antagonists, usually measured perpendicular to the occlusal plane. It is reported either in millimeters, or as a percentage of the total crown length of the mandibular incisors that is overlapped by the maxillary incisors. [Compare with Overjet.]

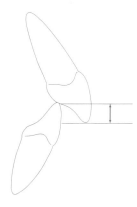

Overbite

Impinging overbite Extremely deep bite with impingement of the mandibular in-

cisors in the mucosa palatal to the maxilla incisors; commonly seen in patients wi severe Class II, Division 2 malocclusions.

Negative overbite See Open bite.

Positive overbite A term indicating th presence of vertical overlap between th maxillary and mandibular anterior teet Positive overbite is a characteristic of th ideal occlusion, but also of deep bite ma occlusions.

Overclosure Reduced vertical dimensio with the teeth in occlusion.

Overcorrection The notion of continuir a certain type of treatment even after an ide relationship has been achieved, in anticip tion of some degree of relapse after the er of active treatment. For example, the ove correction of a typical Class II deep bi malocclusion to an end-to-end anterior rel tionship sometimes is advocated.

Overeruption (Supraeruption, Suprap sition, Supraocclusion) The situatic whereby an unopposed or non-occludir tooth extends beyond the occlusal plane.

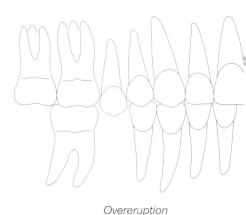

Overeruption

Overjet (Sagittal overbite) The distanc between the labial surface of the mandib lar incisors and the labial aspect of the incis edge of the maxillary incisors, usually me

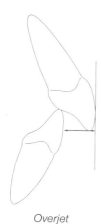

Overjet

sured parallel to the occlusal plane. When not otherwise specified, the term is generally assumed to refer to the most prominent central incisors.

The extent of overjet is determined primarily by the differences of labiolingual position and inclination of the maxillary and mandibular central incisors. Only in a minority of cases is the anteroposterior skeletal relationship reflected directly in the amount of overjet. [Compare with Overbite.]

Buccal overjet The distance between the buccal surfaces of the maxillary posterior teeth and the buccal surfaces of their mandibular antagonists. An unofficial term

sometimes used to indicate whether or not there is a tendency for a posterior crossbite.

Negative overjet (Reverse overjet) A situation usually associated with Class III malocclusions in which the maxillary incisors occlude lingually to the mandibular incisors.

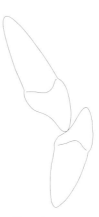

Negative overjet

Positive overjet A term denoting that the maxillary incisors occlude labially to the mandibular incisors, as is seen commonly in Class I or Class II malocclusions.

Overlay archwire See Arch, Overlay.

P

P See Cephalometric landmarks (Hard tissue), Pogonion.

Palatal bar See Arch, Transpalatal.

Palatal crossbite See Crossbite, Palatal.

Palatal plane (ANS-PNS) See Cephalometric lines, Palatal plane.

Palatal rugae The irregular ridges in the masticatory mucosa covering the anterior hard palate.

Palatal sheath See Sheath.

Palatally impinging overbite See Overbite, Impinging.

Palate The structure that serves as the roof of the oral cavity and the floor of the nasal cavity, consisting anteriorly of the hard palate and posteriorly of the soft palate.

Cleft palate See Cleft lip and/or palate.

Hard palate The anterior part of the palate, the osseous framework of which consists of the palatine processes of the maxilla and the horizontal parts of the palatine bones.

Primary palate The embryological structure that forms during the 5th to 7th weeks of human intrauterine life, originating from the fused medial nasal and maxillary processes. The primary palate eventually forms the upper lip, the anterior portion of the maxillary alveolar process and the hard palate anterior to the incisive canal. [Also se Premaxilla.]

Secondary palate The embryologic structure that forms during the 6th–9 weeks of human intrauterine life by fusion the palatine processes (of the maxilla process) at the midline. The anterior parts the palatine processes (palatal shelves) als unite with the nasal septum, eventually form ing the hard palate. In the posterior regio where there is no attachment to the nas septum, the soft palate and uvula eventua ly develop.

Soft palate (Velum) The posterior mobi part of the palate, which is suspended ant riorly from the hard palate. Its sides bler with the pharynx and its posterior portic forms the uvula. In its relaxed position th soft palate is continuous with the roof the mouth. During the process of deglutitic or sucking, as well as during production certain speech sounds, it is elevated, thu separating the nasal cavity and nasophal ynx from the posterior part of the oral cavi and the oral portion of the pharynx.

Palate-splitting appliance See Applianc Haas; Appliance, Hyrax.

Palpation Examination by feeling with one hands; assessment by means of tactile pe ception.

Panoramic radiograph (Orthopantome gram, OPT, "Pan") A radiographic tome gram of the jaws, taken with a specialize machine designed to present a panoramic view of the full circumferential length of the jaws on a single film. Both the film and x-ray machine are located extraorally. When obtaining a radiograph the entire source/film assembly rotates around the patient's head. At the same time, the x-ray source and the film rotate about their own vertical axes in opposite directions to each other. A slit guard present in front of the film allows it to be exposed a portion at a time, so a continuous depiction of bilateral maxillofacial structures is possible on the same film.

The advantage of the technique is that many structures can be seen on one radiograph, reducing radiation exposure. The disadvantages are reduced detail, image distortion, and routine exposure of structures that are not of immediate interest.

[Also known by several proprietary brand names of machines, most of which include "pan" as a part of the name.]

Pantograph A tracking device attached to the mandible and maxilla that enables recording of mandibular movements in three planes of space.

Papilla, Interdental See Interdental papilla.

PAR (Peer assessment rating) index See Index, Peer assessment rating.

Parafunction (Parafunctional activity, Parafunctional habit) Non-physiological activity, including clenching and bruxing, nail-biting, and lip- or cheek-chewing.

Parallel-action pliers (Sargent pliers) See Orthodontic instruments, Parallel-action pliers with cutter.

Parallelism of roots See Root parallelism.

Parasagittal plane See Sagittal plane.

Paresthesia Diminished or abnormal sensation, such as burning, prickling, tingling, or numbness; a common finding following

orthognathic surgery. Almost all patients have some degree of paresthesia of the lower lip over the distribution of the mental nerve immediately following mandibular ramus surgery (e.g. bilateral sagittal split osteotomy). Return of sensation may be rapid, may occur over a few weeks, or may occur gradually over 12 to 18 months. In some instances a permanent degree of paresthesia remains.

Partial glossectomy See Glossotomy.

Partial thickness periodontal graft See Graft, Split thickness periodontal.

Passive torque See Torque, Passive.

Patch of Atherton See Atherton's patch.

Pathognomonic Specifically distinctive characteristic (sign or symptom) of a disease or pathologic condition, on the basis of which a diagnosis of the disease can be made.

Pathologic fracture See Fracture, Pathologic.

Pathologic migration See Migration, Pathologic.

PDGF (Platelet-derived growth factor See Growth factors.

PDL See Periodontal ligament.

Peer assessment rating index See Index, Peer assessment rating.

"Peg-shaped" lateral incisors Atypical, undersized, pointed and tapered crown form of the maxillary permanent lateral incisors.

Pendex appliance See Appliance, Pendulum.

Pendulum appliance See Appliance, Pendulum.

Periapical Pertaining to the area and tissues around the apex of a tooth.

Pericoronitis Acute inflammation of the tissues surrounding the crown of a partially erupted tooth.

Peri-implantitis A term used to describe inflammation around a dental implant.

Perikymata The numerous small transverse ridges and grooves on the surface of the enamel of permanent teeth, representing the rhythmic deposition of enamel. With continued abrasion the surface of the enamel becomes eroded and the perikymata eventually disappear.

Periodontal ligament (PDL) A dense, highly specialized connective tissue situated between the root of a tooth and the alveolar bone. Its principal function is to connect the tooth to the bone while resisting the stress created by the various forces exerted on the teeth. This is achieved by the masses of collagen fiber bundles that follow an undulated course between the bone and the tooth, and by an incompressible gel-like matrix consisting of 70% water (ground substance). The second function of the PDL is to provide sensory input (proprioception) on the level and type of strain that it experiences, partially through specialized sensory receptors. Other than fibers and ground substance, the PDL contains many cells (mainly fibroblasts, epithelial cells and undifferentiated mesenchymal cells), blood vessels and nerves.
Fibers of the PDL The majority of fibers of the periodontal ligament are collagen fibers, mainly a mixture of Type I and Type III. The greatest proportion of the collagen fibers in the PDL are arranged in definite and distinct fiber bundles.
The principal groups of bundles are as follows:
1. The alveolar crest group, attached to the cementum just below the cementoenamel junction and running downward to insert into the rim of the alveolus.

2. The horizontal group, occurring just apical to the alveolar crest group and running at right angles to the long axis of the tooth from cementum to bone just below the alveolar crest.
3. The oblique group, by far the most numerous in the PDL, running from the cementum in an oblique direction, to insert into bone coronally.
4. The apical group, radiating from the cementum around the apex of the root to the bone, forming the base of the socket.
5. The interradicular group, found only between the roots of multirooted teeth and running from the cementum into the bone, forming the crest of the interradicular septum.
At each end, all the principal fibers of the PDL are embedded in cementum or bone. The embedded portion is called a *Sharpey's fiber*.
Other than collagen, the PDL also contains some elastic fibers, consisting of two types of immature elastin, namely oxytalan and eluanin.
Width of the PDL In humans the width of the PDL ranges from 0.15 to 0.38 mm, with its narrowest aspect at the middle third of the root and its widest aspect cervically. Occlusal loading in function affects the width of the PDL. If occlusal forces are within physiologic limits, increased function leads to an increase in width through a thickening of the fiber bundles and an increase in diameter and number of Sharpey's fibers. Unphysiologic situations such as traumatic occlusion typically cause widening of the PDL. Conversely, when function is diminished or absent, the width of the PDL decreases. The fibers are reduced in number and density and they show a tendency to become oriented parallel to the root surface. A widening of the PDL also typically is associated with active orthodontic tooth movement.

Periodontal membrane See Periodontal ligament.

Periodontal trauma See Occlusal trauma.

Periodontitis Inflammation of the supporting tissues of the teeth. Usually a progressive destructive change leading to loss of bone and periodontal ligament.

Periodontium The investing and supporting tissues surrounding the teeth, including the periodontal ligament, alveolar bone and gingiva.

Permanent deformation See Deformation, Permanent.

Permanent dentition See Dentition, Permanent.

Permanent retainer See Retainer, Fixed.

Perpetuating factors Factors that interfere with resolution of, or enhance the progression of, a disease or disorder.

Pg See Cephalometric landmarks (Hard tissue), Pogonion.

Pg' See Cephalometric landmarks (Soft tissue), Soft tissue pogonion.

PG's See Prostaglandins.

PG spring See Orthodontic springs, PG spring.

Pharyngeal flap operation A surgical procedure for lengthening the soft palate by attaching a flap from the posterior pharyngeal wall to it. Depending on the way that the pharyngeal flap is raised, a superiorlybased and an inferiorlybased pharyngeal flap can be distinguished. [Also see Hypernasality; Velopharyngeal insufficiency.]

Philosophy (of treatment) See Treatment philosophy.

Philtral columns Normal ridges in the skin of the central portion of the upper lip, extending bilaterally from the vermilion border of the upper lip to the columella of the nose, and containing the philtrum.

Photoelasticity Engineering technique of stress analysis based on the property of some transparent materials to exhibit patterns of color when viewed with polarized light. These patterns occur as the result of alteration of the polarized light by the internal stresses into waves that travel at different velocities. The patterns that develop consequently are related to the distribution of internal stresses and are called the *photoelastic effect*. A research technique with many orthodontic applications.

Photographic subtraction radiography See Subtraction radiography, Photographic.

Physiologic force See Force, Physiologic.

Physiologic migration See Drift (of teeth).

Physiologic mobility (of the teeth) See Tooth mobility, Physiologic.

Physiologic rest position (of the mandible) The mandibular position assumed when the head is in an upright position and the involved muscles, particularly the elevator and depressor groups, are in equilibrium in tonic contraction, and the condyles are in a neutral, unstrained position.

Physiologic tooth movement Movement of the teeth taking place as part of the natural process from their early stages of development until they become functional at the level of the occlusal plane, and extending to the end of their lifespan in the mouth. The movements teeth make are complex and may be distinguished as *pre-eruptive*, *eruptive* and *post-eruptive*. Superimposed on these is a progression from deciduous to permanent dentition, involving the exfoliation of the deciduous dentition. This categorization of tooth movement merely serves descriptive purposes; it must be recognized that what is being described is a continuous series of events.

Eruptive tooth movement This includes *pre-emergent* and *post-emergent* tooth movement. The mechanism of eruption of deciduous and permanent teeth is thought to be similar, bringing about the axial and occlusal movement of the tooth from its developmental position within the jaw to its final functional position within the occlusal plane. Pre-emergent tooth movement seems to be controlled by a different mechanism than post-emergent tooth movement.

Eruptive movement begins soon after the root begins to form. The PDL also develops only after root formation has been initiated, and once established, it must be remodeled to permit eruptive tooth movement. The remodeling of the PDL fiber bundles is achieved by fibroblasts, which simultaneously degrade and synthesize the collagen fibers as required across the entire extent of the ligament. As the tooth moves occlusally, bone is resorbed occlusal to it and new bone is formed apical to the tooth.

At the time of emergence of the tooth into the oral cavity, its dental follicle fuses with the oral epithelium. Following emergence the tooth erupts rapidly until it approaches the occlusal level (*post-emergent spurt*). Environmental factors such as muscle forces from the tongue, cheeks and lips, as well as forces of contact of the erupting tooth with other erupted teeth [also see "Cone-funnel" mechanism], help determine the final position of the tooth in the dental arch. The effect of thumbsucking on the dentition is an obvious example of environmental determination of tooth position. [See also Post-emergent spurt.]

Post-eruptive tooth movement   Movement of the teeth after they have reached · their functional position in the occlusal plane. The same mechanisms that control post-emergent tooth movement seem to regulate post-eruptive tooth movement in the vertical plane. Post-eruptive tooth movement can be divided into three categories:

1. Vertical movement occurring in concert with jaw growth (*juvenile occlusal equilibrium*). This movement is completed toward the end of the second decade, when jaw growth ceases, and it occurs earlier in girls than in boys. It is related to the growth of the mandibular ramus, which causes the maxilla and mandible to grow apart from each other, permitting further eruptive movement of the teeth. [Also see Occlusal equilibrium, Juvenile.]

2. Movement to compensate for the continuous occlusal wear of the teeth (*adult occlusal equilibrium*). This axial post-eruptive movement occurs even after the apices of the teeth are fully formed. It is demonstrable by the tendency of teeth to overerupt when their antagonist is lost, at any age. [Also see Occlusal equilibrium, Adult.]

3. Movement to compensate for interproximal wear. Wear also occurs at the contact points between teeth on their proximal surfaces, and its extent can be considerable (more than 7 mm in the mandibular dental arch). This interproximal wear is compensated for by a process known as *mesial drift*. The mechanism of this mesial drift is multifactorial and is attributed to the anterior component of the occlusal force, to contraction of the transseptal fibers and/or pressure from the perioral and intraoral soft tissues (cheeks and tongue). [Also see Mesial drift.]

Pre-eruptive tooth movement   Movement of the deciduous and permanent tooth germs within the tissues of the jaw before they begin to erupt. As the deciduous tooth germs grow, the space for them in the developing jaw becomes less, and initially they are "crowded" in the anterior region. This "crowding" usually is alleviated before emergence by growth of the jaws, mainly in the midline, which permits mesial movement of the anterior tooth germs.

The deciduous molar germs gradually increase in size and become displaced distally in association with sagittal growth of the jaws. At the same time, the tooth germs are moving occlusally with the increase in height of the jaws. The permanent anterior tooth germs initially develop on the lingual aspect of their predecessors. From this position they shift considerably as the jaws develop

op (e.g. the incisors eventually come to occupy a position on the lingual aspect of the roots of their predecessors, and the premolar germs are positioned between the divergent roots of the deciduous molars).
In the maxilla, the permanent molar germs initially develop with their occlusal surfaces facing distally, and swing into position only when the maxilla has grown sufficiently to provide space for such movement. In the mandible, the permanent molars develop with their axes showing a mesial inclination, which gradually becomes more vertical.

Physiological occlusion See Occlusion, Functional.

Pierre Robin sequence See Robin sequence.

Piggyback archwire See Arch, Overlay.

"Pigtail" The twisted, cut end of a stainless steel ligature or brass separator that is tucked under the archwire, under a bracket wing, or in the interproximal area for patient comfort.

"Pigtail" attachment (Coil eyelet) A small orthodontic attachment consisting of a pigtail-shaped wire soldered onto a bonding base. "Pigtail" attachments are used mainly as handles for elastic traction. [Also see Attachment, Orthodontic.]

Pin T-shaped orthodontic auxiliary, used mainly in the Begg technique and its modifications. The pins are inserted in the vertical slots of the brackets, and their primary purpose is to retain the archwire in the main slot.

Bi-level pin Used to create an additional slot for a second archwire, which can be inserted between the bi-level pin and the gingival tie-wing of the bracket.

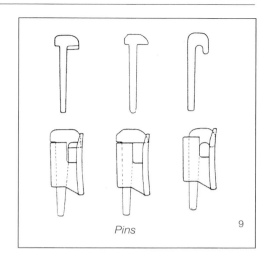

Pins 9

Power pin Used as an attachment to anchor orthodontic elastic bands for the application of traction.

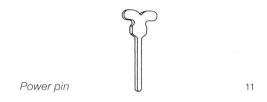

Power pin 11

Pin and ligature wire cutter See Orthodontic instruments, Pin and ligature wire cutter.

Pin-and-tube appliance See Appliance, Pin-and-tube.

Pitchfork instrument See Orthodontic instruments, Ligature director.

Pitting corrosion See Corrosion, Pitting.

PL See Proportional limit.

Placebo Inactive substance, device or measure that is believed by the patient to have an active therapeutic value, but in fact, does not. Placebos sometimes are used in controlled studies to determine the effect of drugs without the influence of bias.

Placebo effect Physical or psychological change in a patient occurring after the administration of a placebo, not directly attributable to any specific property or effect of the substance or therapeutic measure.

Plagiocephalic An individual with an asymmetric skull shape. Plagiocephaly may be produced by unilateral synostosis of the coronal or the lambdoidal suture. [Compare with Trigonocephalic.]

Planar scintigraphy See Emission scintigraphy.

Plaque (Dental plaque, Bacterial plaque) A soft, thin film of adherent non-calcified deposits on the tooth surface that are composed of microorganisms embedded in a matrix formed of bacterial products, salivary constituents and inorganic compounds. The pathogenic microorganisms within the plaque are involved in the etiology of both dental caries and periodontal disease.

Plaster casts (Plaster models) See Orthodontic casts.

Plastic behavior The behavior of a material after its elastic or proportional limit is exceeded.

Plastic bracket See Bracket, Plastic.

Plastic deformation See Deformation, Permanent.

Plate A non-specific term implying a removable orthodontic appliance constructed at least partially of acrylic.

Platelet-derived growth factor (PDGF) See Growth factors.

Platybasia A term denoting a more obtuse than normal cranial base angle (saddle angle, BaSN). [Compare with Basilar kyphosis.]

"Play" of an orthodontic wire in the bracket slot The amount of freedom allowed at the bracket-to-wire interface due to the difference in size between the wire and the bracket slot. The amount of "play" varies depending on the relative size of the bracket and wire and refers to the type of individual movement intended (usually a distinction is made between second-order and third-order clearance). For example, to achieve a certain amount of torquing movement of an individual tooth, more activation (in degrees) is necessary when using a 0.016 x 0.022-inch (0.41 x 0.56-mm) archwire, compared to using an 0.018 x 0.025 inch (0.46 x 0.64-mm) archwire, because of the increased torsional play in the former case. [Also see Second-order clearance, Third-order clearance.]

Pletcher spring See Orthodontic springs, Coil spring, Retraction.

Plication The stitching of folds or tucks in a tissue to reduce its size, as in the retrodiscal tissue of the temporomandibular joint, in an attempt to reposition an anteriorly displaced articular disc and re-establish a physiologic anatomic disc-to-condyle relationship. A type of disc-repositioning surgery.

Plunger cusp See Cusp, Plunger.

Pn See Cephalometric landmarks (Soft tissue), Pronasale.

PNS See Cephalometric landmarks (Hard tissue), Posterior nasal spine.

Po See Cephalometric landmarks (Hard tissue), Porion.

Pog See Cephalometric landmarks (Hard tissue), Pogonion.

Pog' See Cephalometric landmarks (Soft tissue), Soft tissue pogonion.

Pogonion (Pog, P, Pg) See Cephalometric landmarks (Hard tissue), Pogonion.

Point A See Cephalometric landmarks (Hard tissue), A-point.

Point of application One of the four characteristics of vectorial quantities (the other three are *line of action, sense* and *magnitude*). The point on a body where the vector is applied.

Point B See Cephalometric landmarks (Hard tissue), B-point.

Point of dissociation See Burstone's geometry classes, Geometry IV.

Point L See Cephalometric landmarks (Hard tissue), L-point.

Point R See Cephalometric landmarks (Hard tissue), R-point.

Polishing of enamel See Prophylaxis.

Polytetrafluoroethylene (PTFE) See Teflon.

Pontic The part of a restoration that replaces a missing natural tooth.

Porion (Po) See Cephalometric landmarks (Hard tissue), Porion.

Porter arch See Arch, Porter.

Position screw See Fixation screws, Bicortical.

Positioner (Tooth positioner) See Appliance, Positioner.

Positive overbite See Overbite, Positive.

Positive overjet See Overjet, Positive.

Post-emergence eruption See Physiologic tooth movement, Eruptive.

Post-emergent spurt The phase of relatively rapid eruptive movement, from the time a tooth first penetrates the gingiva until it reaches the occlusal level. [See also Physiologic tooth movement; compare with Occlusal equilibrium.]

Posterior attachment (of the articular disc) See Retrodiscal tissue.

Posterior band-removing pliers See Orthodontic instruments, Band-removing pliers.

Posterior bite collapse See Bite collapse.

Posterior crossbite See Crossbite, Posterior.

Posterior debanding pliers See Orthodontic instruments, Band-removing pliers.

Posterior facial height See Cephalometric measurements (Hard tissue), Facial height.

Posterior lower face height See Cephalometric measurements (Hard tissue), Facial height.

Posterior nasal spine (PNS) See Cephalometric landmarks (Hard tissue), Posterior nasal spine.

Posterior non-occlusion See Non-occlusion, Posterior.

Posterior open bite See Open bite.

Posterior rotation (of the mandible) See Mandibular rotation, Clockwise.

Posterior teeth The maxillary and mandibular deciduous molars, premolars and permanent molars.

Posteroanterior cephalometric radiograph See Cephalometric radiograph, Posteroanterior.

Post-eruptive tooth movement See Physiologic tooth movement, Post-eruptive.

Postnormal occlusion See Angle classification, Class II malocclusion.

Postural Related to position.

Postural rest position See Physiologic rest position.

Power arm Extension arm, rigidly fixed on the distogingival or mesiogingival wing of a bracket (most commonly on the canines) to facilitate the application of the force closer to the center of resistance of the tooth during retraction, to reduce the tendency to tip distally. Power arms also can be used for the attachment of intermaxillary elastics.

Power pin See Pin, Power.

PP See Cephalometric lines, Palatal plane.

PPO See Preferred provider organization.

Pr See Cephalometric landmarks (Hard tissue), Prosthion.

Preadjusted appliance See Appliance, Straight-wire.

Pre-angulated bracket See Bracket, Pre-angulated.

Predisposing factors Factors that increase the risk of developing a disease or condition.

Pre-eruptive tooth movement See Physiologic tooth movement, Pre-eruptive.

Preferred provider organization (PPO) A formal agreement between a purchaser of a health benefits program and a defined group of health care practitioners for the delivery of services to a specific patient population, usually as an adjunct to a traditional plan, using discounted fees for cost savings. Preferred provider organizations provide a reduced fee for each service, rather than a fixed fee for all services. Preferred provider organizations allow treatment by a non-PPO physician or dentist, for a higher fee. [Compare with Health maintenance organization (HMO).] [Modified from the AAO Glossary of Dentofacial Orthopedic Terms, 1993.]

Premature loss Loss of a deciduous tooth prior to its normal time of exfoliation, due to extraction or undue resorption of its root. An example of the latter is the situation in which there is severe lack of space in the dental arch for eruption of a permanent incisor, which sometimes results in resorption of the root of not only its predecessor but also of that of the adjacent deciduous tooth.

Premature occlusal contact See Occlusal interference.

Premaxilla The triangular part of the hard palate anterior to the incisive foramen, including the four maxillary incisor teeth, extending in the midline up to the piriform rim. The premaxilla is derived embryologically from the primary palate. It is a separate bone in most animals; however, in humans it generally is not independent of the maxilla, even in the early developmental stages.

Premaxillary segment See Segment, Premaxillary.

Prenormal occlusion See Angle classification, Class III malocclusion.

Prescription (of an appliance) See Appliance prescription.

Presurgical infant orthopedics (PSIO, Presurgical orthopedic treatment, PSOT, Neonatal maxillary orthopedics) Any orthopedic manipulation of the segments of the clefted maxilla in a newborn with complete unilateral or bilateral CLP aiming at establishing a more normal maxillary alveolar arch form or at retracting a protruding premaxilla to facilitate the surgical repair of the lip. This procedure, the value of which is under investigation, usually involves the use of plates (of various designs) in combination with tapes and/or elastics and is either discontinued at the time of lip repair, or in some centers, continued up until the repair of the palate.

resurgical orthodontic treatment Orthodontic treatment in preparation for an orthognathic surgical procedure. The main aims of this treatment are to harmonize the dental arches in size and form, to level the curve of Spee and most importantly to remove the dentoalveolar compensations, so that the discrepancy at the level of the teeth matches the underlying skeletal discrepancy (thus, the occlusion is made "worse" than in the start of treatment). This decompensation gives the surgeon optimal space for the surgical repositioning of the skeletal segments, which should result in the best correction from the standpoint of facial esthetics. [Also see Dentoalveolar compensation; Decompensation.]

resurgical orthopedic treatment See Presurgical infant orthopedics.

re-torqued bracket See Bracket, Pre-torqued.

retreatment records Any records made for the purpose of diagnosis, recording of the patient's history, or treatment planning in advance of therapy.

revalence The number of cases of any disease or condition for a given area and population at a given point in time, as assembled by a descriptive epidemiological investigation of a retrospective nature. It usually is reported as the percentage of positive cases over the total sample screened and expresses the frequency of the disease or condition. [Compare with Incidence.]

reventive orthodontic treatment Any form of treatment aimed at preventing the development of malocclusion by maintaining the integrity of an otherwise normally developing dentition. Typical examples include slicing of deciduous teeth, space maintainers to replace prematurely lost deciduous teeth, or removal of deciduous teeth that fail to shed physiologically, to allow uninhibited eruption of their successors. [Modified from the AAO Glossary of Dentofacial Orthopedic Terms, 1993.]

Primary cartilage Cartilages such as *Meckel's cartilage* (the cartilage of the first branchial arch) and *Reichert's cartilage* (that of the second branchial arch) that precede secondary cartilage in embryological development and have a different histological structure in comparison to the latter. [Compare with Secondary cartilage.]

Primary crowding See Arch length discrepancy, Arch length deficiency.

Primary dentition See Dentition, Deciduous.

Primary occlusal trauma See Occlusal trauma, Primary.

Primary palate See Palate, Primary.

Primate spaces Spaces between the maxillary lateral incisors and canines and the mandibular canines and first deciduous molars. The primate spaces, as other spaces in the deciduous dentition, normally are present from the time that the teeth erupt. [Note: The name comes from the fact that in most non-human primates these spaces are present throughout life to accommodate the characteristically large canines of the opposing arch when the teeth come into occlusion.]

Proclination Anterior (labial) inclination or tipping of anterior teeth. [Compare with Protrusion.]

Proclination arch See Arch, Stopped.

Profile line of Merrifield (Z-line) See Cephalometric lines, Z-line.

Profile type A classification of the profile into convex, straight or concave, depending on the relative anteroposterior position of the soft tissue glabella, subnasale and soft tissue pogonion points. *See illustration next page.*

Prognathic A term used to indicate the situation in which the mandible or the max-

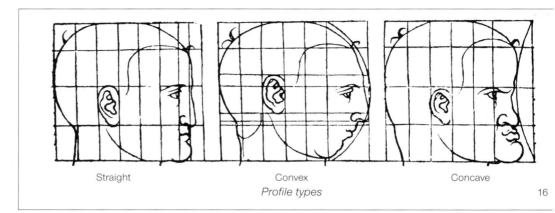

Straight   Convex   Concave

Profile types   16

illa is protrusive (in the anteroposterior plane) in relation to other cranial or facial structures, due to relatively larger size and/or more anterior position. In the classification of facial types, the term is used to connote a prognathic mandible. [See also Facial type; compare with Retrognathic.]

Prognathism   Skeletal protrusion.

Bimaxillary prognathism   Protrusion of both jaws beyond normal limits, in relation to the cranial base and other facial structures.

Mandibular prognathism   Protrusion of the mandible relative to the cranial base and other facial structures, due to a hyperplastic and/or anteriorly positioned mandible.

Maxillary prognathism   Protrusion of the maxilla relative to the cranial base and other facial structures, due to a hyperplastic and/or anteriorly positioned maxilla.

Prognosis   Forecast of the probable course of a disease or a result of therapy.

Progressive posterior torque   See Torque, Progressive posterior.

Prolabium   The central portion of the upper lip, beneath the columella of the nose and

between the philtral columns. The portic of the upper lip that is developed from th primary palate and is part of the premax lary segment in a complete bilateral clet [Also see Segment, Premaxillary.]

Pronasale (Pn)   See Cephalometric land marks (Soft tissue), Pronasale.

Prophylaxis (Polishing of enamel, "Pro phy")   The use of various abrasive mater als such as pumice, silica or zirconium si cate on the enamel to remove plaque, debr and minor exogenous stains from teeth an to produce a smooth, lustrous surface.

Proportional limit (PL)   The point along stress/strain curve beyond which the stres is no longer proportional to strain. Furthe increase of stress past the proportional lim will bring the material to the stage when removal of the stress will not cause complet recovery of the original shape (i.e. residu strain exists). [Compare with Elastic limit.]

Proprioception   A sense providing knowledg of the position of those parts and region of the body containing skeletal muscle: bones and joints. Proprioception als applies to the case of the PDL. [Also se Periodontal ligament.]

Propulsor   See Appliance, Propulsor.

rostaglandins (PG's) Arachidonic acid derivatives that are important mediators of inflammation. Prostaglandins, especially PGE_1 and PGE_2 are thought to play a significant role in orthodontic tooth movement, as they are involved in bone resorption. Research results have shown that local administration of prostaglandins by injection results in acceleration of tooth movement. Acetylsalicylic acid–containing medications that inhibit prostaglandin synthesis are thought to slow down the rate of orthodontic tooth movement.

rosthion (Pr) See Cephalometric landmarks (Hard tissue), Prosthion.

rotective muscle splinting (Reflex muscle splinting) Reflexive contraction of adjacent muscles resulting from a noxious stimulus from a sensory field of a joint, soft tissue, or other structure to prevent movement or provide stabilization of the tissues in the painful area. It differs from muscle spasm in that the contraction is not sustained when the muscle is at rest. [Compare with Muscle spasm.]

roteoglycans A large group of extracellular and cell surface macromolecules that function in regulating cell adhesion, growth, extracellular matrix formation, collagen fibril formation and the binding of growth factors. They are composed of a protein core in which serine-glucine sequences serve as attachment sites for one or more glycosaminoglycan chains.

rotraction (of the maxilla) Orthopedic anterior repositioning of the entire maxillary bone, attempted by extraoral traction appliances such as a face mask. It is reported to be most successful when performed early, and when it is combined with rapid maxillary expansion. Maxillary protraction by distraction osteogenesis also is possible, using intraoral or extraoral devices.

Protraction (of teeth) Anterior (mesial) movement of teeth [usually referring to bodily movement].

Protraction headgear See Appliance, Face mask.

Protrusion The state of being thrust forward, or being anteriorly positioned.

Bimaxillary protrusion See Prognathism, Bimaxillary.

Bimaxillary dentoalveolar (Bialveolar) protrusion Anterior position and labial inclination of the maxillary and mandibular incisors with respect to their supporting bones and the facial profile.

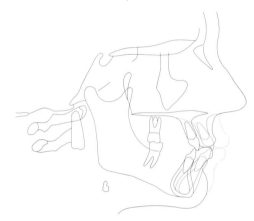

Bimaxillary dentoalveolar protrusion

Dental protrusion Anterior position of a tooth or group of teeth. [Note: The term protrusion does not refer to the inclination of the long axis of the tooth. A tooth can be protrusive but not proclined, if it is positioned too far anteriorly but has a normal inclination.]

Lip protrusion Anterior position of one or both lips relative to the nose and chin or other facial structures.

Protrusion of the mandible See Arthrokinetics of the TMJ.

Protrusive excursion of the mandible See Excursion of the mandible, Protrusive.

Protrusive interference See Occlusal interference, Protrusive.

Proximal Closer to a point of reference.

Proximal segment See Segment, Proximal.

Pseudoankylosis See Adhesion, Intracapsular.

Pseudo-Class III malocclusion An Angle Class III malocclusion caused by an anterior mandibular shift (progenic forced bite) commonly due to an occlusal interference in CO. A functional crossbite also may be present. Treatment usually consists of elimination of the interference by tooth movement or occlusal equilibration. [See also Forced bite, Anterior; Crossbite, Functional; Mandibular shift.]

Pseudocrossbite See Crossbite, Functional.

Pseudoelasticity A non-linear stress-strain behavior of a material during loading and unloading. Often a synonym for superelasticity.

PSIO See Presurgical infant orthopedics.

PSOT See Presurgical infant orthopedics.

Pterygomasseteric sling A structure formed by the combined fibers from the medial pterygoid and masseter muscles, at their attachment on the posterior aspect of the inferior border of the mandible, bilaterally. The pterygomasseteric sling often is stripped away during a BSSO or a TOVRO to increase the potential for stability of the surgical correction, especially in situations where the proximal end of the distal segment is repositioned inferiorly.

Pterygomaxillare See Cephalometric landmarks (Hard tissue), Pterygomaxillary fissure.

Pterygomaxillary disjunction The separation of the maxilla from the pterygoid column (the medial and lateral pterygoid plates) by means of a curved chisel—an important part of all total maxillary osteotomies as well as posterior segmental subapical maxillary procedures.

Pterygomaxillary fissure (PTM) See Cephalometric landmarks (Hard tissue, Pterygomaxillary fissure.

PTFE (Polytetrafluoroethylene) See Teflon

PTM See Cephalometric landmarks (Hard tissue), Pterygomaxillary fissure.

Pubertal growth spurt (Adolescent growth spurt) The increased velocity of physical growth around puberty.

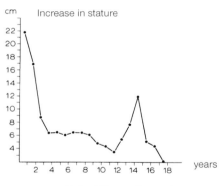

Pubertal growth spurt

Pumice A highly siliceous material of light gray color, produced by volcanic activity. It is used mainly in grit form to polish the tooth enamel prior to placement and after removal of fixed orthodontic appliances.

Pure crown movement See Orthodontic tooth movement, Pure crown movement.

Pure root movement See Orthodontic tooth movement, Pure root movement.

Pure rotation See Orthodontic tooth movement, Pure rotation.

Quad-helix See Appliance, Quad-helix.

Quadrant One of the two halves of each dental arch (mandibular and maxillary) from the midline to the distalmost tooth.

Quadrilateral cephalometric analysis See Cephalometric analysis, Di Paolo.

R

R-point (Registration point) See Cephalometric landmarks (Hard tissue), R-point.

Radio-autography See Autoradiography.

Radiograph (Roentgenogram) An image of a structure or tissue produced on a film by the passage of x-rays. (Sometimes inaccurately referred to as "x-ray.")

Radiolucent Permitting the passage of x-rays with little or no attenuation due to absorption. Appearing darker on a radiograph.

Radiopaque Permitting the passage of x-rays only with considerable attenuation, due to absorption. Appearing lighter on a radiograph.

"Rail" mechanism A theoretical explanation of the transverse expansion of the maxillary dental arch as an adaptation to advancement of the mandibular arch during physiological development or appliance treatment. The mandibular dental arch acts as a rail

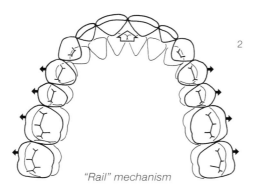

"Rail" mechanism

that through occlusal contacts dictates th buccal movement of the maxillary posteric teeth.

Ramus One of the two posterior vertical po tions of the mandible that are continuou with the mandibular body. Each ramus pre sents two processes at its superior borde the *coronoid* (anterior) and the *condyl* (posterior), that are separated by a deep con cavity, the *sigmoid notch*. The rami serve a attachment areas for the muscles of mast cation and also function to articulate th mandible with the skull.

Range See Working range.

Range of motion (ROM) The range, typicall measured in degrees of a circle, throug which a joint can be extended or flexed. I the case of the TMJ, the range of motio commonly is reported in millimeters rathe than in degrees.

Rapid maxillary expansion (RME) Se Expansion, Rapid maxillary.

Rare-earth magnets See Orthodontic mag nets.

Rare-earth screens See Intensifying screens

Rate of elastic force delivery See Stiffness

Rate of orthodontic tooth movement Th velocity of tooth movement under the influ ence of orthodontic force (usually measure in millimeters per month). The factors tha may influence the rate of orthodontic toot movement are largely unknown. It generally is agreed that the type of desired tooth movement (e.g. tipping versus translation, intrusion versus extrusion) is an important parameter. As well, a large inter-individual variation is recognized.

eaction force See Force, Reaction.

eactive member The part of an orthodontic appliance that is involved directly with anchorage, utilizing teeth that are not to be displaced or to be displaced minimally. [Compare with Active member.]

eactive segment See Segment, Anchorage.

ebonding Replacement of a lost or incorrectly placed bracket or other orthodontic attachment.

ecession, Gingival See Gingival recession.

ecipient site (Host site) The site into which a graft or transplant material is placed. [Compare with Donor site.]

eciprocal anchorage See Anchorage, Reciprocal.

eciprocal clicking See Clicking, Reciprocal.

eciprocal tooth movement The situation in which both the active and the reactive segment of teeth move toward each other

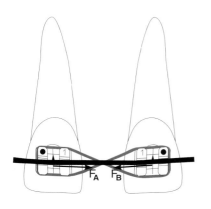

Reciprocal tooth movement

following application of force. In the ideal situation that two segments of equal size are balanced against each other (e.g. closure of a maxillary midline diastema by means of an elastic chain between the central incisors), movement by the same amount should theoretically be observed. [Also see Anchorage, Reciprocal.]

Recovery Change in shape of a material, resulting from the release of internal stresses.

Rectangular loop See Loop, Rectangular.

Rectangular wire See Orthodontic wire, Rectangular.

Recurved spring See Orthodontic springs, Z-.

Reduced tooth mobility See Tooth mobility, Reduced.

Reducing disc See Disc displacement with reduction.

Reduction, Interproximal See Interproximal stripping.

Rees esthetic plane See Cephalometric lines, Rees esthetic plane.

Reference frame See Global reference frame.

Reference line See Cephalometric lines, Reference line.

Referred pain Pain perceived in an area distant to and unrelated to the true site of origin.

Reflex muscle splinting See Protective muscle splinting.

Regeneration, Guided tissue See Guided tissue regeneration (GTR).

Registration, Bite See Bite registration.

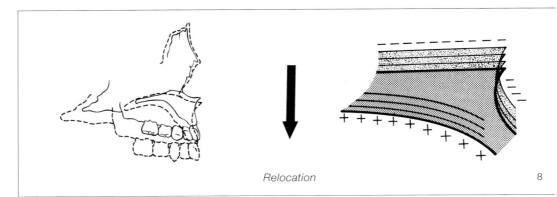

Relocation

8

Registration point (R) See Cephalometric landmarks (Hard tissue), R-Point.

Reichert's cartilage The cartilage of the second branchial arch, the dorsal end of which is closely related to the developing ear, and ossifies eventually to form the stapes of the middle ear and the styloid process of the temporal bone. The portion of cartilage between the styloid process and the hyoid bone regresses, and its perichondrium forms the stylohyoid ligament. The ventral end of Reichert's cartilage ossifies to form the lesser cornu and superior part of the body of the hyoid bone. [Compare with Meckel's cartilage.]

Relapse The partial or full return of certain characteristics of the pretreatment situation following active treatment. The tendency to relapse after an orthodontic correction is the reason why a retention phase routinely follows the active phase of orthodontic treatment. Factors that may be involved in relapse are craniofacial growth; forces acting on the dentition from the orofacial musculature, periodontal tissues and occlusal contacts; the nature and modality by which correction was achieved and the form of retention used. Examples of individual characteristics of malocclusion that are known to be more prone to relapse are rotations of teeth around their long axis, maxillary midline diastemas with frenal involvement and mandibular incisor crowding.

Relaxation See Viscoelastic behavior, Relaxation.

Relaxation splint See Splint, Relaxation.

Relocation A relative movement in space of bony structure, due to bone apposition o one of its surfaces and bone resorption i another. For example, during maxillar growth the palate becomes relocated infer orly by periosteal resorption on the nasa side and periosteal deposition on the ora side. Relocation and remodeling are bon growth mechanisms that are closely relate to one another. [Also see Displacemen (of a bone).]

Remodeling (of bone) A reshaping of th outline of a bone by selective resorptio of bone in some areas of its surface an apposition in other areas. Remodeling c cortical bone involves resorption on on side and apposition on the other, so that i thickness generally is maintained. The term *remodeling* signifies the turnover of alread existing bone (usually superficially) an strictly speaking should be distinguishe from *modeling,* which means the interna change in shape and form of a bone Remodeling is an essential component c the growth process. [Compare with Mc deling (of bone); Relocation.]

Removable appliance See Appliance, R movable.

Removable retainer See Retainer, Removable.

Replantation The replacement of a tooth that has been avulsed, or intentionally luxated, back into its alveolus. Ankylosis is common in replanted teeth, owing to injury to the periodontal ligament.

Repositioned flap See Flap, Repositioned.

Repositioning appliance See Splint, Anterior repositioning.

Reproximation See Interproximal stripping.

Residual ridge See Ridge, Residual.

Residual stress See Stress, Residual.

Resilience The property of a material that represents its ability to store mechanical energy without permanent deformation. [In the everyday practice of orthodontics the term generally is associated with *springiness*.] The resilience of two or more orthodontic wires can be compared by observing the areas under the elastic region of their stress/strain diagrams (provided they are plotted on the same scale). The wire with the larger elastic area under the stress/strain curve has the higher resilience.

Resin-bonded prosthesis A prosthesis that is luted to tooth structure (primarily to the enamel) that has been etched previously to provide micromechanical retention for the resin cement (e.g. a Maryland bridge).

Resin-modified glass-ionomer cement See Orthodontic cement, Resin-modified glass-ionomer.

Resistance, Center of See Center of resistance.

Resorption A loss of substance from tissues that normally are mineralized (e.g. dentin, cementum, bone). The process may be physiologic or pathologic.

Bone resorption See Bone resorption.

External resorption Resorption of mineralized dental tissue beginning on the external surface, as is usually observed at the apex or lateral surface of the root. Principal causative factors include periapical inflammation, tooth reimplantation, orthodontic tooth movement, tumors and cysts, and tooth impaction. Spontaneous resorption sometimes may occur in conjunction with endocrine disorders. External resorption that affects the dentin sometimes is radiographically misdiagnosed as internal resorption.

Frontal resorption (Direct resorption) See Bone resorption, Frontal.

Internal resorption An unusual form of resorption of dental tissues beginning centrally in a tooth, and apparently initiated by an inflammatory process in the pulp. It usually is symptom-free in its early stages.
Histologically, the condition presents a variable degree of resorption of the inner or pulpal surface of the dentin filled by hyperplastic pulp tissue. When it extends to the crown, a pink-hued area representing the hyperplastic pulpal tissue may be visible clinically.

Root resorption Resorption of the roots of the deciduous teeth is a normal, essential and physiologic process. Root resorption of permanent teeth is a common iatrogenic side effect of orthodontic treatment.
Orthodontic tooth movement is possible because of the greater resistance of cementum than bone to resorption. However, even when radiographs show no visible changes in the root surface, most teeth moved orthodontically undergo some degree of loss of cementum or even dentin of their root. This resorption is seen histologically as small lacunae that are repaired rapidly by the formation of new cementum during the period that no active orthodontic force is present. In other words, root remodeling is a constant feature of orthodontic tooth move-

ment at the histological level. When the initially resorbed cementum is not repaired, permanent loss of root structure occurs. Repair of the damaged root does not occur when the attack on the root surface produces large defects, as is usually the case in the area of the root apex.

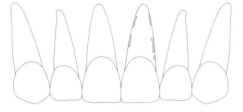

Root resorption

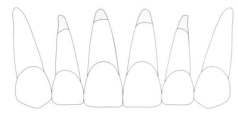

Careful radiographic examination of post-orthodontic individuals shows some loss of root length in nearly every patient. Some teeth are more prone to root resorption than others: maxillary lateral incisors, maxillary central incisors, mandibular incisors, distal root of mandibular first molars, mandibular second premolars and maxillary second premolars (listed in order of severity). In the great majority of patients the amount of root resorption is minimal and clinically insignificant. Occasionally, however, severe root resorption (up to one half of the root length or more) is observed in patients who underwent routine orthodontic therapy.

The factors influencing root resorption after orthodontic treatment still are unclear. Individual susceptibility is considered to play a major role, and some studies suggest that genetic, metabolic, hormonal or other systemic factors may be implicated. Root resorption has been attributed to biomechanical factors such as type of tooth move-

ment, orthodontic force regime and magnitude, distance that a tooth is moved, duration of treatment, type of appliance, contact of apices with cortical bone, intermaxillary elastics, jiggling or round-tripping, but with no conclusive evidence. Finally, factors such as age, sex, occlusal trauma, or type of malocclusion also have yielded equivocal results in the literature.

Pretreatment characteristics considered to be indicators of susceptibility to root resorption are the presence of conical (pipette-shaped) roots with pointed apices, distorted root form (dilaceration), history of trauma, as well as any evidence of root resorption already present prior to orthodontic treatment. However, it is not certain that these factors necessarily are risk factors for severe resorption in all patients.

Undermining resorption (Indirect resorption) See Bone resorption, Undermining.

Rest, Occlusal See Occlusal rest.

Rest position (of the mandible) See Physiologic rest position.

Resultant force See Force, Resultant.

Retainer Any orthodontic appliance, fixed or removable, used to maintain the position of the teeth and stabilize them following orthodontic treatment.

Bonded lingual retainer A wire that is bonded on the lingual surface of the teeth just prior to or after removal of the orthodontic appliances to retain their corrected positions. Bonded lingual retainers are very popular in the mandibular anterior area to provide long-term retention in an attempt to prevent late mandibular incisor crowding. The type of wire used for this purpose ranges from a flexible round multistrand wire to a rigid rectangular stainless steel one. The wire can be bonded on all six mandibular anterior teeth individually, or only on the lingual surface of the canines. Occasionally,

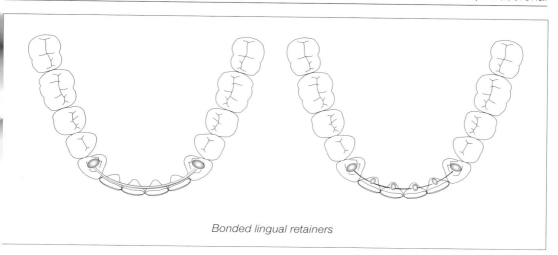

Bonded lingual retainers

the wire can extend to more posterior teeth. The use of maxillary bonded lingual retainers is dependent on the clearance provided by the overbite. One way to overcome this problem is by using *intracoronal retention*. This requires the preparation of cavities within the enamel to receive the retaining wires prior to bonding. Bonded lingual retainers occasionally are used on the maxillary central incisors to prevent relapse of a pre-existing midline diastema.

Canine-to-canine retainer See Retainer, Bonded lingual; Retainer, Essix.

Essix retainer A removable vacuum-formed clear retainer made of thermoplastic copolyester, covering the teeth of one or both arches, from canine to canine. According to J.J. Sheridan, who introduced the appliance, a sheet of the material 0.030 inch (0.75 mm) thick is preferred, for a good combination of flexibility and strength. During the thermoforming process the thickness of the material is reduced from 0.030 inch (0.75 mm) to 0.015 inch (0.38 mm). Despite its limited thickness, the Essix retainer may not be recommended for patients with an open bite tendency, as it only covers the anterior teeth. The risk of swallowing or aspirating the appliance also should be considered.

Fixed retainer (Permanent retainer) A type of retainer that is cemented or bonded to the teeth and thus cannot be removed by the patient. Fixed retainers are a popular choice for long-term retention, as they eliminate the patient cooperation factor. [Also see Retainer, Bonded lingual.]

Hawley retainer One of the most frequently used retaining devices, introduced by C.A. Hawley (1919). It is a removable appliance made of acrylic covering the entire mucosa of the hard palate, or only part of it ("horseshoe" design).
In the original design there were no molar clasps. Today, Adams clasps or sometimes circumferential clasps on the first molars are used to provide retention.
A labial bow of 0.020-inch (0.51-mm) to 0.036-inch (0.90-mm) stainless steel wire (*Hawley* wire) is made to contact the labial surfaces of the four incisors or the six anterior teeth. The labial bow has a U-loop where it crosses the occlusion, usually distal to the canines. When there is interference with the occlusion at this point, the labial bow may alternatively be soldered on the Adams clasps. [Also see Labial bow; Clasp, Adams.] *See illustration next page.*

Intracoronal retainer See Retainer, Bonded lingual.

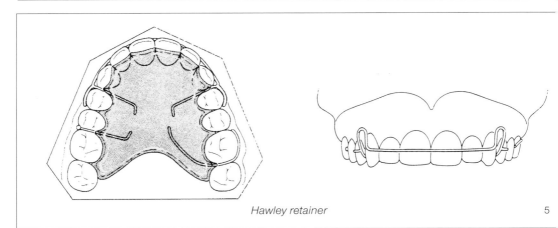

Hawley retainer   5

Permanent retainer See Retainer, Fixed.

Positioner See Appliance, Positioner.

Removable retainer A retainer that is not fixed to the teeth, but can be removed by the patient.

Spring retainer (Barrer retainer) A maxillary or mandibular removable appliance, introduced by H.G. Barrer in 1975. The mandibular appliance is mainly used today. It consists of a single piece of stainless steel wire 0.022 inch (0.56 mm) to 0.029 inch (0.72 mm) in diameter, bent around the six anterior teeth. The wire lies parallel to the incisal edges on the labial side and crosses the occlusion between the canines and premolars, bilaterally. It is bent downward on the labial and lingual surfaces of the canines in the form of U-loops, so that it follows the curvature of the gingiva on these teeth, but without actually contacting it. The ends of the wire overlap in the mid line at the lingual aspect of the incisors. The wire does not touch the surfaces of the teeth and is covered by acrylic on the labial and lingual sides. This forms two bands approximately 4 mm wide, engaging the incisors across the middle third of their crowns. The wire surrounding the canine is free of acrylic and functions as a spring

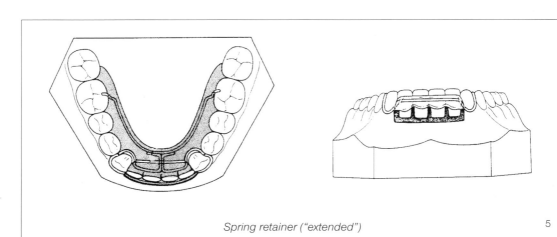

Spring retainer ("extended")   5

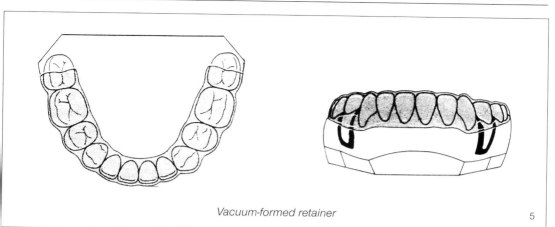

Vacuum-formed retainer 5

which can be appropriately adjusted to activate the appliance.

The greatest disadvantage of the Barrer retainer is its small size. Various modifications to increase its size have been reported, to avoid accidental swallowing or aspiration. The most common modification includes bilateral extensions of the lingual acrylic, terminating with two occlusal rests on the mandibular first molars. [Also see Spring aligner.]

Vacuum-formed retainer A type of removable retainer made of soft or hard clear thermoplastic material that is heated and formed on the patient's plaster model in a vacuum machine. The appliance may cover the entire arch or part of it, and it may also be used for some minor individual tooth corrections, if the teeth are reset prior to its fabrication. Susceptibility of the appliance to fracture (or tear) is a common concern, which is counterbalanced by its esthetic, unobtrusive appearance. [Also see Retainer, Essix.]

Van der Linden retainer A Hawley-type retainer introduced by F.P.G.M. van der Linden, with a modified labial bow made of stainless steel wire 0.028 inch (0.70 mm) in diameter. This labial bow contacts the labial surfaces of the six anterior teeth and is

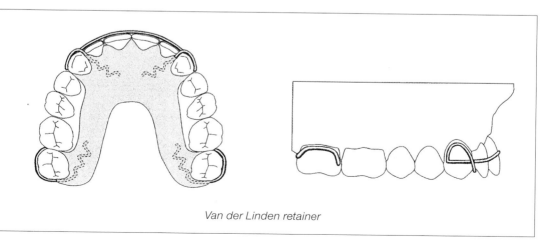

Van der Linden retainer

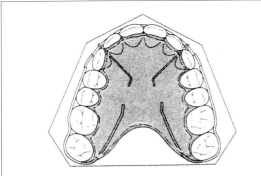 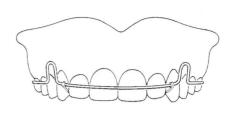

Wrap-around retainer 5

bent back upon itself at the distal aspect of the canines, embracing them in a C-clasp fashion at their cervical regions. When there is inadequate clearance for the labial bow to cross the occlusion mesial to the canines, the crossover wire can be placed distal to them and the recurved C-clasp can be made on the first premolars. These canine clasps provide adequate retention and do not deform by repetitive removal and replacement of the appliance by the patient. Additional C-clasps coming from the distal of the terminal molars are used to enhance retention. The acrylic is relieved from the palatal aspect of the posterior teeth, allowing them to settle in their natural position, as determined by the occlusion. Only the mandibular anterior teeth are contacting the acrylic of the appliance in habitual occlusion. This retainer does not allow adjustment of the anterior tooth position during the retention period due to the design of the labial bow.

Wrap-around (Circumferential) retainer A type of removable retainer sometimes preferred to the Hawley, especially for the maxillary arch, in cases with tight occlusion where there is no space for crossover of the labial bow. It has a Hawley-type acrylic construction and a continuous labial bow that inserts into the acrylic posteriorly to the terminal molars bilaterally, to avoid interference with the occlusion.

Retention The phase following active orthodontic treatment, aimed at stabilization c the achieved orthodontic correction.

Retention clasp See Clasp.

Retraction (of a tooth) Posterior (lingua or distal movement (usually referring to boc ily movement).

Retraction coil spring See Orthodonti springs, Coil spring, Retraction.

Retroclination Lingual inclination or tippin of anterior teeth.

Retrodiscal tissue (Retrodiscal lamina Posterior attachment, Retrodisca pad) The region of loose, highly vascula ized and innervated connective tissue tha is attached to the posterior aspect of th fibrous portion of the articular disc of th temporomandibular joint. This tissue, whic extends to and fills the posterior capsule, i rich in interstitial collagen fibers, adipos tissue, arteries, and elastin, and possesse a venous plexus. The retrodiscal tissue ofte is stretched and interposed between th condyle and the fossa in patients with ante rior or anteromedial disc displacement.

Retrodiscitis The retrodiscal tissues ar highly vascularized and innervated, and a such are unable to tolerate much force. the condyle encroaches on the tissues, breal down and inflammation are likely. Inflammation of the retrodiscal tissues is characterized by constant dull aching pain that often is increased by clenching. If swelling occurs, the condyle may be forced slightly forward, down the posterior slope of the articular eminence. This shift can cause an acute malocclusion, clinically seen as disengagement of the ipsilateral posterior teeth and heavy contact on the contralateral canines. Trauma is the major etiologic factor with retrodiscitis.

Retrognathia See Retrognathism.

Retrognathic A term used to indicate the situation in which the mandible or the maxilla is retrusive (in the anteroposterior plane) in relation to other cranial or facial structures, due to smaller size and/or more posterior position. In the classification of facial types, the term is used to connote a retrognathic mandible. [See also Facial type; compare with Prognathic.]

Retrognathism (Retrognathia) A condition of facial disharmony in which one or both jaws are posterior to normal, in their craniofacial relationships. When the term is mentioned without further clarification, it usually refers to the mandible.

Bimaxillary retrognathism Retrusion of both jaws beyond normal limits in relation to the cranial base and other facial structures.

Mandibular retrognathism Retrusion of the mandible relative to the cranial base and other facial structures, due to a hypoplastic and/or posteriorly positioned mandible.

Maxillary retrognathism Retrusion of the maxilla relative to the cranial base and other facial structures due to a hypoplastic and/or posteriorly positioned maxilla.

Retrusion Posterior location. The term commonly is used to express a posterior position of teeth with regard to a certain reference plane. [When referring to jaws the term *retrognathism* is more appropriate.]

Bimaxillary retrusion See Retrognathism, Bimaxillary.

Bimaxillary dentoalveolar (Bialveolar) retrusion Posterior position of the maxillary and mandibular incisors with respect to their supporting bones and the facial profile.

Dental retrusion Posterior position of a tooth or group of teeth. [Note: The term *retrusion* does not refer to the inclination of the long axis of the tooth. A tooth can be retrusive without being retroclined, if it is positioned too far posteriorly but has a normal inclination.]

Lip retrusion Posterior position ("flatness") of one or both lips relative to the nose and chin or other facial structures.

Retrusion of the mandible See Arthrokinetics of the TMJ.

Reversal lines (of bone) Approximately half of the cortical plate of the facial and cranial bones is formed by the outer surface (i.e. the periosteum) and the remaining half by the inner surface (i.e. the endosteum). Reversal lines are lines that represent the interface between endosteally and periosteally produced bone layers. They also indicate the demarcation between resorptive and depository growth fields, and can be used to identify the layers of bone that were produced first on one side and then on the other, as the direction of growth turned about (reversal of growth).

Reverse curve of Spee See Curve of Spee, Reverse.

Reverse functional appliance See Appliance, Class III functional.

Reverse loop See Loop, Closed.

Reverse overjet See Overjet, Negative.

Reverse-pull headgear See Appliance, Face mask.

Reverse swallow See Swallow, Tongue-thrust.

Reversible treatment Any therapy that does not cause permanent change.

Rheumatoid arthritis See Arthritis, Rheumatoid.

Rheumatoid factor (RhF) Antigamma globulin antibodies found in the serum of most patients with rheumatoid arthritis, but also occurring in a small percentage of apparently normal individuals and in individuals with other collagen vascular diseases, chronic infections and noninfectious diseases.

Rhinolalia aperta See Hypernasality.

Rhinolalia clausa See Hyponasality.

Ribbon-arch appliance See Appliance, Ribbon-arch.

"Ribbonwise" A rectangular archwire fitting in the bracket slot with its large dimension perpendicular to the occlusal plane (rotated 90° about its long axis, compared to the regular edgewise wire). [Also see Appliance, Ribbon-arch.]

Ricketts' esthetic line (E-line) See Cephalometric lines, E-line.

Ricketts' facial axis See Cephalometric lines, Facial axis of Ricketts.

Ricketts' facial axis angle See Cephalometric measurements (Hard tissue), Facial axis angle of Ricketts.

Ridge A projecting structure; a long, narrow, raised crest.

Alveolar ridge The part of the maxilla or mandible that contains the alveolar processes.

Key ridge A radiographic anatomical landmark commonly appearing on a lateral cephalometric radiograph. It represents the lower contour of the zygomatic bony ridge, situated between the maxillary tuberosity and the canine fossa.

Marginal ridges Elevated convex crests that form the mesial and distal occlusal margins of posterior teeth and the lingual surface margins of anterior teeth.

Residual ridge (Edentulous ridge) The bony ridge remaining after disappearance of the alveoli from the alveolar process, following removal or loss of the teeth.

Ridge augmentation Any procedure designed to increase the height or thickness of the residual alveolar ridge, usually by grafting bone or other bone substitutes.

Riedel plane See Cephalometric lines, Riedel plane.

RIF See Fixation (Surgical), Rigid internal.

Rigid body A body that does not change its shape or size under the action of forces. This is a theoretical concept, as all real bodies experience some degree of deformation when subjected to forces. When such changes in size or shape are negligible compared with the overall dimensions of a body, then rigidity can be assumed.

Rigid fixation (RIF) See Fixation (Surgical), Rigid internal.

Risk factor Any factor that causes an individual or a group to be vulnerable to a disease or condition, resulting in an increased incidence or severity for the susceptible population.

RME See Expansion, Rapid maxillary.

Robin sequence (Robin anomalad, Pierre Robin syndrome) A condition described by the well-recognized triad of mandibular micrognathia, glossoptosis and cleft of the secondary palate, often accompanied by severe nasorespiratory distress in the neonatal period. Named after the French oral pathologist P. Robin, although many earlier reports on the same anomaly were published by others. Birth prevalence estimates range from 1:2,000 to 1:30,000.

It is advocated that the term "Robin sequence" is not really a diagnostic entity, but rather a nonspecific complex of symptoms that can occur *sui generis*, as a component of various syndromes (e.g. Stickler syndrome, velocardiofacial syndrome, fetal alcohol syndrome) or in association with various anomalies that are not currently recognized as specific syndromes.

It is not clear whether the mandibular micrognathia plays a role in the pathogenesis of the cleft palate, as has been suggested, nor is there agreement on the etiology of the micrognathia. Theories range from a positional mechanical compression of the mandible against the sternum in utero restricting normal mandibular growth to metabolic or genetic etiology. If the respiratory obstruction and feeding difficulty of the infants is marked, tracheostomy, nasotracheal intubation or tongue-lip adhesion may be necessary. The severe mandibular micrognathia may improve somewhat in the first months of life (what has been termed *catch-up growth*) but the mandible does not reach normal dimensions. Early treatment with distraction osteogenesis may assist in early removal of the tracheostomy.

Roentgenogram See Radiograph.

ROM See Range of motion.

Root amputation The removal of a root from a multirooted tooth.

Root movement, Pure See Orthodontic tooth movement, Pure root movement.

Root parallelism One of the objectives of orthodontic treatment, achieved mainly by controlling the angulation (second-order, tip) of teeth.

Root planing Smoothing of the rough and infected root surface of a tooth following subgingival scaling or curettage.

Root proximity Close approximation of roots of adjacent teeth.

Root resection Surgical removal of a portion of the root of a tooth. It usually is performed in teeth with incomplete endodontic treatment, in conjunction with a retrograde apical seal procedure, to eliminate infection.

Root resorption See Resorption, Root.

Root springs See Orthodontic springs, Root.

Root torque See Torque, Root.

Rostral In the direction of the back. [Compare with Ventral.]

Rotation, Center of See Center of rotation.

Rotation (of the condyle) The initial phase of condylar movement, which does not involve translation. Rotation occurs primarily between the condyle and the inferior surface of the disc (inferior joint space).

Rotation (of the mandible) See Mandibular rotation.

Rotation (of a tooth) See Orthodontic tooth movement, Pure rotation.

First-order rotation Rotation of a tooth around its long axis; rotation in the x-z plane, around the y-axis. [Also see Orthodontic tooth movement, Pure rotation.]

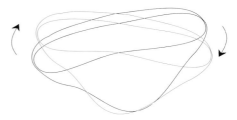

First-order rotation

Second-order rotation (Mesiodistal tipping) Rotation of a tooth around the labiolingual (x-)axis (when referring to an incisor), or around the buccolingual (z-)axis (when referring to a posterior tooth), thereby causing a change in its angulation.

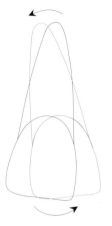

Second-order rotation

Third-order rotation (Labiolingual or buccolingual tipping) Rotation of a tooth around its mesiodistal axis (i.e. around the z-axis when referring to an incisor, or around the x-axis when referring to a posterior tooth), thereby causing a change in its inclination.

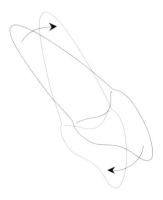

Third-order rotation

Rotation spring See Orthodontic springs Rotation.

Rotation wedge An orthodontic auxiliar made of rubber or stainless steel (*Steine* rotation wedge), which is used when a sma degree of rotation of a tooth still is neces sary, but there is no more activation left i the wire (e.g. when bracket placement not ideal), and the clinician wants to avoi placing a bend. The wedge is attached o the side of the bracket that needs to b moved in a lingual direction, and subse quently the archwire is ligated tightly on th opposite aspect of the bracket with a stain less steel ligature, so that the wedge i squeezed between the archwire and th tooth. Because of their mode of action wedges require a rigid archwire and are nc effective with flexible wires.

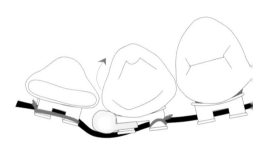

Rotation wedge

Round-tripping Movement of teeth in a direc tion opposite to that in which they wer moved in an earlier stage of orthodonti treatment. It is thought to increase the ris of root resorption significantly and thu should be avoided, if possible. Howeve strictly speaking, round-tripping of teeth i an almost inevitable phenomenon in every day clinical orthodontics, irrespective c force regimen and appliance used. All toot movements actually consist of a series c minute opposite tipping movements ("jig gling"). This translates into continuous reve sal of the root surfaces that sustain com pression and tension, which at the histolog ical level is equivalent to round-tripping. Th same also may occur due to the relaps tendency of teeth during the intervals in which the intermittent force of, e.g. a headgear, is not active. [Also see "Jiggling."]

Round wire See Orthodontic wire, Round.

RPE See Expansion, Rapid maxillary.

Rubber bands See Orthodontic elastics.

Rugae See Palatal rugae.

S

S See Cephalometric landmarks (Hard tissue), Sella.

S-line (Esthetic plane of Steiner) See Cephalometric lines, S-line.

Saddle angle See Cephalometric measurements (Hard tissue), Cranial base angle.

Safety release module Component of a headstrap, of various designs, allowing immediate release if pulled by excessive force, to reduce the risk of injury.

Sagittal appliance See Appliance, Sagittal.

Sagittal overbite See Overjet.

Sagittal plane (Parasagittal plane) Any vertical plane that passes through the body parallel to the median plane and divides the body into left and right parts. [See also Median plane.]

Sagittal split osteotomy See Osteotomy, Bilateral sagittal split.

Sargent pliers See Orthodontic instruments, Parallel-action pliers with cutter.

Sassouni cephalometric analysis See Cephalometric analysis, Sassouni.

Scalar A physical quantity consisting only of a number (magnitude) and a physical unit of measurement (e.g. temperature). [Compare with Vectorial.]

Scalene muscles See Muscle, Scalene.

Scaling Removal of plaque and calculus from the surface of a tooth by means of a scale

Subgingival scaling Removal of plaqu and calculus from surfaces of a tooth apica to the gingival margin, usually accumulate in periodontal pockets or pseudopockets.

Supragingival scaling Removal c plaque and calculus from surfaces of tooth coronal to the gingival margin.

Schwarz appliance See Appliance, Schwarz

Scintigraphy See Emission scintigraphy.

Scissors-bite See Crossbite, Scissors-bite.

Screen, Intensifying See Intensifying screen

Screen, Oral See Appliance, Oral screen.

Seating lug A small strip of stainless stee welded on the palatal or lingual aspect c orthodontic bands to facilitate their seating and/or removal. They sometimes can have

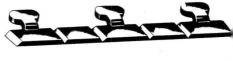

Seating lug

extensions that are used as hooks for orthodontic elastics. Seating lugs occasionally are removed after the band is fitted, for reasons of patient comfort.

Second branchial arch syndrome See Hemifacial microsomia.

Second order See Angulation.

Second-order bends See Bends, Second-order.

Second-order clearance The angle through which an engaged archwire may be tipped within the bracket slot (with reference to the long axis of the slot) before making contact with the occlusal and gingival slot walls at its mesialmost and distalmost aspects. [Also see "Play" of an orthodontic wire in the bracket slot; compare with Third-order clearance.]

Second-order rotation See Rotation (of a tooth), Second-order.

Second transitional period The period during which the deciduous canines and molars are replaced by their successors.

Secondary cartilage Cartilages like those of the mandibular condyle and symphysis (which contribute to the development of the mandible) and the zygomatic (malar) cartilage (which contributes to the development of the maxilla). These cartilages are distinguished from the primary cartilages histologically (as their cells are larger, with less intercellular matrix) and embryologically (as they develop at a later stage). Secondary cartilages generally are more responsive to changes in mechanical stress than primary cartilages. [Compare with Primary cartilage.]

Secondary crowding See Arch length discrepancy, Arch length deficiency.

Secondary occlusal trauma See Occlusal trauma, Secondary.

Secondary palate See Palate, Secondary.

Sectional appliance See Mechanics, Segmental arch.

Sectional archwire See Archwire, Sectional.

Sectional mechanics See Mechanics, Segmental arch.

Segment A portion of a larger body or structure.

Active segment The segment of teeth that is to be moved. [Also see Mechanics, Segmental arch.]

Anchorage segment (Reactive segment) The segment of teeth that provides anchorage for the movement of the active segment. [Also see Mechanics, Segmental arch.]

Buccal stabilizing segment An anchorage segment set up by connecting a number of posterior teeth with a passively engaged rigid rectangular wire.

Distal segment 1. When referring to teeth, the more distally (posteriorly) lying dental segment.
2. When referring to segments after an osteotomy such a BSSO, the segment farther away from the head (bearing the teeth and alveolar process), as opposed to the proximal segments (bearing the rami and the condyles).

Greater segment In a unilateral cleft, the maxillary alveolar segment on the non-cleft side.

Lesser segment In a unilateral cleft, the maxillary alveolar segment on the side of the cleft.

Premaxillary segment In a complete bilateral cleft, the anterior segment that is separated from the maxilla (encompassing the median part of the maxillary alveolar process and teeth and the prolabium) and is attached to the nasal septum. [Also see Premaxilla.]

Proximal segment When referring to segments after an osteotomy such as a bilateral sagittal split osteotomy (BSSO), the segments closer to the head (bearing the rami and condyles), as opposed to the distal segment (bearing the teeth and alveolar process).

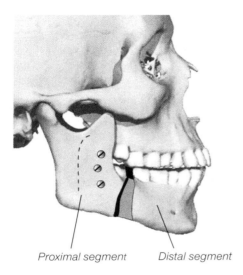

Proximal segment   *Distal segment*

Segmental appliance See Mechanics, Segmental arch.

Segmental arch mechanics See Mechanics, Segmental arch.

Segmental archwire See Archwire, Sectional.

Segmental surgery Surgical mobilization and repositioning of one or more alveolar segments of either the maxilla or mandible containing the respective teeth.

Self-ligating bracket See Bracket, Self-ligating.

Sella (S) See Cephalometric landmarks (Hard tissue), Sella.

Sella-Nasion line (SN) See Cephalometric lines, Sella-Nasion.

Sense One of the four characteristics of vectorial quantities. The sense of a vector shows the orientation to which the vector acts and is connoted by an arrowhead. [Not to be confused with the *direction* of the vector which is the line along which it is active irrespective of orientation.]

Sensitivity (of a test) An indication of the capability of a test to accurately yield positive results when applied to patients known to have a disease. Sensitivity is calculated by the following formula:
Sensitivity = TP/(TP + FN) x 100% where:
TP = True positives (the number of subjects with the disease, correctly identified by the test)
FN = False negatives (the number of subjects with the disease, incorrectly classified by the test as disease-free). [Compare with Specificity.]

Sentalloy See Nickel-titanium alloy.

Separating elastic See Separator, Elastic.

Separating spring See Separator, Spring-clip.

Separation An orthodontic procedure aiming at slightly loosening the tight interproximal contacts between teeth to create space for the fitting of orthodontic bands. This is achieved by the use of various kinds of separators.

Separator A device used to create separation between adjacent teeth. There are different kinds, but the principle is the same with any type of separator used: the separator is inserted so it can force or wedge the teeth apart, and it is left in place long enough for initial tooth movement to occur (usually for a week) so banding can be performed by the next patient visit. Separators also can be used to create space in which clasps or crossover wires of removable appliances (e.g. Fränkel appliance) will fit.

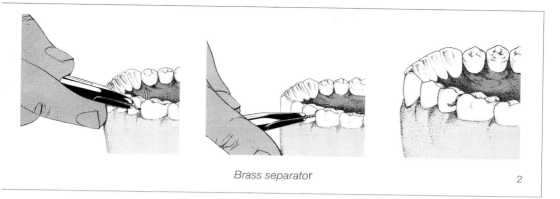

Brass separator

2

Brass separator A piece of soft 0.020-inch (0.51-mm) brass wire, bent in the shape of a hook. The flattened edge of the hook is passed beneath the interproximal contact and slid around it. The two free ends of the separator wire then are grasped with a pair of Mathieu pliers or a hemostat and twisted tightly, so a separating force is created. The twisted end of the separator ("pigtail") is cut to a length of approximately 3 mm and tucked in the interproximal area.

Elastic separator ("Donut") Elastomeric ring of varying thickness that is placed around the interproximal contact point to create the necessary separation over time. The elastomeric ring is stretched with the help of special pliers or by pulling apart two pieces of dental floss threaded through it, while it is forced through the contact. An elastic separator (as any separator) can cause problems if lost into the interproximal space because they usually are radiolucent,

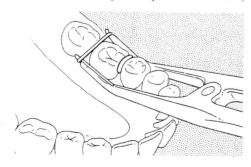

Elastic separator   5

so their position and number should be noted in the chart at the time of placement and the area thoroughly inspected in case of a missing separator at the banding appointment.

Maxian elastic separator This type of separator resembles a wide rubber band with thick, rolled edges. They are obtained in strips and cut to size by the operator, to accommodate the various teeth. The two rolled edges are stretched apart, making the interconnecting rubber thin enough to be forced into the interproximal space. Maxian separators are capable of producing rapid separation (they are recommended to be placed 30 minutes before band fitting) but can be quite painful for the patient.

Spring-clip separator A spring made of 0.020-inch (0.51-mm) stainless steel wire that carries a small helix. The spring is grasped with a plier next to the helix, at the base of its shorter leg. The bent-over end of the longer leg is placed in the lingual embrasure between the two teeth to be separated and the spring is pulled open so the shorter leg can slip beneath the contact, with the helix on the vestibular side. Stainless steel spring separators are tolerated easily by the patient, but they tend to come loose and may fall out as separation of the teeth occurs. *See illustration next page.*

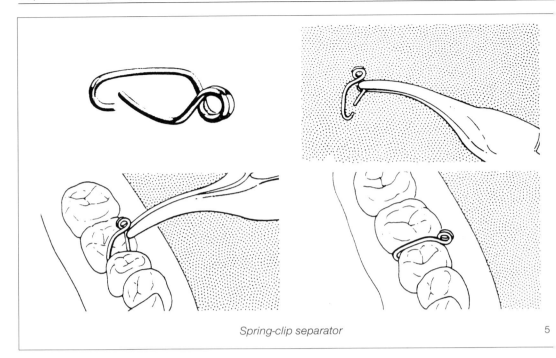

Spring-clip separator 5

Separator pliers See Orthodontic instruments, Elastic separator pliers.

Sequential bonding See Bonding, Sequential.

Serial extraction A planned sequence of selective, timed extraction of deciduous and subsequently permanent teeth, with the objective of relieving severe crowding early and facilitating the eruption of remaining teeth into improved positions. Close supervision and control of ensuing eruption are essential to avoid unfavorable sequelae, such as closure of the spaces by mere mesial migration or tipping of the posterior teeth. Comprehensive orthodontic treatment is almost always required for space management, control of the tipping and increase of overbite usually induced by the procedure, and for other malrelationships that may be present. Serial extraction is preferably performed on patients with minimal overbite, symmetrical buccal segments and a Class I molar relationship. It is often

indicated in patients with large tooth siz rather than small bony bases. [Compare wit Guidance of eruption.] [Modified from th AAO Glossary of Dentofacial Orthopedi Terms, 1993.]

Serrated amalgam-plugger See Orth dontic instruments, Serrated amalgan plugger.

Setback (of the mandible) An orthogn thic surgical procedure aiming at sagitt (anteroposterior) reduction of the mandibl A mandibular setback most often is pe formed through a bilateral sagittal sp ramus osteotomy (BSSO) or a transor vertical ramus osteotomy (TOVRO), but variety of different osteotomy procedure also are available for certain situation [Compare with Advancement of the ma dible.]

Settling Even with the most meticulous ar precise positioning, it is very likely th some teeth will not be in their most stab position during the finishing stage of treatment with a rectangular archwire. Shortly after the appliances have been removed, the teeth "settle" into position by re-establishing occlusal contacts with their antagonist and adjacent teeth until an equilibrium is reached.

Settling can be facilitated during the finishing stages of treatment by replacing the heavy rectangular archwires with light round ones that provide some freedom for movement of the teeth, possibly with the added use of some light posterior vertical elastics. Some clinicians prefer to remove part of the fixed appliances (usually from the posterior teeth) a few weeks prior to the insertion of retainers, to allow for some spontaneous settling of the teeth into their final occlusion.

Setup, Bracket See Bracket setup.

Setup, Diagnostic See Diagnostic setup.

Shape memory A property of certain alloys (such as some nickel-titanium alloys) that will permit shaping at a higher temperature, followed by a deformation at a lower temperature and return to the original shape by reheating.

Sharpey's fibers See Periodontal ligament, Fibers.

Shear The internal resistance to a force trying to slide one portion of a body over another. [Also see Stress, Shear.]

Shear deformation A change in shape as a result of shear stress. (In the finite element example, shear deformation of a rectangular element would cause it to assume the shape of a parallelogram.)

Shear stress See Stress, Shear.

Sheath An orthodontic attachment in the form of a tube, usually welded to the lingual or palatal surface of molar bands for insertion of fixed/removable palatal arches

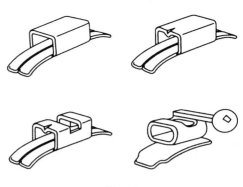

Sheaths 11

(e.g. TPA, Quad-helix) or mandibular lingual arches. A sheath is designed to accept a 0.030-inch (0.76-mm) or 0.036-inch (0.90-mm) round wire doubled upon itself. Sheaths sometimes carry gingivally directed ball hooks to allow ligation of the wire in place and/or latch indents *(Dillon dimples)* to increase retention of the wire in the sheath. [Also see Dillon dimple.]

Shedding See Exfoliation.

Shield, Soft tissue See Soft tissue shield.

Shield, Vestibular See Appliance, Vestibular shield.

Shift, Mandibular See Mandibular shift.

Shift, Midline See Midline discrepancy.

SI See International System of Units.

Siamese bracket See Bracket, Twin.

Side-winder spring See Appliance, Tip-edge.

Sign (of a disease or disorder) Objective evidence of the disease or disorder, as perceived by an examiner. [Compare with Symptom.]

Simple tipping See Orthodontic tooth movement, Tipping (Uncontrolled).

Single bracket See Bracket, Single.

Single clicking See Clicking, Single.

Single-contrast arthrography See Arthrography of the TMJ, Single-contrast.

Single-jaw surgery See Orthognathic surgery, Single-jaw.

Single-piece maxillary osteotomy See Osteotomy, One-piece maxillary.

Single-space arthrography See Arthrography of the TMJ, Single-space.

Single-width bracket See Bracket, Single.

Sintering A process by which a preformed body is densified, through diffusion of its particles into each other, usually at high temperatures. The process is very common in the manufacturing of ceramic brackets, rare earth magnets and also some metal brackets.

Six keys of occlusion The six morphological characteristics of an optimal occlusion, as determined by L.F. Andrews in a study of 120 casts of non-orthodontic individuals with excellent occlusion, which constituted the basis for the development of the straight-wire appliance. The six keys are:
1. Molar relationship The distal surface of the distobuccal cusp of the maxillary first permanent molars occludes (makes contact) with the mesial surface of the mesiobuccal cusps of the mandibular second permanent molars. The mesiobuccal cusp of the maxillary first permanent molars falls within the groove between the mesial and middle cusps of the mandibular first permanent molars.
2. Crown angulation (Mesiodistal "tip") The gingival portion of the long axis of the crown of each tooth is distal to the incisal (or occlusal) portion. The degree of this "mesial

tip" depends on the type of tooth. [The angulation of the long axis of the crown of the tooth is considered, rather than that of the long axis of the entire tooth.]
3. Crown inclination (Labiolingual or buccolingual inclination) [The inclination of the long axis of the crown of the tooth is considered, rather that of the long axis of the entire tooth.] The long axes of the crowns of the maxillary and mandibular incisors are labially inclined to a degree sufficient to resist overeruption of their antagonists. This labial inclination allows proper distal positioning of the contact points of the maxillary teeth in relation to the respective contact points of their mandibular antagonists, permitting ideal occlusion of the posterior crowns. In the case of the maxillary canines and posterior teeth a lingual crown inclination exists, which is relatively constant and similar from the canines through the second premolars, and is slightly more pronounced in the molars. The mandibular posterior teeth have a similar lingual crown inclination that increases progressively from the canines through the second molars.
4. Rotations No rotations are present.
5. Spaces No interdental spaces exist, but rather tight contacts between the teeth.
6. Occlusal plane The plane of occlusion is either flat, or a mild curve of Spee is present.

Skeletal Pertaining to the osseous framework of the body.

Skeletal crossbite See Crossbite, Skeletal.

Skeletal malocclusion A malocclusion that is due to a discrepancy between the maxilla and mandible, or between them and the cranial base.

Sleep apnea See Obstructive sleep apnea.

Slenderizing See Interproximal stripping.

Slicing (of teeth) The removal of tooth material from the mesial and/or distal aspect of deciduous canines and molars to allow the adjacent permanent teeth to attain better positions in the dental arch during or after

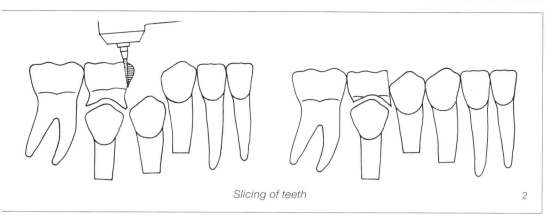

Slicing of teeth

2

emergence. With this procedure, the use of the available leeway space to relieve crowding in the anterior region can be maximized.

Slide in centric See Mandibular shift.

Sliding condylar movement See Translation of the condyle.

Sliding mechanics See Mechanics, Sliding.

Sling, Pterygomasseteric See Pterygomasseteric sling.

Slot, Bracket See Bracket slot.

Slot engagement See Bracket slot engagement.

Slow maxillary expansion See Expansion, Slow maxillary.

Sls See Cephalometric landmarks (Soft tissue), Superior labial sulcus.

Sm See Cephalometric landmarks (Hard tissue), B-point.

SME See Expansion, Slow maxillary.

Smile line See Tooth-to-lip relationship.

SN See Cephalometric lines, Sella-Nasion line.

Sn See Cephalometric landmarks (Soft tissue), Subnasale.

SNA angle See Cephalometric measurements (Hard tissue), SNA angle.

SNB angle See Cephalometric measurements (Hard tissue), SNB angle

SnPg-CMe See Cephalometric measurements (Soft tissue), Lower face-throat angle.

Soft palate See Palate, Soft.

Soft tissue glabella See Cephalometric landmarks (Soft tissue), Soft tissue glabella.

Soft tissue landmarks, Cephalometric See Cephalometric landmarks, Soft tissue.

Soft tissue measurements, Cephalometric See Cephalometric measurements, Soft tissue.

Soft tissue menton See Cephalometric landmarks (Soft tissue), Soft tissue menton.

Soft tissue nasion See Cephalometric landmarks (Soft tissue), Soft tissue nasion.

Soft tissue pogonion See Cephalometric landmarks (Soft tissue), Soft tissue pogonion.

Soft tissue shield (Vestibular shield, Buccal shield) Component of a removable or functional orthodontic appliance aimed at keeping the lips or cheeks away from the alveolar process and teeth. In this way a stretching of the periosteum is created in the area of the apical base that is supposed to stimulate its growth. In addition, the dental arches are free of the forces from the surrounding soft tissues. [Also see Appliance, Fränkel.]

Soldering An operation in which metallic parts are joined by means of a filler metal having a melting temperature below that of the parts to be joined (in general lower than 450°C), which wets the parent metals. [When a filler metal (braze) with a melting temperature above 450°C is used, the process is termed *brazing*.] The parent metals do not participate by fusion in making the joint.

Somatic Pertaining to the body, as a distinction from the mind or psyche. Pertaining to the structures of the body wall (e.g. skeletal tissue) in contrast to visceral structures.

Somatic swallow See Swallow, Somatic.

Space maintainer (Space-retaining appliance) An orthodontic appliance, fixed or removable, used to control the arch length, usually following the early loss of a deciduous tooth (most commonly a second or first deciduous molar) until the eruption of its successor.

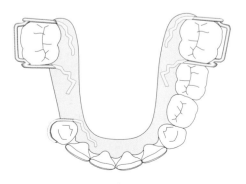

Removable space maintainer

"Band and bar" space maintainer A fixed space maintainer consisting of a bar across the edentulous space. The bar is soldered onto bands on both or one of the teeth adjacent to the space.

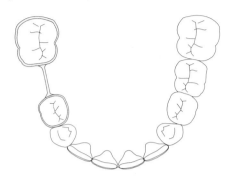

"Band and bar" space maintainer

"Band and loop" space maintainer A cantilever-type of fixed space maintainer that consists of a band cemented to (usually) the tooth posterior to the edentulous space and a loop of wire across the edentulous space abutting the anterior tooth. An occlusal rest also can be soldered on the anterior end of the loop to avoid gingival dislodgment of the appliance due to the forces of mastication and subsequent mesial tipping of the posterior tooth, which would result in loss of space.

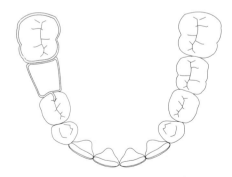

"Band and loop" space maintainer

"Distal shoe" space maintainer A type of fixed band and loop space maintainer indicated especially when a second decid

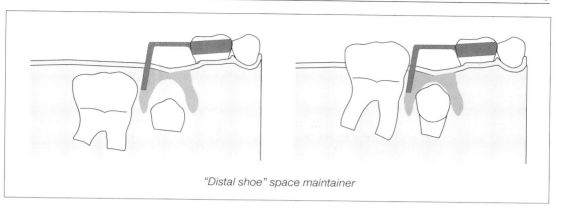

"Distal shoe" space maintainer

uous molar (usually mandibular) is lost before eruption of the first permanent molar. The appliance consists of a metal or plastic guide plane ("blade" or "distal shoe") that is meant to guide the permanent molar eruption. The loop carrying the intra-alveolar distal shoe is soldered on a band on the first primary molar. To be effective, the distal shoe must extend into the alveolar process so that it contacts the permanent first molar approximately 1 mm below its mesial marginal ridge, at or before its emergence from the bone.

Lingual arch space maintainer A lingual arch is indicated for space maintenance when multiple deciduous posterior teeth are missing and the mandibular permanent incisors have erupted. A conventional lingual arch, contacting the cingula of the mandibular incisors while staying approximately 1 to 1.5 mm away from the soft tissue laterally, can prevent anterior movement of the posterior teeth and posterior movement of the anterior teeth. It can be soldered to bands on the primary second or permanent first molars, or it can be of a fixed/removable design.

Space regainer (Space-regaining appliance) Orthodontic appliance used to regain space lost by the premature reduction of arch circumference via extraction, exfoliation or caries. Space regaining is more effective when the space loss is recent

and small and may be accomplished with varying types of appliances.

Coil-spring space regainer A cantilever-type space regainer consisting of a band, cemented to the tooth distal to the edentulous space, that is equipped with a buccal and lingual horizontal tube. In these fits a U-crib, loaded by two compressed coil springs. The reciprocal force generated by the spring-loaded U-crib upon insertion tips the adjacent teeth away from the edentulous area, regaining some space.

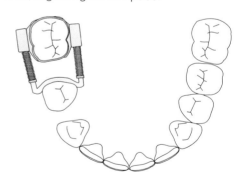

Coil-spring space regainer

Space-retaining appliance See Space maintainer.

Spacing See Arch length discrepancy, Arch length excess.

"Spaghetti" elastics See Orthodontic elastics, Vertical.

Spasm (of muscle) See Muscle spasm.

SPE See Expansion, Slow maxillary.

Specificity (of a test) An indication of the capability of a test to yield negative results accurately, when applied to subjects known to be free of disease. Specificity is calculated by the following formula:
Specificity = TN/(TN + FP) x 100%
where:
TN = True negatives (the number of healthy subjects correctly identified by the test)
FP = False positives (the number of healthy subjects incorrectly classified by the test as having the disease). [Compare with Sensitivity.]

Spee, Curve of See Curve of Spee.

Speed appliance (SPEED system) See Appliance, SPEED.

SPEED bracket See Appliance, SPEED.

Spinal plane See Cephalometric lines, Palatal plane.

Splint Any apparatus, appliance or device employed to provide stabilization or support of teeth or bones, or generally to resist motion or displacement of fractured or injured structures.

Anterior repositioning splint (Anterior repositioning appliance) An interocclusal device that encourages the mandible to assume a position more anterior than the intercuspal position, in an attempt to eliminate the signs and symptoms (e.g. clicking) associated with disc derangement disorders.
The alteration of the mandibular position is not permanent, but only temporary, so as to give the retrodiscal tissues a chance to adapt to the re-established condyle-disc relationship. Once tissue adaptation has

occurred, the appliance is discontinued.
The appliance typically is made of hard acrylic and can be used in either arch (more commonly in the maxilla). A guiding ramp in the anterior aspect of the appliance dictates the new mandibular position. The appliance provides even contacts with all the teeth of the opposing arch.

Bruxism splint See Nightguard.

Diagnostic splint (De-programming splint, Flat occlusal splint) An appliance used to "de-program" the neuromuscular reflex system from its adaptation to the existing occlusal conditions. This is performed to diagnose the true centric relation position in patients where a CR-CO discrepancy is suspected, due to mandibular posturing, muscle splinting etc.
The appliance typically is fabricated from hard acrylic, and the surface that is meant to contact the teeth of the opposing arch usually is flat.

Final surgical splint See Splint, Surgical.

Gelb splint A type of anterior repositioning, partial coverage mandibular splint. The splint consists of two acrylic parts covering the occlusal surface of the mandibular posterior teeth, connected by a metal bar on the lingual aspect of the mandibular incisors. Slight indexing of the occlusal surfaces of the maxillary teeth is used to maintain the anterior position of the mandible. The standard mode of retention is two ball clasps mesial to the mandibular first permanent molars.

Intermediate surgical splint See Splint, Surgical.

Relaxation splint (Stabilization splint, Muscle relaxation splint) An interocclusal device that usually is fabricated for the maxillary arch and provides an occlusal relationship that is considered optimal for the patient. The treatment goal with such an appliance is to eliminate any orthopedic instability or incoordination between the occlusion and the joints. It is advocated for patients with parafunction (bruxism) or stress-related muscle hyperactivity. The use of such an appliance also is advocated in patients with retrodiscitis secondary to trauma.

A maxillary appliance design usually is preferred. The appliance is constructed so that there are full occlusal contacts in centric relation. It also is adjusted carefully, so as to allow smooth and gentle anterior guidance on protrusion and canine guidance on lateral mandibular excursions. The occlusal surface of the appliance should be as flat as possible, with no imprints of the mandibular teeth.

The patient is instructed to wear the appliance according to the disorder that is being treated. When bruxism is the problem, nighttime wear is essential, whereas daytime use may not be as important. When the disorder is retrodiscitis, the appliance may need to be worn full-time.

Surgical splint (Surgical wafer) The surgical splint is a thin, horseshoe-shaped, interocclusal acrylic wafer that is constructed on the basis of the occlusion established from the model surgery. It is used during the operation to provide positive indexing between the teeth, specifying the desired maxillomandibular occlusal relationship. Without such a splint, it may be difficult to make a judgment in the operating room about the precision of the intended final jaw position and occlusion. Splints also are thought to increase the potential for stability of the surgical correction, especially in the case of a multiple-piece maxillary procedure.

Surgical splints are about 1 to 2 mm thick and usually carry small holes bilaterally through which ligatures can be threaded to fixate the splint to the maxillary dental arch (or to both arches, if IMF is used).

When a single-jaw procedure is performed, only one surgical splint is necessary, which will determine the final relationship between the teeth of the two jaws (*final splint*).

However, when a 2-jaw procedure is to be performed, an extra splint (*intermediate splint*) is necessary. The intermediate splint is used after the maxillary osteotomy but prior to the mandibular procedure, in order to provide a reference for the final maxillary position, based on the centric relation of the mandible. After the maxilla has been fixated in its final position, the mandibular osteotomy is performed and the final splint is used to determine the final position of the mandibular distal segment. [Also see Model surgery; Segment, Distal.]

Splinting (of muscles) See Protective muscle splinting.

Splinting (of teeth) The joining together of two or more teeth to immobilize them (e.g. after trauma or considerable periodontal attachment loss) and to increase resistance to applied force, by enlarging the effective root surface area. Splinting may be temporary or permanent.

Split-palate appliance See Appliance, Expansion; Expansion, Slow maxillary.

Split thickness periodontal graft See Graft, Split thickness periodontal.

Spot welding See Welding, Spot.

Spring aligner An active form of the spring retainer used to correct mild mandibular incisor crowding in untreated individuals or in patients with post-orthodontic relapse. The spring aligner is made on a model on which the teeth (usually the incisors) have been cut out and reset in an ideal position.

Interproximal mandibular incisor stripping is recommended at the time of insertion of the appliance to facilitate achievement of the desired correction. The creation of artificial undercuts, by adding composite at the mesial half of the labial surface of the mandibular canines, can enhance retention. [Also see Retainer, Spring; Undercuts, Artificial.]

Spring retainer See Retainer, Spring.

Springback The recovery exhibited by an orthodontic wire, loop, or spring upon its unloading (deactivation) from a state at or beyond its elastic limit. The springback is given by the ratio YS/E, which is approximately equal to the maximum elastic strain, or working range of the wire. (The formal expression from materials science for springback is PL/E.) Because the unloading curve from the permanent deformation range for typically behaving orthodontic wire alloys (i.e. other than nickel-titanium alloys) is parallel to the elastic loading curve, the value of YS/E represents the approximate amount of elastic strain released by the archwire upon unloading (*clinically useful springback*).

Spring-clip separator See Separator, Spring-clip.

Spurt, Growth See Pubertal growth spurt.

Spurt, Post-emergent See Post-emergent spurt.

Square wire See Orthodontic wire, Square.

ss See Cephalometric landmarks (Hard tissue), A-point.

St See Cephalometric landmarks (Soft tissue), Stomion.

Stabilization appliance See Splint, Relaxation.

Stabilization splint See Splint, Relaxation.

Stabilizing wire See Archwire, Stabilizing.

Stainless steel The most popular wire alloy for clinical orthodontics because of its outstanding combination of mechanical properties, corrosion resistance in the oral environment, and cost. The wires used in orthodontics are composed principally of iron (approximately 70%), 17% to 20% chromium, 8% to 12% nickel and 0.08% maximum carbon. These are the "18-8" stainless steels, so designated because of the respective percentages of chromium and nickel in the alloys. Chromium is the element that gives stainless steel its corrosion resistance, whereas nickel enhances its ductility.
Heat treatment can be used to eliminate residual stresses that might cause fracture during manipulation of stainless steel wires.

Stainless steel ligature See Ligature, Stainless steel.

Stainless steel wire See Stainless steel.

Standard edgewise appliance See Appliance, Edgewise.

Static fatigue failure See Fatigue failure, Static.

Static friction See Friction.

Statically determinate/indeterminate force system See Force system, Statically determinate/indeterminate.

Statics The branch of mechanics that considers forces on bodies that are either at rest or have a constant velocity along a straight line.

Steep mandibular plane A high value of the mandibular plane angle.

Steiner cephalometric analysis See Cephalometric analysis, Steiner.

Steiner ligature-tying pliers See Orthodontic instruments, Steiner ligature-tying pliers.

Steiner rotation wedge See Rotation wedge.

Steiner's esthetic plane (S-line) See Cephalometric lines, S-line.

Step bends See Bends, Step.

Sternocleidomastoid muscle See Muscle, Sternocleidomastoid.

Sti See Cephalometric landmarks (Soft tissue), Stomion inferius.

Stiffness (Rate of elastic force delivery) The ratio of change in load to accompanying change in deformation of an orthodontic wire, when it is activated within its elastic limit. The inverse of the property of flexibility. Stiffness of a material is expressed by the modulus of elasticity (the slope of the initial linear part of the load/deformation diagram). Wire stiffness is dependent on two fundamental factors: 1) the composition and structure of the wire alloy (which determines its modulus of elasticity) and 2) the wire segment geometry, i.e. the size and shape of the cross-section and the length of the particular segment.

Still's disease See Arthritis, Juvenile rheumatoid.

STO See Surgical prediction tracing.

Stöckli-Teuscher activator See Appliance, Teuscher-Stöckli activator/headgear combination.

Stomatognathic system The complex of all the structures of the mouth and jaws, involved in a variety of functions such as speech, respiration, deglutition and mastication.

Stomion (St) See Cephalometric landmarks (Soft tissue), Stomion.

Stomion inferius (Sti) See Cephalometric landmarks (Soft tissue), Stomion inferius.

Stomion superius (Sts) See Cephalometric landmarks (Soft tissue), Stomion superius.

Stop, Archwire See Archwire, stop.

Stop bends See Bends, Stop.

Stop, Occlusal See Occlusal rest.

Stopped arch See Arch, Stopped.

Straight-pull headgear See Headgear, Straight-pull.

Straight-wire appliance See Appliance, Straight-wire.

Straight-wire bracket See Appliance, Straight-wire; Bracket, Pre-angulated; Bracket, Pretorqued.

Strain (ε) The consequence of stress, expressing the internal distortion of a body produced by a load on it. Relative deformation of a body subjected to external load, defined as dimensional change (deformation, Δd) divided by the original dimension d ($\varepsilon = \Delta d/d$). Commonly expressed as a percentage (%).

Strength (of a material) The stress that is necessary to cause fracture (*fracture strength*) or a specified amount of deformation (*yield strength, ultimate tensile strength*).

Stress (σ) The internal response of a body to the application of external forces to it, defined as force (load) per unit area ($\sigma = F/A$).

Compressive stress Stress created by two sets of forces with the same line of action and senses towards each other.

Residual stress Internal stress remaining between parts of a solid body after the applied stress is removed.

Shear stress Stress created by two sets of non-coplanar forces with parallel lines of action and opposite sense. Equal to shearing force per unit of shearing area. [Also see Shear.]

Tensile stress Stress created by two sets of forces with the same line of action and senses away from each other.

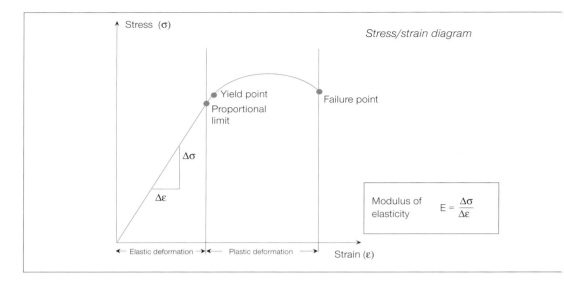

Stress corrosion See Corrosion, Stress.

Stress raiser An irregularity on the surface or in the interior of an object that causes applied stress to concentrate at a localized area of the object. Other things being equal, the sharper the stress raiser, the greater the localized stress around it.

Stress relief A heat-treatment process intended to reduce the magnitudes of residual stresses that are "locked in" an orthodontic wire due to plastic deformation.

Stress/strain diagram   (Stress/strain curve) A common means by which materials can be compared. The information usually is obtained by subjecting a specimen of the material to tension in special testing machines that can monitor the applied load and change in length continuously. By plotting stress along the vertical axis and strain along the horizontal axis, a stress/strain diagram can be constructed that is characteristic of the material. Initially, there often is a straight linear portion on the curve. If the stress is removed from the material while in this portion of the curve, complete recovery of the initial shape of the specimen will result. This part of the curve

is called the *elastic region of behavior* (*elastic range*). When the specimen is stressed beyond the elastic range, permanent deformation will take place. In other words, removal of the stress while in this portion of the curve will not cause recovery of the initial shape of the specimen. This part of the curve is called the *plastic region of behavior* (*plastic range*). Continued tensile load on the specimen will eventually cause it to fracture.

Stripping (of teeth) See Interproximal stripping.

Strips, Abrasive See Abrasive strips.

Sts See Cephalometric landmarks (Soft tissue), Stomion superius.

Study casts See Orthodontic casts, Study.

Study models See Orthodontic casts, Study.

Subdivision See Angle classification, "Subdivisions."

Subepithelial connective tissue graft See Graft, Subepithelial connective tissue.

Subgingival scaling See Scaling, Subgingival.

Subluxation (of the TMJ) Incomplete condylar dislocation during wide jaw opening (usually accompanied by a joint sound), during which the joint surfaces remain in partial contact.

Subluxation (of a tooth) 1. The intentional movement of a tooth within its alveolus by means of forceps, sometimes performed in an effort to release the ankylosis of a tooth. **2.** The traumatic injury to a tooth that does not result in complete removal from its alveolus but increases its mobility beyond physiologically observed levels.

Submucous cleft palate A congenital cleft in the bone or soft tissue underlying the mucous membrane of the palate. In the case of a submucous cleft of the soft palate, the defect is a lack of continuity in the musculature of the soft palate. In submucous clefts of the hard palate, the posterior nasal spine characteristically is absent. Submucous clefts also are called *occult* clefts, because they are not readily seen on cursory examination.

Subnasale (Sn) See Cephalometric landmarks (Soft tissue), Subnasale.

Subperiosteal implant See Implant, Subperiosteal.

Subspinale (ss) See Cephalometric landmarks (Hard tissue), A-point.

Subtraction radiography A technique of eliminating background anatomical structures from an image to bring out the differences between the pre- and post-procedure radiographic images.

Digital subtraction radiography A radiographic image subtraction technique in which the pre- and post-procedure radiographic images are subtracted from each other within the computer memory and the resulting subtracted image is displayed on the monitor.

Photographic subtraction radiography A radiographic image subtraction method in which a mask film (negative) is made of the pre-procedure radiograph. When this mask film is superimposed and viewed over the post-procedure film, the resultant image is a subtraction image containing the difference (or contrast medium) between the pre- and post- procedure radiographs.

Succedaneous teeth (Successional teeth) Those permanent teeth that have predecessors, which includes all permanent teeth except the molars.

"Sunday" bite A situation in which patients with a skeletal Class II jaw relationship habitually position their mandible in a more anterior position, making the occlusion appear "better" than it really is.

Superelasticity A remarkable property of some alloys that exhibit a reversible elastic deformation characterized by a distinct nonlinear relationship between load and deflection. This is seen as a characteristic plateau-like appearance of the stress/strain curve during loading and unloading. In superelastic alloys, such as certain nickel-titanium alloys, martensitic transformation can be induced by the application of mechanical stress (e.g. bending). [See also Martensitic transformation; Nickel-titanium alloy.] *See illustration next page.*

Superimposition The process of placing two images upon each other, registering on structures that remain relatively stable during the time period separating the two images, to evaluate the changes brought about by growth and/or treatment. In orthodontics, most commonly applies to cephalometric tracings or occlusograms.

Superior joint space (Superior joint compartment) The intra-articular space

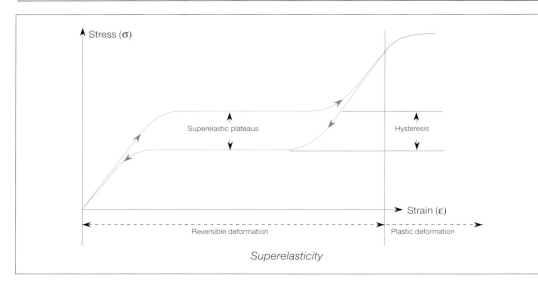

Superelasticity

between the head of the superior surface of the articular disc of the TMJ and the mandibular fossa of the temporal bone that is involved in the translational movement of the condyle during the later stages of opening movement. [Also see Joint, Temporomandibular.]

Superior labial sulcus (Sls) See Cephalometric landmarks (Soft tissue), Superior labial sulcus.

Superior prosthion See Cephalometric landmarks (Hard tissue), Prosthion.

Supernumerary teeth (Hyperodontia) Teeth in excess of 20 in the deciduous dentition, or 32 in the permanent dentition. Supernumerary teeth often have abnormal or atypical shape and may interfere with the eruption of adjacent unerupted permanent teeth. [Compare with Hypodontia.]

Superoinferior The global direction perpendicular to the transverse plane of the dentofacial complex or the occlusal plane of one dental arch; the superior direction/sense is upward, and the inferior direction/sense is downward.

Supporting cusp See Cusp, Functional.

Supracontact See Occlusal interference.

Supradentale See Cephalometric landmarks (Hard tissue), Prosthion.

Supraeruption See Overeruption.

Supragingival scaling See Scaling, Supragingival.

Suprahyoid muscles See Muscle, Suprahyoid.

Supramentale (sm) See Cephalometric landmarks (Hard tissue), B-point.

Supraocclusion See Overeruption.

Supraposition See Overeruption.

Surface roughness A parameter influencing the coefficient of friction (μ) between bracket and archwire during orthodontic tooth movement by sliding mechanics. It may also influence plaque accumulation on the orthodontic appliances and teeth, as well as the degree of corrosion of metallic appliances. Surface roughness of various brackets and wires can be estimated by using methods such as specular reflectance, which involves quantification of the amount of light that is reflected back from a surface. A very smooth surface reflects much of the light shone on it in a narrow pattern, whereas a rough surface scatters the light and reflects it back in a more dispersed pattern.

Surgery, Model See Model surgery.

Surgery, Mucogingival See Mucogingival surgery.

Surgery, Orthognathic See Orthognathic surgery.

Surgical archwires See Archwire, Surgical.

Surgical exposure (of a tooth) Surgical uncovering of an unerupted or impacted tooth, which may involve a mucosal flap with or without removal of alveolar bone to access the tooth. Following exposure, and depending on its location, the tooth either is left to erupt spontaneously, or an attachment is bonded on it and traction is applied to guide it into the arch. [Also see Forced eruption.]

Surgical fixation See Fixation.

Surgical prediction tracing (Surgical treatment objective, STO) A visual projection of the changes in osseous, dental and soft tissue relationships, as a result of an orthognathic surgical procedure in combination with orthodontic treatment. An STO is constructed by specific manipulation of a lateral cephalometric tracing to relocate the underlying structures into a more favorable position, based on clinical assessment and cephalometric analysis. The same principles applying to the lateral cephalometric prediction tracing may be employed with posteroanterior (P-A) cephalometrics. [Also see Visual treatment objective.]

Surgical splint See Splint, Surgical.

Surgical treatment objective (STO) See Surgical prediction tracing.

Surgical wafer See Splint, Surgical.

Surgically assisted rapid maxillary expansion See Expansion, Surgically assisted rapid maxillary.

Surgically assisted RPE See Expansion, Surgically assisted rapid maxillary.

Suture Fibrous joint between those bones of the cranium that are formed by intramembranous ossification. These periosteum-lined areas do not contain cartilage but fibrous connective tissue and in the mature state they allow no movement of the joined parts.

At birth, the sutures between the flat bones of the skull as well as their points of intersection, the *fontanels*, are rather wide and contain loose connective tissue. This contributes to increased flexibility that allows a considerable amount of deformation of the head as it passes through the birth canal.

Sutures also play an important role in postnatal craniofacial growth and development. Their function is to permit the skull and face to accommodate growing organs such as the eyes and brain. When two bones are separated (e.g. the skull bones are forced apart by the growing brain) bone forms at the sutural margins with successive waves of new bone cells differentiating from the suture's osteogenic layer.

Continuous apposition of bone along the edges of the cranial bones gradually reduces the sutural spaces, which eventually fuse in adult life. Mature sutures show a variety of intricate interdigitating patterns and contain minimal connective tissue.

SWA See Appliance, Straight-wire.

Swallow The act of deglutition. It begins with the swallow-preparatory positioning of the bolus within the mouth, followed by its passage from the mouth to the pharynx and through the hypopharyngeal sphincter.

In the first (voluntary) phase, the chewed food or liquid is placed between the tongue and the anterior palate, the circumoral and tongue muscles being most active.

The preliminary phase is followed by the bolus being propelled posteriorly by the tongue against the palate and into the pharynx and opening of the pharynx, while the hyoid bone is raised by the mylohyoid muscles and the soft palate is elevated to allow the palatopharyngeal muscles to constrict so that the passage of the nasal cavity may be closed. While the tongue propels the bolus, the maxillary and mandibular teeth come in contact and the larynx is raised, with the glottis being closed to interrupt respiration. The bolus is forced over and around the epiglottis, through the hypopharynx and into the esophagus.

The entire process is accomplished within approximately 1 second. The center for swallowing is situated in the floor of the fourth ventricle.

Infantile swallow (Visceral swallow) The swallowing pattern of infants, which is closely related to their mode of feeding. Reflex suckling (small nibbling movements of the lips) action of the facial and circumoral muscles of the infant aid in stimulating the smooth muscle of the breast to squirt milk into the mouth. Following that, the tongue is grooved and placed anteriorly, in contact with the lower lip and between the gum pads, to allow the milk to flow posteriorly into the pharynx and esophagus. This sequence of events determines the characteristics of infantile swallowing pattern, which are: active contractions of the musculature of the lips, a tongue tip brought forward into contact with the lower lip, and little activity of the posterior tongue or pharyngeal musculature. The suckling reflex and the infantile mode of swallowing normally disappear after the first year of life.

Somatic swallow (Mature swallow, Teeth-together swallow) The adult pattern of deglutition, characterized by a cessation of lip activity (i.e. relaxed lips), the placement of the tongue tip against the palatal aspect of the alveolar process behind the maxillary incisors, and the posterior teeth brought into occlusion during swallowing. The transition from an infantile to a mature swallowing pattern is made difficult, as long as sucking habits persist.

Tongue-thrust swallow (Reverse swallow, Teeth-apart swallow) A swallowing pattern normally in the transition between infantile and mature swallow. It is characterized by various degrees of lip activity and an anterior placement of the tongue behind the maxillary anterior teeth, or between the maxillary and mandibular teeth. It is considered to be closely related to sucking habits. When a tongue-thrust swallow is retained for a long period, it may play a role in the creation or maintenance of an anterior open bite.

Symphysis See Mandibular symphysis.

Symptom (of a disease or disorder) Subjective indications of a disease or disorder, as reported by the patient. [Compare with Sign.]

Syndrome See Malformation syndromes.

Syngeneic graft See Graft, Isologous.

Synovial joint See Joint, Synovial.

System of Axes See Global reference frame.

Système Internationale d'Unités (SI) See International System of Units.

T

T-loop See Loop, T-.

Tarnish The process by which a metal surface is dulled in brightness or discolored through the formation of a chemical film (such as the formation of black oxides and sulfides on silver). Tarnish should be differentiated from corrosion, as it is observable as a surface discoloration on a metal, or even as a slight loss of the surface finish (luster). In the oral cavity tarnish often occurs from the formation of hard and soft deposits on the surface of a restoration (e.g. plaque, calculus). As well, surface discoloration may arise on a metal in the oral cavity, from the formation of thin films such as oxides, sulfides and chlorides. Thus, it usually is an early indication of corrosion.

Tartar See Calculus.

Taurodontism A dental shape anomaly (observed mainly in molars) in which the furcation is displaced apically. This results in relative elongation of the body and pulp chamber, and in shortening of the roots. Affected teeth may lack the usual constriction at the cementoenamel junction found in normal teeth.
The term comes from the Greek words *tauros* (bull) and *odous* (tooth). It was developed by A. Keith in 1913 to describe the apparent similarity in form and structure between these teeth and those of cud-chewing ungulates. Taurodontism can occur in both deciduous and permanent dentitions, although it is more common in the latter. It has been found to occur either as an isolated, singular trait or in association with syndromes and anomalies including amelogenesis imperfecta, Down syndrome, Klinefelter syndrome, ectodermal dysplasia and hypodontia.

Teardrop loop See Loop, Tear-drop.

Technique A treatment method or procedure, based on a certain school of thought, using certain appliances or treatment modalities in specific ways and in a particular sequence. Numerous different techniques are employed worldwide in the everyday practice of orthodontics (e.g. the straight-wire technique, the Begg technique). [For a discussion of various techniques, please see Appliance.]

Teeth-apart swallow See Swallow, Tongue-thrust.

Teeth-together swallow See Swallow, Somatic.

Teflon (PTFE, Polytetrafluoroethylene) The material with the lowest coefficient of friction. Teflon-coated stainless steel ligatures and archwires are available as a means for reducing frictional resistance to tooth movement with sliding mechanics.

Telecanthus A soft tissue measurement reflecting increased distance between the medial canthi of the eyelids, a common finding in patients born with conditions such as Waardenburg syndrome or Down syndrome. [Compare with Orbital hypertelorism.]

Telescoping bite See Crossbite, Telescoping bite.

Temporal fossa See Glenoid fossa.

Temporalis muscle See Muscle, Temporalis.

Temporomandibular articulation See Joint, Temporomandibular.

Temporomandibular disorders (TMD, Craniomandibular disorders, CMD) A collective term embracing a number of clinical problems that involve the masticatory musculature, the temporomandibular joint (TMJ) and associated structures, or both. Temporomandibular disorders have been identified as a major cause of nondental pain in the orofacial region and are considered to be a subclassification of musculoskeletal disorders.
Although TMD traditionally were considered as one syndrome [see Costen's syndrome], current research supports the view that TMD are a cluster of related disorders in the masticatory system that have many common symptoms. The most common presenting symptom is pain, usually localized in the muscles of mastication, the preauricular area, and/or the TMJ. The pain usually is aggravated by chewing or other jaw function. In addition to complaints of pain, patients with these disorders frequently have limited or asymmetric mandibular movement and TMJ sounds that are most frequently described as clicking, popping, grating or crepitus. Other common patient complaints include jaw ache, earache, headache and facial pain. Non-painful masticatory muscle hypertrophy and abnormal occlusal wear associated with oral parafunction, such as bruxism (jaw clenching and tooth grinding), may be related problems. Pain or dysfunction due to non-musculoskeletal causes such as otolaryngologic, neurologic, vascular, neoplastic or infectious disease in the orofacial region is not considered a primary temporomandibular disorder, even though musculoskeletal pain may be present. However, TMD often coexist with other craniofacial and orofacial pain disorders.

Temporomandibular joint (TMJ) See Joint, Temporomandibular.

Tendon Strong, flexible and inelastic band of fibrous tissue attaching muscle to bone.

TENS See Transcutaneous electric nerve stimulation.

Tensile stress See Stress, Tensile.

Tension The deformation experienced by a body that is subjected to two sets of forces applied along the same line of action and with opposite sense, tending to increase the characteristic length of that body.

Tension-type headache Dull, aching, pressing, usually bilateral headache of mild to moderate intensity. When severe, it may include photophobia or rarely nausea. It may be intermittent, lasting from minutes to days, or chronic without remission.

Teratogen An agent that may cause birth defects when present in the fetal or embryonic environment. Included under such a definition are a wide array of drugs; chemicals; and infectious, physical and metabolic agents that may affect the intrauterine environment of the developing fetus adversely. Such factors may operate by exceedingly heterogeneous pathogenic mechanisms to produce alterations of form and function (including growth, learning and behavior disorders) as well as embryonic or fetal death.

Terminal attachments The orthodontic attachments (brackets or tubes) on the distal-most teeth in the arch, bilaterally.

Terminal closing clicking See Clicking, Late-closing.

Terminal molars The distalmost erupted molars in the arch.

Terminal opening clicking See Clicking, Late-opening.

Terminal plane The distal proximal surface of the maxillary and mandibular second deciduous molars (being the distal terminal plane of the deciduous dentition). The relationship between the maxillary and mandibular terminal planes in the early mixed dentition is thought to determine, to a degree, the eventual relationship between the (at the time still unerupted) maxillary and mandibular first permanent molars.

Distal step A situation in which the terminal plane of the mandibular second deciduous molar is situated posteriorly to that of the maxillary second deciduous molar. This situation is thought to be predisposing to, but not necessarily predictive of, a Class II relationship of the (at the time, still unerupted) first permanent molars.

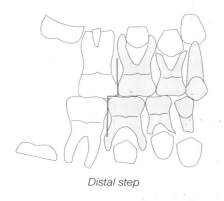

Distal step

Flush terminal plane An end-to-end relationship between the distal proximal surfaces of the maxillary and mandibular

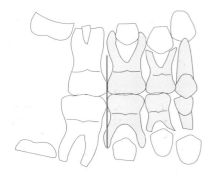

Flush terminal plane

second deciduous molars, usually leading to a Class I or Class II relationship between the (at the time, still unerupted) maxillary and mandibular first permanent molars.

Mesial step A situation in which the terminal plane of the mandibular second deciduous molar is situated anteriorly to that of the maxillary second deciduous molar. Depending on the severity of the mesial step, this relationship is thought to predispose to (but is, strictly speaking, not predictive of) either a Class I or a Class III relationship of the (at the time, still unerupted) maxillary and mandibular first permanent molars.

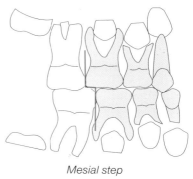

Mesial step

Tertiary crowding See Arch length discrepancy, Arch length deficiency.

Teuscher-Stöckli activator See Appliance, Teuscher-Stöckli activator/headgear combination.

TGF-β See Growth factors.

Theories of tooth eruption See Tooth eruption mechanisms.

Theory, Differential force See Differential force theory.

Theory, Functional matrix See Functional matrix theory.

Theory, Normal occlusion See Extraction vs. non-extraction debate.

Theory, Optimal force See Optimal force theory.

Theory, "Wedge" See "Wedge" theory.

Third order See Inclination.

Third-order bends See Bends, Third-order.

Third-order clearance The angle through which an engaged rectangular archwire may be rotated about its longitudinal axis (placed in torsion) before the edges of the wire make diagonal contacts with the occlusal and gingival walls of the bracket slot. [Also see "Play" of an orthodontic wire in the bracket slot; compare with Second-order clearance.]

Third-order rotation See Rotation (of a tooth), Third-order.

Thread, Elastic See Elastomeric modules, Elastomeric thread.

Three-jaw pliers See Orthodontic instruments, Triple-beaked pliers.

Three-quarter clasp See Clasp, Circumferential.

Threshold The minimum level of stimulus required to produce a result.

Threshold of force required for tooth movement The minimum magnitude of force necessary to produce orthodontic tooth movement (a theoretical concept).

Through-the-bite elastics See Orthodontic elastics, Crossbite.

Thumbsucking appliance See Appliance, Crib.

Thumbsucking habit (Finger-sucking habit) A habit that is considered normal during infancy, but if prolonged can lead to malocclusion. As a general rule, sucking habits during the deciduous dentition have little if any long-term effect. However, if these habits persist beyond that time, they are likely to affect the position of the teeth, creating or aggravating existing malocclusion.

The typical characteristic changes associated with sucking habits include flaring or spacing of the maxillary incisors, anterior open bite, forward maxillary position and narrow maxillary arch. The above presumably are caused by a combination of direct pressure on the teeth by the thumb or finger, as well as an alteration in the pattern of resting cheek and lip pressures.

Tie Term used to indicate fastening of a ligature around a bracket, or placement and ligation of an archwire in place. [Also see Ligature.]

Tie-back A stop, hook or loop, soldered, crimped or bent into an archwire, usually at some point anterior to the molar tubes, so that the archwire can be tied to the molar attachments by means of stainless steel or elastic ligatures. *See illustration next page.*

Tie-wings (of a bracket) See Bracket wings.

Tinnitus Subjective ringing, buzzing, or roaring sound in the ear.

"Tip" See Angulation.

Tip-back bends See Bends, Tip-back.

Tip bends See Bends, Second-order.

Tip-Edge appliance See Appliance, Tip-Edge.

Tip-forward bends See Bends, Tip-forward.

Tipping See Orthodontic tooth movement, Tipping.

Titanium A material with numerous applications in dentistry, primarily because of its excellent biocompatibility (as a result of its stable oxide layer), and its mechanical properties. As well, its ability to achieve osseointegration has made titanium very popular in implantology. In orthodontics titanium is

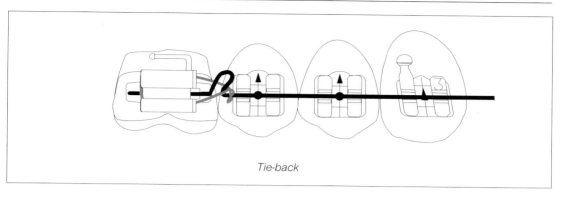

Tie-back

used mainly as alloys for archwires, and more recently by Dentaurum also for brackets (which are especially useful for patients with nickel hypersensitivity who react to the nickel in conventional stainless steel brackets). [Also see Beta-titanium alloy; Nickel-titanium alloy.]

Titanium-molybdenum alloy (TMA) See Beta-titanium alloy.

TMA wire See Beta-titanium alloy.

TMD See Temporomandibular disorders.

TMJ See Joint, Temporomandibular.

Toe-in bends See Bends, Toe-in.

Tomography Radiographic imaging technique capable of generating structural images of the internal body within a predetermined cross-sectional plane of tissues, while eliminating or blurring images of structures lying in other planes.
This involves movement of the x-ray tube and film, which are connected so as to rotate about a pivot. They move in opposite directions about a stationary object so that there is a fixed plane about which there is no relative movement between them. This plane is referred to as the *tomographic cut*. Structures in adjacent planes are blurred due to movement and therefore not visualized.

Computerized tomography (CT, Computer-assisted tomography, CAT scan) Computerized tomographic imaging method that employs a narrowly collimated radiographic beam that passes through the body and is recorded by an array of scintillation detectors. These detectors convert the information into a grey scale image. A computer then can calculate tissue absorption within the film images, reflecting the densities of various structures.
With the appropriate instrumentation, the computer can synthesize three-dimensional images by reformatting a series of axial and coronal scans (3D-CT). By setting the appropriate attenuation values (which reflect the different tissue densities) it is possible to display both soft tissues and bone (or just bone) on the same tomogram.

Tongue crib See Appliance, Crib.

Tongue interposition Habitual placement of the tongue between the maxillary and mandibular teeth.

Tongue-thrust See Swallow, Tongue-thrust.

Tongue-tie See Ankyloglossia.

Tooth eruption The movement of a tooth during the final stages of odontogenesis in an axial and occlusal direction, from its developmental position within the jaw (crypt) to its final functional position in the occlusal plane.

Eruptive movement of a tooth starts soon after its root begins to form. In the stage of eruption prior to emergence into the oral cavity, the bone overlying the crown of the erupting tooth is resorbed, as are the roots of its deciduous predecessor (if applicable) and the tooth moves in the direction where the path has been cleared.

After its emergence into the mouth the tooth erupts rapidly until it approaches the occlusal plane and is subjected to the occlusal forces. [See Post-emergent spurt.] At that point, its eruption slows down and eventually a dynamic equilibrium is reached once the tooth is in complete function. Subsequently, the teeth continue to erupt at a rate that parallels the rate of vertical growth of the mandibular ramus. [See Occlusal equilibrium, Juvenile.]

Tooth eruption continues throughout adult life at a slow rate, to compensate for the loss of tooth material due to wear and to maintain the vertical dimension of the face to a reasonable degree, unless wear is excessive. [Also see Occlusal equilibrium, Adult; Physiologic tooth movement.]

Tooth eruption, Forced See Forced eruption.

Tooth eruption mechanisms The mechanism of tooth eruption is not clearly understood; most investigations have concluded that eruption is a multifactorial process in which cause and effect are difficult to separate. Some theories attempting to explain the mechanisms of tooth eruption are:

1. The root elongation theory, which supports the idea that root growth is responsible for occlusal movement of the crown.

2. The hydrostatic pressure theory (vascular theory), according to which local increases in tissue fluid pressure in periapical tissues push the tooth occlusally.

3. The alveolar bone growth theory, according to which apposition of bone to the crypt beneath the erupting tooth, and resorption of bone occlusal to it, is what causes the tooth to rise into functional occlusion.

4. The pulp theory, which states that the pulp produces a propulsive force generated by extrusion of pulp due to growth of dentin, by interstitial pulp growth, or by hydraulic effects within the pulpal vasculature. This results in an eruptive force because of pressure gradients that are greater below the tooth than above it.

5. The periodontal ligament theory, according to which the mechanism for tooth eruption lies within the periodontal ligament, possibly related to the contractility of collagen fibers.

6. The dental follicle theory, which states that tooth eruption largely is a function of bone resorption above the erupting tooth (forming its eruption pathway), in combination with intense osteoblastic activity below it, both of which are controlled by the dental follicle.

The above listed theories are not necessarily mutually exclusive; in fact there is reasonable evidence that tooth eruption is regulated by a different mechanism in the pre-emergent and post-emergent stages. Physiological factors such as hormonal fluctuations also seem to play an important role.

Tooth mobility Visually perceptible movement of a tooth within its alveolar socket upon application of a force on its crown.

Increased mobility (Hypermobility) Increased tooth mobility is associated with various physiologic phenomena such as tooth eruption (due to incomplete maturation of the periodontal ligament), pregnancy (as a result of the hormonal influences on collagen and the vascular structures of the PDL tissues) and orthodontic treatment (due to remodeling of the PDL tissues during tooth movement). Pathologic conditions related to increased tooth mobility are trauma from occlusion and periodontal disease.

Physiologic (Normal) mobility The limited amount of tooth displacement allowed by the resilience of an intact and healthy periodontal ligament and by the bending potential of the alveolar bone, when a light or moderate force is applied to the crown of a tooth.

Reduced mobility (Hypomobility)
Tooth mobility below the physiologic levels can be found in cases of ankylosis. In such situations there is no intra-socket tooth displacement and any movement of the tooth can be attributed to elastic deformation of the alveolar bone. [Also see Ankylosis.]

Tooth movement   See Orthodontic tooth movement, Physiological.

Tooth positioner   See Appliance, Positioner.

Tooth size discrepancy (Bolton discrepancy)   Incongruity between the sums of the mesiodistal tooth sizes of sets of corresponding maxillary and mandibular teeth, as determined by the Bolton analysis.
A discrepancy could involve the *overall ratio* (which encompasses all permanent teeth except the second and third molars) or the *anterior ratio* (which includes the six anterior teeth of each jaw) and is identified as a maxillary or mandibular excess or deficiency. Only deviations that are larger than two standard deviations are considered to be of potential clinical significance.
A tooth size discrepancy may cause difficulties in achieving an ideal overjet and overbite or arriving at a good intercuspation during the final stages of orthodontic treatment. Different ways to address such a problem include extraction of teeth in the arch with the excess tooth material (usually one mandibular incisor), interproximal stripping, compromising the angulation of some teeth so they can occupy a larger or a smaller space in the arch, or increasing the mesiodistal tooth size in the arch with the deficiency in tooth material (build-ups). [Also see Bolton analysis.]

Tooth-to-lip relationship   For optimal esthetics, it is considered desirable that approximately 2 to 4 mm of the maxillary central incisors be uncovered by the upper lip at rest (in other words, the upper lip should cover roughly $2/3$ of the maxillary central incisor crown length at rest). Similarly, in an esthetically pleasing smile, the upper lip is raised

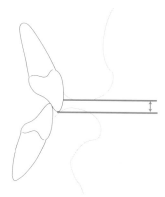

Tooth-to-lip relationship

approximately to the level of the cementoenamel junction of the incisors, so that the full crowns of the maxillary incisors are shown.
Excessive gingival exposure on smiling ("gummy" smile) is considered unesthetic, as is inadequate maxillary incisor exposure on smiling ("edentulous" smile). The tooth-to-lip relationship is an important parameter in orthodontic treatment planning, which to a great extent determines the type of incisor movement desired.

Torque   Type of activation placed into a rectangular (or square) orthodontic archwire by twisting it around its long axis, with the purpose of achieving a rotation of the tooth (or group of teeth) around the x- (mesiodistal) axis. The intended type of torquing movement is accomplished largely by movement of the root of the tooth in the labiolingual or buccolingual direction (e.g. buccal root torque, labial crown torque), with no or minimal movement of the crown in the opposite direction. The type of bends placed in an archwire to produce torque are classified in Tweed's coordinate system as *third-order bends*.
The term *torque* often (though strictly speaking, incorrectly) is used as a substitute for the term *inclination*. [See also Orthodontic springs, Torquing spring].

Active torque Activation for labiolingual or buccolingual root movement of a tooth or group of teeth, brought about by actively placing a torsional bend into an archwire with rectangular or square cross-section. [Compare with Torque, Passive.]

Continuous posterior torque A torquing activation placed unilaterally or bilaterally at one point on the archwire for the entire buccal segment, as described by C.H. Tweed. This can be performed by holding the archwire with two pairs of pliers very close to each other, and by twisting appropriately so that a torquing bend is placed at a specific point on the archwire.

The choice of term is somewhat unfortunate, as in this case the torquing activation is mainly "felt" by the tooth immediately distal to the bend. The teeth lying more posteriorly along the archwire will probably "feel" minimal torquing activation, until the inclination of the tooth distal to the bend has actually changed as a result of the torque. [Compare with Torque, Progressive posterior.]

Crown torque Change of inclination by movement of the crown, with relatively little movement of the root (termed *buccal* or *lingual/palatal* crown torque, depending on the direction of movement).

Passive torque Activation for labiolingual or buccolingual root movement of a tooth or group of teeth without actively placing twisting bends on the archwire. Passive torque is a consequence of tooth inclination and the resulting corresponding orientation of the bracket slot in relation to the rectangular (or square) archwire. [Compare with Torque, Active.]

Progressive posterior torque A torquing activation placed unilaterally or bilaterally over the entire buccal segment, as described by C.H. Tweed. This can be performed by holding the archwire with one pair of pliers (or with the fingers), e.g. distal to the canine bracket and with another pair of pliers close to the end of the wire, and by twisting appropriately. In this way the torquing activation is distributed over all the teeth engaged on that part of the archwire. [Compare with Torque, Continuous posterior.]

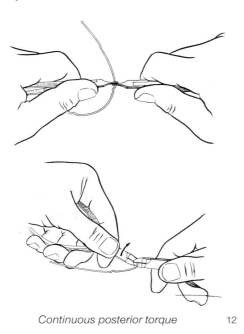

Continuous posterior torque   12

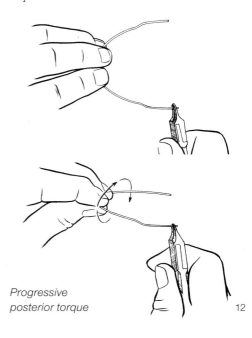

Progressive posterior torque   12

Root torque Change of inclination of a tooth by movement of the root, with relatively little movement of the crown (termed *buccal* or *lingual/palatal* root torque, depending on the direction of movement).

Torquing auxiliary See Orthodontic springs, Torquing.

Torquing bends See Bends, Third-order.

Torquing key See Orthodontic instruments, Torquing key.

Torquing spring See Orthodontic springs, Torquing.

Torsion The type of deformation of a body that is twisted about its long axis, be it elastic (reversible) or plastic (irreversible).

Torsional mechanical couples A combination of two mechanical couples with opposite senses applied at a certain distance from each other along the length of a wire to place torsional deformation (torque) in it. In practice, this is accomplished by holding a wire with two pliers (or a plier and a torquing key) and twisting in opposite directions.

Torsiversion A type of malposition of a tooth that is rotated about its long axis (not related to torque as described above).

Torticollis Contracted state of cervical muscles producing twisting of the neck and an unnatural head posture.

Torus A bulging bony prominence occurring at the midline of the hard palate (*torus palatinus*) or on the lingual aspect of the mandible in the canine-premolar area, bilaterally (*torus mandibularis*).

Total facial height See Cephalometric measurements (Hard tissue), Facial height.

Total maxillary osteotomy See Osteotomy, One-piece maxillary.

Total non-occlusion See Non-occlusion, Total.

Total rotation (of the mandible) See Mandibular rotation, Total.

Toughness The total amount of energy required to fracture a material. It is a measure of resistance to fracture. Toughness can be measured by calculating the total area under the stress/strain curve from zero stress to the fracture stress. Toughness depends on strength and ductility. The higher the strength and the higher the ductility (total plastic strain) the greater the toughness. Thus, a tough material is generally strong, whereas a strong material is not necessarily tough.

TOVRO See Osteotomy, Transoral vertical ramus osteotomy.

Towne's projection Fronto-occipital, plain film radiographic projection of the skull, obtained with the patient in the supine position and with the chin depressed. It allows visualization of the occipital and petrous bones, as well as the mandibular condyles.

TPA (Transpalatal arch) See Arch, Transpalatal.

Tr See Cephalometric landmarks (Soft tissue), Trichion.

Tracing, Cephalometric See Cephalometric tracing.

Traction Force delivered by a component of an appliance that previously has been activated by elastically extending its characteristic length (e.g. the stretching of an elastic module). [Compare with Decompression.]

Transcranial radiograph Plain film projection of the contralateral temporomandibular joint from a superior-posterior angulation. This technique demonstrates oblique views of the glenoid fossa and the mandibular condylar head.

Transcutaneous electric nerve stimulation (TENS) Low-voltage electrical stimulation used as a form of therapy.

Transfer tray A template usually made of silicone or vinyl material, used for transferring the exact position of orthodontic attachments from a plaster cast to the patient's mouth. [Also see Bonding, Indirect.]

Transforming growth factor β (TGF-β) See Growth factors.

Transition The replacement of the deciduous teeth by the permanent ones.

Transition temperature The temperature at which a transformation occurs between different crystalline structures of a material. In the case of nickel-titanium alloys, it is the temperature at which a transformation occurs between the martensite and austenite crystalline structures. This temperature varies between products and depends on the proportion of nickel to titanium as well as the addition of other metals, such as cobalt or copper. [Also see Martensitic transformation; Nickel-titanium alloy.]

Transitional dentition See Dentition, Mixed.

Transitional period, First; Second See First transitional period; Second transitional period.

Translation (of a bone) See Displacement (of a bone).

Translation (of the condyle) Condylar movement occurring during protrusion or lateral excursion of the mandible, or mouth opening beyond the initial phase. It involves primarily the superior aspect of the disc and the articular fossa and eminence (superior joint space).

Translation (of a tooth) See Orthodontic tooth movement, Translation.

Transoral vertical ramus osteotomy (TOVRO) See Osteotomy, Transoral vertical ramus.

Transosteal implant See Implant, Transosteal.

Transpalatal arch See Arch, Transpalatal.

Transpalatal elastics See Orthodontic elastics, Transpalatal.

Transpharyngeal radiograph Plain film projection taken with the mouth open and with the center beam passing through the contralateral sigmoid notch, to show bony detail of the neck and head of the condyle.

Transplantation (of a tooth) See Autotransplantation of a tooth.

Transposition Abnormality of tooth alignment in which two adjacent teeth have erupted in interchanged positions in the dental arch. The maxillary canines are the teeth most commonly involved in transpositions.

Transseptal fibers See Gingival fibers, Transseptal.

Transverse plane (Horizontal plane) Any plane passing through the body at right angles to both the median and the frontal plane, dividing the body into upper and lower parts. *See illustration next page.*

Trapezius muscle See Muscle, Trapezius.

Trauma from occlusion See Occlusal trauma.

Trauma, Occlusal See Occlusal trauma.

Traumatic occlusion See Occlusal trauma.

Treacher Collins syndrome (Mandibulofacial dysostosis) An autosomal dominant condition, generally characterized by bilateral and (usually) symmetrical abnormalities of structures of the first and second branchial arches and the nasal placode. The birth prevalence is in the range of 1 in 25,000 to 1 in 50,000 live births. The clinical characteristics include a severe-

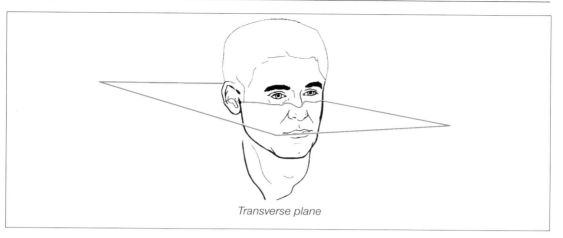

Transverse plane

ly convex facial profile with a prominent dorsum of the nose and a markedly retrognathic mandible and chin. The face is narrow, with hypoplastic supraorbital rims and zygomas. The lateral canthi of the eyes are positioned inferiorly (*antimongoloid slant of the palpebral fissures*). The most characteristic finding is marked hypoplasia of the cheekbones, accompanied by deficiency of the overlying soft tissues. There often is (75%) a coloboma in the outer third of the lower eyelid, the inner aspect of which (medial to the coloboma) has few eyelashes. The external ears can be absent, malformed or malposed, and hearing is impaired as a result of variable degrees of hypoplasia of the external auditory canals and middle ear ossicles. Intelligence is not inherently affected.

The maxilla and mandible also are characteristically hypoplastic, with variable effects on the TMJs and the muscles of mastication. The mandible is retrognathic, with deep antegonial notching, and the rami often are deficient, with malformed condyles. This typically results in a Class II anterior open bite malocclusion and a steep (clockwise rotated) occlusal plane.

Multiple surgical procedures are necessary for the correction of the above deformities, including zygomatic, orbital and TMJ reconstruction with bone grafts; ear and nose reconstruction; as well as bimaxillary orthog-

nathic surgery or distraction osteogenesis. [Also see Antegonial notch; Coloboma.]

Treatment philosophy A term that has come to signify an individual's school of thought with regards to his favored techniques and modalities. [Also see Technique.]

Treatment plan The sequence of procedures planned for the treatment of a patient, after a diagnosis is established.

Treatment technique See Technique.

Treatment time The period of duration of active orthodontic treatment.

Tri-helix See Appliance, Tri-helix.

Triangular elastics See Orthodontic elastics, Vertical.

Tribology The study of friction and of the variables associated with it.

Trichion (Tr) See Cephalometric landmarks (Soft tissue), Trichion.

Trigger point Any cutaneous or muscular area that when stimulated brings about an acute neuralgic or referred musculoskeletal pain, respectively. [See also Myofascial trigger point.]

Trigonocephalic An individual with a triangular skull shape. Trigonocephaly may be produced by premature synostosis of the metopic (interfrontal) suture. [Compare with Plagiocephalic.]

Trimmer See Model trimmer.

Trimming (of an appliance) See Appliance trimming.

Triple-beaked pliers See Orthodontic instruments, Triple-beaked pliers.

Trismus (Mandibular trismus) Muscle spasm of the masticatory muscles specifically causing limited mouth opening.

Trisomy 21 See Down syndrome.

True horizontal line See Cephalometric lines, True horizontal.

True rotation (of the mandible) See Mandibular rotation, Total.

True vertical line See Cephalometric lines, True vertical.

Tube (Molar tube) The part of a molar attachment that receives an orthodontic wire, being either directly bonded to the tooth or welded to a band. Tubes are in essence "closed" brackets, into which the archwire is threaded (usually from the mesial), without the need for ligation. They typically are made of stainless steel.

Auxiliary tube A second tube (in addition to the main tube) incorporated in a molar attachment that can be used for the insertion of segmental loops, auxiliary springs, overlay or intrusive arches etc.

Convertible tube A molar tube whose buccal wall ("cap") can be removed by using the appropriate instrument, transforming it into a bracket. Convertible tubes on the first permanent molars are very useful in situations in which continuous archwire mechanics is used to align severely malpositioned or under-erupted second molars. In such cases converting the tubes of the first molars into brackets allows insertion of a continuous wire with steps, or springs (loops) bent between the first and second molars that otherwise would be impossible. [Also see Conversion of a tube into a bracket.]

Headgear tube A large tube incorporated in some first molar attachments that can be used for insertion of a headgear facebow. When no extraoral appliance is used, headgear tubes also may serve as extra slots for insertion of auxiliary or overlay arches. [Also see Arch, Overlay.]

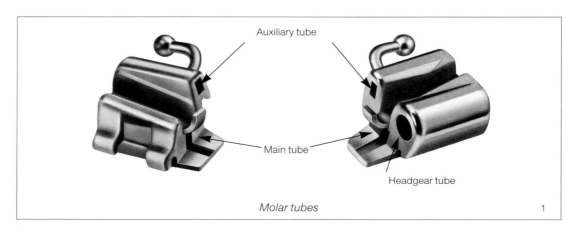

Molar tubes

Main tube The part of a molar attachment that receives the main archwire.

Tuberosity The most distal aspect of the maxillary alveolar process, bilaterally.

Turret See Orthodontic instruments, Turret.

Tweed arch-adjusting pliers See Orthodontic instruments, Tweed arch-adjusting pliers.

Tweed cephalometric analysis See Cephalometric analysis, Tweed.

Tweed loop-forming pliers See Orthodontic instruments, Tweed loop-forming pliers.

Tweed orthodontic coordinate system See Bends.

Tweed triangle See Cephalometric analysis, Tweed.

Twin arch appliance See Appliance, Twin arch.

Twin block appliance See Appliance, Twin block.

Twin bracket See Bracket, Twin.

Twin wire appliance See Appliance, Twin arch.

Twinning Complete division of a single tooth bud to create two separate teeth. [Compare with Fusion; Gemination; Concrescence.]

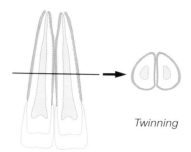

Twinning

Two-by-four appliance See Appliance, Two-by-four.

Two-jaw surgery See Orthognathic surgery, Bimaxillary.

Type A anchorage See Anchorage, Maximum.

Type B anchorage See Anchorage, Moderate.

Type C anchorage See Anchorage, Minimum.

Types of tooth movement See Orthodontic tooth movement.

U

U-bow activator See Appliance, U-bow activator.

"Ugly duckling" stage A stage of dental development at the end of the first transitional period, first recognized by B.H. Broadbent. The "ugly duckling" stage generally is characterized by a midline diastema between the maxillary permanent central incisors and distal tipping and flaring of the crowns of the maxillary permanent lateral incisors. This is associated with the position of the maxillary permanent canines, which are developing in close proximity to the labiodistal aspect of the apices of the lateral incisors. As the canines continue to erupt, the lateral incisors upright and eventually the spaces are closed spontaneously.

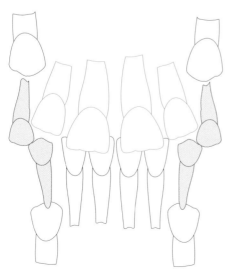

"Ugly duckling" stage

UI-to-AP distance See Cephalometric measurements (Hard tissue), UI-to-AP distance.

Ultrasonography Diagnostic ultrasound imaging relies on high-frequency mechanical vibrations that are transmitted through the tissues. These are produced by a transducer constructed of a piezoelectric material, which converts electrical signals into sound waves. The sound waves are transmitted into the tissues as a series of pulses. Those sound waves that are reflected back from the tissues are received by the transducer and reconverted into electrical signals for processing into an image. The image is displayed on a monitor and recorded. The frequencies used for diagnostic ultrasound range from 1 to 20 MHz (typically 3 to 7 MHz), well above the audible range.

Air and bone do not transmit ultrasound waves readily, hence limiting the usefulness of ultrasound imaging in the maxillofacial region. It is, however, of value in the examination of soft tissues and space-occupying lesions within them.

No detectable, hazardous biological effects have as yet been demonstrated with ultrasound below a certain threshold (the vast majority of such diagnostic apparatuses operate below this threshold level).

Uncontrolled tipping See Orthodontic tooth movement, Tipping (Uncontrolled).

Underbite (Underjet) A non-technical term for negative overjet.

Undercuts Areas that provide mechanical retention for placement of dental materials or appliances.

Artificial undercuts "Simulated" undercuts created by bonding small amounts of composite resin on the labial or buccal surface of teeth to facilitate the retention of clasps or other parts of a removable appliance.

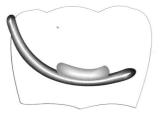

Bonded artificial undercut

Natural undercuts Curved portions or inclines on the natural surfaces of teeth that could be used to provide retention for orthodontic appliances.

Undereruption (Infraeruption) A situation in which a tooth (or group of teeth) is positioned below the occlusal plane because its eruption never was completed, e.g. due to lack of space, a deleterious habit, overeruption of an antagonist, or ankylosis during eruption.
Undereruption sometimes is difficult to distinguish from infraposition. [Compare with Infraposition.]

Underjet See Underbite.

Undermining resorption See Bone resorption, Undermining.

Unilateral Occurring on one side only. [Compare with Bilateral.]

Universal appliance See Appliance, Universal.

Universal pliers See Orthodontic instruments, Adams pliers.

University of Michigan Growth Study See Michigan Growth Study.

Unloading of a joint See Decompression of a joint.

Up-down elastics See Orthodontic elastics, Vertical.

Upper jaw See Maxilla.

Upper lip length See Cephalometric measurements (Soft tissue), Upper lip length.

Uprighting Changing the angulation of a mesially or distally tipped tooth to a more vertical angulation.

Molar uprighting Orthodontic tooth movement aiming at correction of the variable mesial tipping and extrusion (as well as rotation, in the maxilla) that molars tend to undergo in the absence of the teeth mesial to them. Control of the vertical (as well as the transverse) dimension often is a challenge during such treatment.

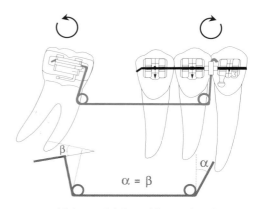

Molar uprighting with equal and opposite moments

Uprighting spring See Orthodontic springs, Uprighting.

Utility arch See Arch, Utility.

Uvula, Bifid See Bifid uvula.

V

V-bends See Bends, V-.

"V" principle (of growth) The "V" principle is an important facial growth mechanism, since many facial and cranial bones have a "V" configuration or "V"-shaped regions. According to this concept, which was described by D.H. Enlow, a "V"-shaped bone grows by resorption on the outer surface of the "V" and apposition on its inner side. Thus, the "V" moves away from its narrow end and enlarges in overall size simultaneously.

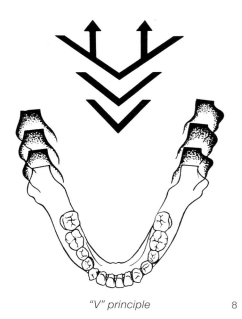

"V" principle   8

Vacuum-formed retainer See Retainer, Vacuum-formed.

Van Beek appliance See Appliance, Van Beek.

Van der Linden retainer See Retainer, Van der Linden.

Vectorial A physical quantity characterized by a point of application, direction (line of action), sense (orientation) and magnitude in terms of physical units of measurement. A typical example of a vectorial quantity is force. [Compare with Scalar.]

Velopharyngeal insufficiency (Velopharyngeal incompetence, VPI) Anatomic (structural) or functional deficiency of the soft palate or superior pharyngeal constrictor muscle, resulting in inability to provide adequate velopharyngeal closure during speech, with a consequent hypernasal voice quality. Velopharyngeal insufficiency is a frequent finding in patients with a history of cleft palate, for which a pharyngeal flap operation often is performed. [Also see Hypernasality; Pharyngeal flap operation.]

Velum See Palate, Soft.

Ventral Towards the front. [Compare with Rostral.]

"Vertical" case See "High angle" case.

Vertical dimension A term commonly employed referring to facial height. [Also see Cephalometric measurements (Hard tissue), Facial height.]

Vertical elastics See Orthodontic elastics, Vertical.

Vertical growth pattern Craniofacial growth in a predominantly downward direction. Usually associated with long anterior face height, steep mandibular plane and minimal overbite.

Vertical loop See Loop, Vertical.

Vertical maxillary excess (VME) Excessive development of the maxilla in the vertical dimension, most commonly associated with Class II skeletal malocclusions. Unesthetic gingival exposure during smiling ("gummy smile") is a common sign that, however, must be differentiated from that occurring because of an absolutely short upper lip. The treatment for VME is maxillary impaction by orthognathic surgery.

Vertical overbite See Overbite.

"Vertical patient" See "High-angle" patient.

Vertical plane Any plane perpendicular to the transverse plane (sagittal or frontal plane).

Vertical-pull headgear See Headgear, Vertical-pull.

Vertical slot See Bracket slot, Vertical.

Vestibular shield (Vestibular screen) See Appliance, Vestibular shield.

Vestibule The part of the oral cavity bounded by the oral surfaces of the cheeks and lips and the labial and buccal aspects of the alveolar processes and teeth.

Videofluoroscopy A cineradiographic diagnostic method with various applications, e.g. for examination of the velopharyngeal area during speech. After the x-rays pass through the subject, they are projected onto a fluorescent screen instead of a film, so the immediate image of the subject in motion can be viewed. The image is electronically intensified and recorded by a video camera.

Visceral swallow See Swallow, Infantile.

Viscoelastic material Having both elastic and viscous properties.

Viscoelastic behavior (Viscoelasticity) The characteristic property of some materials to exhibit time-dependent behavior during loading. This means that the strain developed within the material is dependent on the rate of application of stress on it. More generally, the response of a viscoelastic material depends on the rate of load application and on how long the load is applied. Viscoelasticity does not occur in materials with elastic behavior in which the response to load application is both independent of time and completely reversible. Two aspects of the time-dependent behavior of viscoelastic materials are creep and relaxation.

Creep Gradual increase in strain (permanent deformation) of a material as a result of long-term constant load at stresses in the elastic region below the yield stress.

Relaxation The decay (relief) of stress within a material after it has been subjected to permanent deformation. The result of it is change in shape or contour of the material due to rearrangement of its atomic or molecular positions. The state of relaxation increases with an increase in temperature. For example, after a stainless steel wire has been bent, it may tend to straighten out if it is heated to a high temperature.

Viscoelasticity See Viscoelastic behavior.

Viscous Resistant to flow (referring to a fluid).

Visual treatment objective (VTO) A treatment planning and communication aid that may be used to define the tooth movements and/or surgical changes required to achieve the desired facial goals. Essentially it consists of the patient's pretreatment lateral cephalometric tracing, modified to demonstrate the changes that are anticipated in the course of treatment. This can be accomplished either manually, or with the help of a computer program. Since growth prediction and the effects of treatment on growth are relatively inaccurate, a VTO of a growing child often is only a rough estimate of the actual outcome, nevertheless it can be a helpful tool in arriving at a final treatment plan. Visual treatment objectives performed for orthognathic surgical treatment planning are sometimes referred to as *STOs* (*Surgical Treatment Objectives*). [See Surgical prediction tracing.]

The construction of a VTO is somewhat abstract and requires a trial and error process. It can be very helpful in exploring various treatment options, but it is important, once a plan is determined, that the clinician goes back and makes sure that it is the product of a logical and practical approach to the problem. The VTO is linked directly to, and evaluated in conjunction with, the occlusogram. [Also see Occlusogram.]

VME See Vertical maxillary excess.

VPI See Velopharyngeal insufficiency.

VTO See Visual treatment objective.

W

W-arch See Arch, Porter.

Wafer, Surgical See Splint, Surgical.

Wassmund osteotomy See Osteotomy, Anterior maxillary segmental.

Wax bite See Bite registration.

Wear, Occlusal See Attrition.

Wear facet A flat polished or concave area on the surface of a tooth produced by repeated physiologic or parafunctional occlusal contact or prematurity. [Also see Attrition.]

Wedge, Rotation See Rotation wedge.

"Wedge" theory A concept based on the notions that the mandible is a class III lever and that the vertical position of the mandible and the face height are determined by the occlusion. According to this theory, any pure distal movement of posterior teeth will result in rocking the mandible open (clockwise rotation), whereas when the distalmost occlusal contacts are moved forward (e.g. by mesial movement of the posterior teeth) this may have the opposite effect of decreasing the facial height by allowing the mandible to rotate in a counterclockwise direction. Extraction of the maxillary and mandibular second molars aiming at reduction or correction of an anterior open bite is based on the same theory. The validity of the theory is questionable, as is the long-term stability of any such changes in the orientation of the mandibular plane.

Weingart pliers See Orthodontic instruments, Weingart utility pliers.

Weldability Having the capability of being joined by the passage of a strong electric current or by the use of laser energy.

Welding An operation by which two or more metal surfaces are united, by means of heat and/or high compressive forces, in such a way that there is continuity of the nature of the material between these parts. The use of a filler material, the melting temperature of which is of the same order as that of the parent material, is optional.

Laser welding Welding procedure by which two pieces of metal are connected through the use of heat generated by a laser beam. The advantage of laser welding is that the generated heat is localized in a confined area, and thus it has a low thermal influence on the parts being joined.

Spot welding The form of welding most commonly used in orthodontics. The joining of metals by means of pressure and heat generated by the passage of electric current. No filler metal is used. If a pulse of sufficient voltage and duration is applied by means of copper electrodes, melting will begin at the interface between the parts, which will spread out to form a weld.

WFO See World Federation of Orthodontists.

Whiplash See Flexion-extension injury.

White spot lesion (Decalcification) Initial symptom of a carious lesion representing a subsurface demineralization. A common side effect of orthodontic treatment in patients with compromised oral hygiene. White spot lesions also may occur in areas where there is inadequate bonding material between the bracket base and the enamel creating a space, or in instances of badly fitted bands where there is space between the band and the tooth surface. Such defects can be repaired, at least partially, by fluoride treatment.

Width of the PDL See Periodontal ligament, Width.

Wilson, Curve of See Curve of Wilson.

Wilson loop See Loop, Wilson.

Wings (of a bracket) See Bracket wings.

Wire cross-section See Archwire cross-section.

Wits appraisal See Cephalometric measurements (Hard tissue), Wits appraisal.

Wits cephalometric analysis See Cephalometric measurements (Hard tissue), Wits appraisal.

Wolff's law of bone remodeling A book published in 1892 by J. Wolff [original title: "Das Gesetz der Transformation der Knochen"] presenting his observation that bone reacts to mechanical functional stress through an adaptive process resulting in a change of its external and internal architecture to better withstand this stress. According to Wolff, the trabecular pattern of a bone is related to stress trajectories and thus can be correlated with its function in a mathematical way.

Woodside activator See Appliance, Harvold-Woodside activator.

Work-hardening See Hardening, Work-hardening.

Working casts See Orthodontic casts, Working casts.

Working range (Range, Maximum elastic strain) The maximum deformation (deflection) of an orthodontic wire or spring within its elastic range.

Working side (Functioning side, Laterotrusive side) The side toward which the mandible moves during a lateral excursion.

Working side contact See Occlusal contact, Working side.

World Federation of Orthodontists (WFO) An organization of orthodontic specialists formed by 69 orthodontic organizations from 62 countries at the Fourth International Orthodontic Congress in San Francisco, California, USA, on May 15, 1995. The purpose of the WFO is to advance the art and science of orthodontics throughout the world.

Woven bone See Bone, Woven.

Wrap-around retainer See Retainer, Wrap-around.

Wunderer osteotomy See Osteotomy, Anterior maxillary segmental.

Wylie cephalometric analysis See Cephalometric analysis, Wylie.

X

X-bite Abbreviation for crossbite. [See Cross-bite.]

X-ray Electromagnetic radiation, produced when electrons strike a target under high voltage in a vacuum. The term "x-ray" is sometimes used incorrectly as a synonym for radiograph.

Xenogenic graft See Graft, Heterologous.

Y

Y-axis See Cephalometric lines, Y-axis.

Yield point The point on a stress/strain curve at which 0.1% or 0.2% permanent deformation has occurred to a body (e.g. an orthodontic wire) under the influence of a load. (In other words, the point on a stress/strain curve where there is appreciable plastic deformation [0.1% or 0.2% is arbitrarily selected.]) [Also see Stress/strain diagram.]

Yield strength (YS) A property that represents the stress value at which a small amount of permanent deformation has occurred. A value of either 0.1% or 0.2% of permanent deformation is usually selected and is referred to as the *percent offset*. The yield strength of a material always is slightly higher than the elastic limit. A material with a high yield strength is more resistant to permanent deformation than a material with a low yield strength. The yield strength of a material increases proportionally to the amount of work-hardening that it is subjected to.

Young's modulus of elasticity (E) See Modulus of elasticity.

YS See Yield strength.

Z

Z-angle (of Merrifield) See Cephalometric measurements (Soft tissue), Z-angle.

Z-line (Profile line of Merrifield) See Cephalometric lines, Z-line.

Z-spring See Orthodontic springs, Z-.

Zig-zag elastics See Orthodontic elastics, Vertical.

Zinc oxide-eugenol cement (ZOE) See Orthodontic cement, Zinc oxide-eugenol.

Zinc phosphate cement See Orthodontic cement, Zinc phosphate.

ZOE cement See Orthodontic cement, Zinc oxide-eugenol.

Zygomatic bone (Malar bone, Cheek bone) A roughly diamond-shaped bone on either side of the face that forms the prominence of the cheek, the lateral wall and floor of the orbit and parts of the temporal and infratemporal fossae. It articulates with the frontal bone, maxilla, zygomatic process of the temporal bone and greater wing of the sphenoid bone. At birth, the bone may be divided by a horizontal suture into a superior and an inferior part.

Selected references

Aelbers CM, Dermaut LR. Orthopedics in orthodontics: Part I, Fiction or reality—a review of the literature. Am J Orthod Dentofac Orthop 1996; 110:513–9.

Albers DD. Ankylosis of teeth in the developing dentition. Quintessence Int 1986; 17:303–8.

Altenburger E, Ingervall B. The initial effects of the treatment of Class II, division 1 malocclusions with the van Beek activator compared with the effects of the Herren activator and an activator-headgear combination. Eur J Orthod 1998; 20:389–97.

Al Yami EA, Kuijpers-Jagtman AM, van 't Hof MA. Assessment of biological changes in a non-orthodontic sample using the PAR index. Am J Orthod Dentofac Orthop 1998; 114:224–8.

American Association of Orthodontists. Glossary of Dentofacial Orthopedic Terms. AAO, 1993.

American Board of Orthodontics—past, present, and future. Am J Orthod Dentofac Orthop 1996; 110:108–10.

American Sleep Disorders Association. Practice parameters for the treatment of snoring and obstructive sleep apnea with oral appliances. Sleep 1995; 18:511–3.

Anderson D, Popovich F. Relation of cranial base flexure to cranial form and mandibular position. Am J Phys Anthropol 1983; 61:181–7.

Andreasen GF, Zwanziger D. A clinical evaluation of the differential force concept as applied to the edgewise bracket. Am J Orthod 1980; 78:25–40.

Andreasen GF, Hilleman TB. An evaluation of 55 cobalt substituted Nitinol wire for use in orthodontics. J Am Dent Assoc 1971; 82:1373–5.

Andreasen JO, Andreasen FM. Textbook and Color Atlas of Traumatic Injuries of the Teeth (3rd edition). Munksgaard, Copenhagen, 1994.

Andrews LF. The six keys to normal occlusion. Am J Orthod 1972; 62:296–309.

Andrews LF. Straight Wire, the Concept and Appliance. LA Wells Co., San Diego, 1989.

Angle EH. The latest and best in orthodontic mechanisms. Dent Cosmos 1928; 70:1143–58.

Anusavice KJ (ed.). Phillips' Science of Dental Materials (10th edition). WB Saunders Co., Philadelphia, 1996.

Asbell MB. A brief history of orthodontics. Am J Orthod Dentofac Orthop 1990; 98:176–83.

Asbell MB. A brief history of orthodontics. Am J Orthod Dentofac Orthop 1990; 98:206–13.

Ash MM, Ramfjord S. Occlusion (4th edition). WB Saunders Co., Philadelphia, 1995.

Athanasiou AE (ed.). Orthodontic Cephalometry. Mosby-Wolfe, London, 1995.

Atherton JD. The gingival response to orthodontic tooth movement. Am J Orthod 1970; 58: 179–186.

Atherton JD, Kerr NW. Effect of orthodontic tooth movement upon the gingivae. An investigation. Br Dent J 1968; 124:555–60.

Ayala Perez C, de Alba JA, Caputo AA, Chaconas SJ. Canine retraction with J hook headgear. Am J Orthod 1980; 78:538–47.

Bazakidou E, Nanda RS, Duncanson MG Jr, Sinha P. Evaluation of frictional resistance in esthetic brackets. Am J Orthod Dentofac Orthop 1997; 112:138–44.

Becker A. The Orthodontic Treatment of Impacted Teeth. Martin Dunitz, London, 1998.

Bednar JR, Gruendeman GW, Sandrik JL. A comparative study of frictional forces between orthodontic brackets and arch wires. Am J Orthod Dentofac Orthop 1991; 100:513–22.

Begg PR, Kesling PC. Begg Orthodontic Theory and Technique (3rd edition). WB Saunders, Philadelphia, 1977.

Bell WH (ed.). Modern Practice in Orthognathic and Reconstructive Surgery. WB Saunders Co., Philadelphia, 1992.

Bench RW. The quad helix appliance. Sem Orthod 1998; 4:231–7.

Bennett JC, McLaughlin RP. Orthodontic Treatment Mechanics and the Preadjusted Appliance. Wolfe Publishing, London, 1993.

Berger JL. The SPEED appliance: a 14-year update on this unique self-ligating orthodontic mechanism. Am J Orthod Dentofac Orthop 1994; 105:217–223.

Berkowitz S (ed.).Cleft Lip and Palate: Perspectives in Management. Singular Publishing Group, Inc., San Diego, 1996.

Bernstein L. Edward H. Angle versus Calvin S. Case: extraction versus nonextraction. Part I. Historical revisionism. Am J Orthod Dentofac Orthop 1992; 102:464–70.

Bernstein L. Edward H. Angle versus Calvin S. Case: extraction versus nonextraction. Historical revisionism. Part II. Am J Orthod Dentofac Orthop 1992; 102:546–51.

Björk A. The use of metallic implants in the study of facial growth in children: method and application. Am J Phys Anthropol 1968; 29:243–54.

Björk A, Skieller V. Normal and abnormal growth of the mandible. A synthesis of longitudinal cephalometric implant studies over a period of 25 years. Eur J Orthod 1983; 5:1–46.

Blackwood HO 3rd. Clinical management of the Jasper Jumper. J Clin Orthod 1991; 25:755–60.

Block MS, Hoffman DR. A new device for absolute anchorage in orthodontics. Am J Orthod Dentofac Orthop 1995; 107:251–258.

Boersma H. Eenvoudige Orthodontische Therapie (4e druk). Samsom Stafleu, Alphen aan de Rijn, 1989.

Bolender CJ, Bounoure GM, Barat Y (eds.). Extraction Versus Nonextraction. SID Publisher, Paris, 1995.

Boucher's Clinical Dental Terminology (4th edition). Mosby-Year Book, St. Louis, 1993.

Bourauel C, Fries T, Drescher D, Plietsch R. Surface roughness of orthodontic wires via atomic force microscopy, laser specular reflectance, and profilometry. Eur J Orthod 1998; 20:79–92.

Boyne PJ, Sands NR. Secondary bone grafting of residual alveolar and palatal clefts. J Oral Surg 1972; 30:87–92.

Brattström V, McWilliam J, Larson O, Semb G. Craniofacial development in children with unilateral clefts of the lip, alveolus, and palate treated according to four different regimes. I. Maxillary development. Scand J Plast Reconstr Hand Surg 1991; 25:259–67.

Braun S, Hnat WP, Johnson BE. The curve of Spee revisited. Am J Orthod Dentofac Orthop 1996; 110:206–10.

Braun S, Marcotte MR. Rationale of the segmented approach to orthodontic treatment. Am J Orthod Dentofac Orthop 1995; 108:1–8.

Broadbent BH. A new x-ray technique and its application to orthodontia. Angle Orthod 1931; 1:45–60.

Broadbent JM. The sagittal appliance. Funct Orthod 1986; 3:38–9.

Broadbent BH Sr, Broadbent BH Jr, Golden WH. Bolton Standards of Dentofacial Developmental Growth. The CV Mosby Co., St. Louis, 1975.

Browne RM, Edmondson HD, John Rout PG. Atlas of Dental and Maxillofacial Radiology and Imaging. Mosby-Wolfe, London, 1995.

Burgett FG. Trauma from occlusion: periodontal concerns. Dent Clin North Am 1995; 39:301–11.

Burstone CJ. Integumental contour and extension patterns. Angle Orthod 1959; 29:93–104.

Burstone CJ. Lip posture and its significance in treatment planning. Am J Orthod 1967; 53:262–84.

Burstone CJ. The segmented arch approach to space closure. Am J Orthod 1982; 82:361–78.

Burstone CJ, James RB, Legan H, Murphy GA, Norton LA. Cephalometrics for orthognathic surgery. J Oral Surg 1978; 36:269–77.

Burstone CJ, Koenig HA. Force systems from an ideal arch. Am J Orthod 1974; 65:270–89.

Burstone CJ, Koenig HA. Creative wire bending—the force system from step and V bends. Am J Orthod Dentofac Orthop 1988; 93:59–67.

Burstone CJ, Pryputniewicz R. Holographic determination of centres of rotation produced by orthodontic forces. Am J Orthod 1980; 77:396–409.

Burstone CJ, Qin B, Morton JY. Chinese Ni Ti wire: a new orthodontic alloy. Am J Orthod 1985; 87:445–52.

Cameron CA. Informed consent in orthodontics. Semin Orthod 1997; 3:77–93.

Canut JA, Arias S. A long-term evaluation of treated Class II division 2 malocclusions: a retrospective study model analysis. Eur J Orthod 1999; 21:377–86.

Carels C, van der Linden FPGM. Concepts on functional appliances' mode of action. Am J Orthod Dentofac Orthop 1987; 92:162–68.

Carlson DS (ed.). Orthodontics in an aging society. Monograph #22, Craniofacial Growth Series. Center for Human Growth and Development, The University of Michigan, Ann Arbor, 1989.

Carlson DS, Goldstein SA (eds.). Bone biodynamics in orthodontic and orthopedic treatment. Vol. 27, Craniofacial Growth Series. Center for Human Growth and Development, The University of Michigan, Ann Arbor, 1991.

Carter LM, Yaman P. Dental Instruments. The CV Mosby Co., St. Louis, 1981.

Case CS. The question of extraction in orthodontics (reprinted). Am J Orthod 1964; 50:658–91.

Chemello PD, Wolford LM, Buschang PH. Occlusal plane alteration in orthognathic surgery—Part II: Long-term stability of results. Am J Orthod Dentofac Orthop 1994; 106:434–40.

Clark GT, Seligman DA, Solberg WK, Pullinger AG. Guidelines for the treatment of temporomandibular disorders. J Craniomand Disord Facial Oral Pain 1990; 4:80–7.

Clark WJ. Twin Block Functional Therapy: Applications in Dentofacial Orthopaedics. Mosby-Wolfe, London, 1995.

Cohen ES, Jr. (Ed.). Atlas of Cosmetic and Reconstructive Periodontal Surgery (2nd edition). Lea & Febiger, Philadelphia, 1994.

Cohen MM Jr. The Robin anomalad - its nonspecificity and associated syndromes. J Oral Surg 1976; 34:587–93.

Cohen MM Jr. Syndrome designations. J Med Genet 1976; 13:266–70.

Cohen MM Jr. Syndromology's message for craniofacial biology. J Maxillofac Surg 1979; 7:89–109.

Cohen MM Jr. A critical review of cephalometric studies of dysmorphic syndromes. Proc Finn Dent Soc 1981;77:17–25.

Contasti GI, Legan HL. Biomechanical guidelines for headgear application. J Clin Orthod 1982; 16:308–312.

Dahl EH, Zachrisson BU. Long-term experience with direct-bonded lingual retainers. J Clin Orthod 1991; 25:619–30.

Darendeliler MA, Darendeliler A, Mandurino M. Clinical application of magnets in orthodontics and biological implications: a review. Eur J Orthod 1997; 19:431–42.

Daskalogiannakis J, McLachlan KR. Canine retraction with rare earth magnets: An investigation into the validity of the constant force hypothesis. Am J Orthod Dentofac Orthop 1996; 109: 489–95.

Davidovitch Z (ed.). The Biological Mechanisms of Tooth Eruption and Root Resorption. EBSCO Media, Birmingham, 1988.

Davidovitch Z (ed.). Biological Mechanisms of Tooth Eruption, Resorption and Replacement by Implants. The Harvard Society for the Advancement of Orthodontics, Boston, 1994.

Davidovitch Z, Nicolay OF, Ngan PW, Shanfield JL. Neurotransmitters, cytokines and the control of alveolar bone remodeling in orthodontics. Dent Clin North Am 1988; 32:411–435.

Davidovitch Z, Norton LA (eds.). Biological Mechanisms of Tooth Movement and Craniofacial Adaptation. The Harvard Society for the Advancement of Orthodontics, Boston, 1996.

Dellinger EL. Active vertical corrector treatment: Long-term follow-up of anterior open bite treated by intrusion of posterior teeth. Am J Orthod Dentofac Orthop 1996; 110:145–54.

Denison TF, Kokich VG, Shapiro PA. Stability of maxillary surgery in openbite versus non-openbite malocclusions. Angle Orthod 1989; 59:5–10.

Dental Standards Committee. British Standard Glossary of Dental Terms. British Standards Institution, London, 1983.

Dermaut LR, Aelbers CM. Orthopedics in orthodontics: Part II, Fiction or reality—a review of the literature. Am J Orthod Dentofac Orthop 1996; 110:667–71.

Dermaut LR, van den Eynde F, de Pauw G. Skeletal and dento-alveolar changes as a result of headgear activator therapy related to different vertical growth patterns. Eur J Orthod 1992; 14:140–6.

Di Paolo RJ. An individualized approach to locating the occlusal plane. Am J Orthod Dentofac Orthop 1987; 92:41–5.

Di Paolo RJ, Philip C, Maganzini AL. The quadrilateral analysis: an individualized skeletal assessment. Am J Orthod 1983; 83:19–32.

Dorland's Illustrated Medical Dictionary (28th edition). WB Saunders Co., Philadelphia, 1994.

Downs WB. Variations in facial relations: their significance in treatment and prognosis. Am J Orthod 1948; 34:812–40.

Downs WB. The role of cephalometrics in orthodontic case analysis and diagnosis. Am J Orthod 1952; 38:162–82.

Downs WB. Analysis of the dento-facial profile. Angle Orthod 1956; 26:191–212.

Drescher D, Bourauel C, Schumacher HA. Frictional forces between bracket and archwire. Am J Orthod Dentofac Orthop 1989;96:397–404.

Edwards JG. A study of the periodontium during orthodontic rotation of teeth. Am J Orthod 1968; 54:441–61.

Edwards JG. A long-term prospective evaluation of the circumferential supracrestal fiberotomy in alleviating orthodontic relapse. Am J Orthod Dentofac Orthop 1988; 93:380–7.

Ellis E 3rd. Modified splint design for two-jaw surgery. J Clin Orthod 1982; 16:619–22.

Ellis E 3rd, McNamara JA Jr. Components of adult Class III open-bite malocclusion. Am J Orthod 1984; 86:277–90.

Ellis E 3rd, McNamara JA Jr, Lawrence TM. Components of adult Class II open-bite malocclusion. J Oral Maxillofac Surg 1985; 43:92–105.

Enlow DH (ed.). Facial Growth (3rd edition). WB Saunders Co., Philadelphia, 1990.

Epker BN, Fish LC. Surgical-orthodontic correction of open-bite deformity. Am J Orthod 1977; 71: 278–99.

Epker BN, Turvey T, Fish LC. Indications for simultaneous mobilization of the maxilla and mandible for correction of dentofacial deformities. Oral Surg 1982; 54:369–81.

Epker BN, Stella JP, Fish LC. Dentofacial Deformities: Integrated Orthodontic and Surgical Correction (2nd edition). The CV Mosby Co., St. Louis, 1995.

Farkas LG (ed.). Anthropometry of the Face (2nd edition). Raven Press, New York, 1994.

Fiorelli G, Melsen B. Biomechanics in Orthodontics CD-ROM, version 1.1. Libra Ortondonzia, Arezzo, 1995.

Ford KB, McGahan JP. Cephalic index: its possible use as a predictor of impending fetal demise. Radiology 1982; 143:517–8.

Fotis V, Melsen B, Williams S, Droschl H. Vertical control as an important ingredient in the treatment of severe sagittal discrepancies. Am J Orthod 1984; 86:224–32.

Franchi L, Baccetti T, McNamara JA Jr. Treatment and posttreatment effects of acrylic splint Herbst appliance therapy. Am J Orthod Dentofac Orthop 1999; 115:429–38.

Fränkel R. A functional approach to orofacial orthopaedics. Br J Orthod 1980; 7:41–51.

Fränkel R, Fränkel C. Orofacial Orthopedics with the Function Regulator. Karger, Basel, 1989.

Gawley JR, Gawley RJ. Treatment with the universal appliance. Am J Orthod 1971; 59:156–64.

Gelb H (ed.). New Concepts in Craniomandibular and Chronic pain Management. Mosby-Wolfe, London, 1994.

Gianelly AA. Distal movement of the maxillary molars. Am J Orthod Dentofac Orthop 1998; 114: 166–72.

Gianelly AA, Bednar JR, Dietz VS. A bidimensional edgewise technique. J Clin Orthod 1985; 19: 418–21.

Gjessing P. Biomechanical design and clinical evaluation of a new canine-retraction spring. Am J Orthod 1985; 87:353–62.

Gjessing P. Controlled retraction of maxillary incisors. Am J Orthod Dentofac Orthop 1992;101:120–31.

Gjessing P. A universal retraction spring. J Clin Orthod 1994; 28:222–42.

Gorlin RJ, Cohen MM Jr, Levin SL (eds.). Syndromes of the Head and Neck (3rd edition). Oxford University Press, New York, 1990.

Gorman CJ Jr. Lingual orthodontics. Dent Clin North Am 1997; 41:111–25.

Gottlieb EL, Nelson AH, Vogels DS 3rd. 1996 JCO Study of orthodontic diagnosis and treatment procedures. Part 1. Results and trends. J Clin Orthod 1996; 30:615–29.

Graber TM, Neumann B. Removable Orthodontic Appliances (2nd edition). WB Saunders, Philadelphia, 1984.

Graber TM, Rakosi T, Petrovic AG. Dentofacial Orthopedics with Functional Appliances (2nd edition). Mosby—Year Book, St. Louis, 1997.

Graber TM, Vanarsdall RL, Jr. (eds.). Orthodontics—Current Principles and Techniques. Mosby—Year Book, St. Louis, 1994.

Grayson BH, Santiago PE. Treatment planning and biomechanics of distraction osteogenesis from an orthodontic perspective. Sem Orthod 1999; 5:9–24.

Greenbaum KR, Zachrisson BU. The effect of palatal expansion therapy on the periodontal supporting tissues. Am J Orthod 1982; 81:12–21.

Haack DC, Weinstein S. The mechanics of centric and eccentric cervical traction. Am J Orthod 1958; 44:346–57.

Haas AJ. Long-term posttreatment evaluation of rapid palatal expansion. Am J Orthod 1980; 50:189–217.

Halazonetis DJ, Katsavrias E, Spyropoulos MN. Changes in cheek pressure following rapid maxillary expansion. Eur J Orthod 1994; 16: 295–300.

Hamula W. Modified mandibular Schwarz appliance. J Clin Orthod 1993; 27:89–93.

Hamula DW, Hamula W, Sernetz F. Pure titanium orthodontic brackets. J Clin Orthod 1996; 30: 140–4.

Hanson GH. The SPEED system: a report on the development of a new edgewise appliance. Am J Orthod 1980; 78:243–65.

Harris R, Griffin CJ. Tooth eruption and migration theories [letter]. Oral Surg Oral Med Oral Pathol 1985; 60:604.

Harvold EP. The asymmetries of the upper facial skeleton and their morphological significance. Europ Orthod Soc Trans 1961; 63–9.

Harvold EP. Some biological aspects of orthodontic treatment in the transitional dentition. Am J Orthod 1963; 49:1–14.

Harvold EP. The Activator in Interceptive Orthodontics. The CV Mosby Co., St. Louis, 1974.

Haymond CS, Stoelinga PJW, Blijdorp PA, Leenen RJ, Merkins NM. Surgical orthodontic treatment of anterior skeletal open bite using small plate internal fixation. Int J Oral Maxillofac Surg 1991; 20:223–7.

Heasman PA, Millett DT, Chapple IL. The Periodontium and Orthodontics in Health and Disease. Oxford University Press, Oxford, 1996.

Henderson D. A Colour Atlas and Textbook of Orthognathic Surgery. Wolfe Medical Publications Ltd., London, 1985.

Hickham JH. Directional forces revisited. J Clin Orthod 1986; 20:626–37.

Hickham JH. Maxillary protraction therapy: diagnosis and treatment. J Clin Orthod 1991; 25: 102–13.

Hilgers JJ. The pendulum appliance for Class II non-compliance therapy. J Clin Orthod 1992; 26:706–14.

Holdaway RA. A soft tissue cephalometric analysis and its use in orthodontic treatment planning. Part I. Am J Orthod 1983; 84:1–28.

Holdaway RA. A soft tissue cephalometric analysis and its use in orthodontic treatment planning. Part II. Am J Orthod 1984; 85:279–93.

Hollender L, Rönnerman A, Thilander B. Root resorption, marginal bone support and clinical crown length in orthodontically treated patients. Eur J Orthod 1980; 2:197–205.

Howe RP, McNamara JA, Jr. Clinical management of the bonded Herbst appliance. J Clin Orthod 1983; 17:456–63.

Howes AE. A polygon portrayal of coronal and basal arch dimensions in the horizontal plane. Am J orthod 1954; 40:811–31.

Hunter WS, Carlson DS (eds.). Essays in honor of Robert E. Moyers. Volume 24, Craniofacial Growth Series. Center for Human Growth and Development, The University of Michigan, Ann Arbor, 1991.

Hussels W, Nanda RS. Analysis of factors affecting angle ANB. Am J Orthod 1984; 85:411–23.

Hussels W, Nanda RS. Clinical application of a method to correct angle ANB for geometric effects. Am J Orthod Dentofac Orthop 1987; 92:506–10.

Isaacson RJ, Lindauer SJ, Davidovitch M. The ground rules for archwire design. Sem Orthod 1995; 1:3–11.

Jablonski S. Illustrated Dictionary of Dentistry. WB Saunders Co., Philadelphia, 1982.

Jacobs JD, Sinclair PM. Principles of orthodontic mechanics in orthognathic surgery cases. Am J Orthod 1983; 84:399–407.

Jacobson A. The "Wits" appraisal of jaw disharmony. Am J Orthod 1975; 67:125–38.

Jacobson A. Application of the "Wits" appraisal. Am J Orthod 1976; 70:179–89.

Jacobson A. Radiographic Cephalometry: From Basics to Videoimaging. Quintessence Publishing Co., Chicago, 1995.

Jacobson A, Caufield PW. Introduction to Radiographic Cephalometry. Lea and Febiger, Philadelphia, 1985.

Jarabak JR, Fizzell JA. Technique and Treatment with Light-Wire Edgewise Appliances (2nd edition). The CV Mosby Co., St. Louis, 1972.

Jasper JJ, McNamara JA Jr. The correction of interarch malocclusions using a fixed force module. Am J Orthod Dentofac Orthop 1995; 108:641–50.

Johnston LE Jr (ed.). New Vistas in Orthodontics. Lea and Febiger, Philadelphia, 1985.

Johnston MC. Developmental biology of the mouth, palate and pharynx. In: Tewfik TL, Derkaloussian VM (eds.). Congenital Anomalies of the Ears, Nose and Throat. Oxford University Press, New York, 1997.

Jones KL. Smith's Recognizable Patterns of Human Malformations (5th edition). WB Saunders Co., Philadelphia, 1997.

Kapila S, Angolkar P, Duncanson MG, Jr., Nanda RS. Effect of wire size and alloy on bracket-wire friction. J Dent Res 1989; 68:386.

Kapila S, Sachdeva R. Mechanical properties and clinical applications of orthodontic wires. Am J Orthod Dentofac Orthop 1989; 96:100–9.

Kapila S, Angolkar PV, Duncanson MG, Jr., Nanda RS. Evaluation of friction between edgewise stainless steel brackets and orthodontic wires of four alloys. Am J Orthod Dentofac Orthop 1990; 98:117–26.

Kesling PC, Rocke RT, Kesling CK. Treatment with Tip-Edge brackets and differential tooth movement. Am J Orthod Dentofac Orthop 1991; 99:387–401.

Khier SE, Brantley WA, Fournelle RA. Bending properties of superelastic and nonsuperelastic nickel-titanium orthodontic wires. Am J Orthod Dentofac Orthop 1991; 99:310–8.

Kimmel SS. A disclusion appliance to eliminate occlusally generated TMD symptoms prior to, and during fixed orthodontic therapy. J Gen Orthod 1994; 5:5–11.

Kirveskari P, Alanen P, Jämsä T. Association between craniomandibular disorders and occlusal interferences. J Prosthet Dent 1989; 62:66–9.

Kokich VG. Esthetics: the ortho-perio-restorative connection. Sem Orthod 1996; 2:21–30.

Kokich VG. Interdisciplinary management of single-tooth implants. Sem Orthod 1997; 3:45–72.

Krüger E. Lehrbuch der chirurgischen Zahn-, Mund- und Kieferheilkunde, Teil I und II. Quintessenz Verlags-GmbH, Berlin, 1993.

Kula K, Phillips C, Gibilaro A, Proffit WR. Effect of ion implantation of TMA archwires on the rate of orthodontic sliding space closure. Am J Orthod Dentofac Orthop 1998; 114:577–80.

Kurol J, Franke P, Lundgren D, Owman Moll P. Force magnitude applied by orthodontists. An inter- and intra-individual study. Eur J Orthod 1996; 18:69–75.

Kurol J, Magnusson BC. Infraocclusion of primary molars: a histologic study. Scand J Dent Res 1984; 92:564–76.

Kusters ST, Kuijpers-Jagtman AM, Maltha JC. An experimental study in dogs of transseptal fiber arrangement between teeth which have emerged in rotated or non-rotated positions. J Dent Res 1991; 70:192–7.

Kusy RP, Andrews SW, Norling BK. Sputter coating and ion implantation of model orthodontic appliances. J Dent Res 1989; 68:386.

Kusy RP, Whitley JQ. Coefficients of friction for archwires in stainless steel and polycrystalline alumina bracket slots. I. The dry state. Am J Orthod Dentofac Orthop 1990; 98:300–312.

Kusy RP, Whitley JQ, Ambrose WW, Newman JG. Evaluation of titanium brackets for orthodontic treatment: Part I, The passive configuration. Am J Orthod Dentofac Orthop 1998; 114:558–72.

Kusy RP, Whitley JQ, Mayhew MJ, Buckthal JE. Surface roughness of orthodontic archwires via laser spectroscopy. Angle Orthod 1988; 58:33–45.

Lee CF, Proffit WR. The daily rhythm of tooth eruption. Am J Orthod Dentofac Orthop 1995; 107:38–47.

Lee JH, Park JB, Andreasen GF, Lakes RS. Thermomechanical study of Ni-Ti alloys. J Biomed Mater Res 1988; 22:573–88.

Legan HL, Burstone CJ. Soft tissue cephalometric analysis for orthognathic surgery. J Oral Surg 1980; 38:744–51.

Lehman JA, Haas AJ. Surgical-orthodontic correction of transverse maxillary deficiency. Dent Clin North Am 1990; 34:385–95.

Lehman R, Hulsink JH. Treatment of Class II malocclusion with a headgear-activator combination. J Clin Orthod 1989; 23:430–3.

Lewis S. Cephalic index and how it may be of relevance in radiography of the petrous bone. Radiography 1984; 50:180–4.

Linder-Aronson S. Respiratory function in relation to facial morphology and the dentition. Angle Orthod 1979; 6:59–71.

Lindhe J, Karring T, Lang NP (eds.). Clinical Periodontology and Implant Dentistry (3rd edition). Munksgaard, Copenhagen, 1998.

Lindsten R, Kurol J. Orthodontic appliances in relation to nickel hypersensitivity. A review. J Orofac Orthop 1997; 58:100–8.

Little RM. The irregularity index: a quantitative score of mandibular anterior alignment. Am J Orthod 1975; 68:554–63.

Little RM. The effects of eruption guidance and serial extraction on the developing dentition. Pediatr Dent 1987; 9:65–70.

Little RM, Riedel RA, Artun J. An evaluation of changes in mandibular anterior alignment from 10 to 20 years postretention. Am J Orthod Dentofac Orthop 1988; 93:423–8.

Little RM, Riedel RA, Stein A. Mandibular arch length increase during the mixed dentition: postretention evaluation of stability and relapse. Am J Orthod Dentofac Orthop 1990; 97:393–404.

Little RM, Wallen TR, Riedel RA. Stability and relapse of mandibular anterior alignment - first premolar extraction cases treated by traditional edgewise orthodontics. Am J Orthod 1981; 80:349–65.

Livieratos FA, Johnston LE Jr. A comparison of one-stage and two-stage nonextraction alternatives in matched Class II samples Am J Orthod Dentofac Orthop 1995; 108:118–31.

Lundström A, Lundström F, Lebret LML, Moorrees CFA. Natural head posture and natural head orientation: basic considerations in cephalometric analysis and research. Eur J Orthod 1995; 17:111–20.

Macdonald KE, Kapust AJ, Turley PK. Cephalometric changes after the correction of class III malocclusion with maxillary expansion/facemask therapy. Am J Orthod Dentofac Orthop 1999; 116:13–24.

Magnusson T, Enbom L. Signs and symptoms of mandibular dysfunction after introduction of experimental balancing-side interferences. Acta Odontol Scand 1984; 42:129–35.

Marchac D (ed.). Craniofacial Surgery. Springer-Verlag, Berlin, 1987.

Marks SC Jr., Schroeder HE. Tooth eruption: theories and facts. Anat Rec 1996; 245:374–93.

Mason RM. Orthodontic perspectives on orofacial myofunctional therapy. Int J Orofacial Myology 1988; 14:49–55.

McCarthy JG, Schreiber J, Karp N, Thorne CH, Grayson BH. Lengthening the human mandible by gradual distraction. Plast Reconstr Surg 1992; 89:1–8.

McCormick SU, Grayson BH, McCarthy JG, Staffenberg D. Effect of mandibular distraction on the temporomandibular joint: Part 2, Clinical study. J Craniofac Surg 1995; 6:364–7.

McCulloch KJ, Mills CM, Greenfeld RS, Coil JM. Dens evaginatus from an orthodontic perspective: report of several clinical cases and review of the literature. Am J Orthod Dentofac Orthop 1997; 112:670–5.

McNamara JA Jr. A method of cephalometric evaluation. Am J Orthod 1984; 86:449–69.

McNamara JA Jr. Orthodontic treatment and temporomandibular disorders. Oral Surg Oral Med Oral Pathol Oral Radiol Endod 1997; 83:107–17.

McNamara JA Jr (ed.). Nasorespiratory function and craniofacial growth. Monograph #9, Craniofacial Growth Series. Center for Human Growth and Development, The University of Michigan, Ann Arbor, 1979.

McNamara JA Jr (ed.). Esthetics and the treatment of facial form. Volume 28, Craniofacial Growth Series. Center for Human Growth and Development, The University of Michigan, Ann Arbor, 1993.

McNamara JA Jr, Brudon WL. Orthodontic and Orthopedic Treatment in the Mixed Dentition. Needham Press, Ann Arbor, Mich., 1993.

McNamara JA Jr, Seligman DA, Okeson JP. Occlusion, orthodontic treatment and temporomandibular disorders. J Orofacial Pain 1995; 9:73–90.

McNamara JA Jr, Trotman C-A (eds.). Orthodontic treatment: management of unfavorable sequelae. Volume 31, Craniofacial Growth Series. Center for Human Growth and Development, The University of Michigan, Ann Arbor, 1995.

McNamara JA Jr, Turp JC. Orthodontic treatment and temporomandibular disorders: is there a relationship? Part 1: Clinical studies. J Orofac Orthop 1997; 58:74–89.

McNeill C. Current Controversies in Temporomandibular Disorders. Quintessence Publishing Co., Chicago, 1991.

McNeill C (ed.). Temporomandibular Disorders. Quintessence Publishing Co., Chicago, 1994.

Melsen B (ed.). Current Controversies in Orthodontics. Quintessence Publishing Co., Chicago, 1991.

Melsen B. Biological reaction of alveolar bone to orthodontic tooth movement. Angle Orthod 1999; 69:151–8.

Melsen B, Bonetti G, Giunta D. Statically determinate transpalatal arches. J Clin Orthod 1994; 28:602–6.

Melsen B, Bosch C. Different approaches to anchorage: a survey and an evaluation. Angle Orthod 1997; 67:23–30.

Melsen B, Fiorelli G, Bergamini A. Uprighting of lower molars. J Clin Orthod 1996; 33:640–5.

Merrifield LL. The profile line as an aid in critically evaluating facial esthetics. Am J Orthod 1966; 52:804–22.

Miethke RR, Behm-Menthel A. Correlations between lower incisor crowding and lower incisor position and lateral craniofacial morphology. Am J Orthod Dentofac Orthop 1988; 94:231–9.

Miller PD Jr. A classification of marginal tissue recession. Int J Periodontics Restorative Dent 1985; 5:8–13.

Mitchell L. An Introduction to Orthodontics. Oxford University Press, Oxford, 1996.

Molina F, Ortiz Monasterio F. Mandibular elongation and remodeling by distraction: a farewell to major osteotomies. Plast Reconstr Surg 1995; 96:825–40.

Molina F, Ortiz Monasterio F, de la Paz Aguilar M, Barrera J. Maxillary distraction: aesthetic and functional benefits in cleft lip-palate and prognathic patients during mixed dentition. Plast Reconstr Surg 1998; 101:951–63.

Moore KL. The Developing Human (3rd edition). WB Saunders Co., Philadelphia, 1982.

Moss ML. The functional matrix. In: Kraus B, Reidel R (eds.). Vistas in Orthodontics. Lea and Febiger, Philadelphia, 1962, p. 85–98.

Moss ML. Genetics, epigenetics and causation. Am J Orthod 1981; 80:366–75.

Mouradian WE. Making decisions for children. Angle Orthod 1999; 69:300–5.

Moyers RE. Handbook of Orthodontics (4th edition). Year Book Medical Publishers Inc., Chicago, 1988.

Moyers RE, van der Linden FPGM, Riolo ML, McNamara JA Jr (eds.). Standards of human occlusal development. Monograph #5, Craniofacial Growth Series. Center for Human Growth and Development, The University of Michigan, Ann Arbor, 1976.

Mulligan TF. Common Sense Mechanics. CSM Publishing Co., Phoenix, 1982.

Nanda R (ed.). Biomechanics in Clinical Orthodontics. WB Saunders Co., Philadelphia, 1997.

Nanda SK, Sassouni V. Planes of reference in roentgenographic cephalometry. Angle Orthod 1965; 35:311–9.

Nelson S, Broadbent BH, Hans MG. The demographics of Dr. Geoffrey Walker's cephalometric collection. Am J Orthod Dentofac Orthop 1997; 111:646–9.

Ngan P, Hagg U, Yiu C, Merwin D, Wei SH. Treatment response to maxillary expansion and protraction. Eur J Orthod 1996; 18:151–68.

Nikolai RJ. Bioengineering Analysis of Orthodontic Mechanics. Lea & Febiger, Philadelphia, 1985.

Norton LA, Burstone CJ (eds.). The Biology of Tooth Movement. CRC Press, Boca Raton, Florida, 1989.

O'Brien WJ (ed.). Dental Materials and Their Selection (2nd edition). Quintessence Publishing Co., Chicago, 1997.

Odman J, Lekholm U, Jemt T, Thilander B. Osseointegrated implants as orthodontic anchorage in the treatment of partially edentulous adult patients. Eur J Orthod 1994; 16:187–201.

Okeson JP. Management of Temporomandibular Disorders and Occlusion (3rd edition). Mosby-Year Book, St. Louis, 1993.

Orthlieb JD. The curve of Spee: understanding the sagittal organization of mandibular teeth. Cranio 1997; 15:333–40.

Owen AH 3rd. The maxillary sagittal appliance: a clinical study. Am J Orthod Dentofac Orthop 1987; 91:271–85.

Owman-Moll P, Ingervall B. Effect of oral screen treatment on dentition, lip morphology, and function in children with incompetent lips. Am J Orthod 1984; 85:37–46.

Pancherz H. The mechanism of Class II correction in Herbst appliance treatment. Am J Orthod 1982; 82:104–13.

Perez MM, Sameshima GT, Sinclair PM. The long-term stability of LeFort I maxillary downgrafts with rigid fixation to correct vertical maxillary deficiency. Am J Orthod Dentofac Orthop 1997; 112:104–8.

Peterson LJ, Ellis E 3rd, Hupp JR, Tucker MR (eds.). Contemporary Oral and Maxillofacial Surgery (3rd edition). Mosby-Year Book, St. Louis, 1997.

Peterson L, Spencer R, Andreasen G. Comparison of friction resistance for nitinol and stainless steel wire in edgewise brackets. Quintessence Int 1982; 13:563–71.

Phillips C, Medland WH, Fields HW Jr, Proffit WR, White RP Jr. Stability of surgical maxillary expansion. Int J Adult Orthod Orthognath Surg 1992; 7:139-46.

Pilon JJ, Kuijpers-Jagtman AM, Maltha JC. Magnitude of orthodontic forces and rate of bodily tooth movement: an experimental study. Am J Orthod Dentofac Orthop 1996; 110:16–23.

Pini Prato G, Clauser C, Tonetti MS, Cortellini P. Guided tissue regeneration in gingival recessions. Periodontol 2000 1996; 11:49–57.

Polley JW, Figueroa AA. Management of severe maxillary deficiency in childhood and adolescence through distraction osteogenesis with an external, adjustable, rigid distraction device. J Craniofac Surg 1997; 8:181–5.

Popovich F, Thompson GW. Craniofacial templates for orthodontic case analysis. Am J Orthod 1977; 71:406–420.

Posnick JC, Tompson B. Modification of the maxillary Le Fort I osteotomy in cleft-orthognathic surgery: the unilateral cleft lip and palate deformity. J Oral Maxillofac Surg 1992; 50:666–75.

Poswillo D.E. The aetiology and pathogenesis of craniofacial deformity. Development 1988;103 Suppl.:207–12.

Proffit WR, Fields HW Jr. Contemporary Orthodontics (2nd edition). Mosby—Year Book, St. Louis, 1993.

Proffit WR, Fields HW Jr. Contemporary Orthodontics (3rd edition). Mosby—Year Book, St. Louis, 1999.

Proffit WR, White RP Jr. Surgical Orthodontic Treatment. Mosby—Year Book, St Louis, 1991.

Proffit WR, Phillips C, Tulloch JFC, Medland P. Surgical versus orthodontic correction of skeletal Cl II malocclusion in adolescents: Effects and indications. Int J Adult Orthod Orthognath Surg 1992; 7:209–220.

Proffit WR, Turvey TA, Phillips C. Orthognathic surgery: A hierarchy of stability. Int J Adult Orthod Orthognath Surg 1996; 11:191–204.

Rakosi T, Jonas I, Graber TM. Orthodontic diagnosis. Color Atlas of Dental Medicine. Thieme Medical Publishers, New York, 1993.

Ranly DM. A Synopsis of Craniofacial Growth (2nd edition). Appleton and Lange, Norwalk, Connecticut, 1988.

Ranta R. A review of tooth formation in children with cleft lip/palate. Am J Orthod Dentofac Orthop 1986; 90:11–8.

Razdolsky Y, Sadowsky C, BeGole EA. Occlusal contacts following orthodontic treatment: a follow-up study. Angle Orthod 1989; 59:181–5.

Reidel R. The relation of maxillary structures to the cranium in malocclusion and in normal occlusion. Angle Orthod 1952; 22:142–5.

Reitan K. Some factors determining the evaluation of forces in orthodontics. Am J Orthod 1957; 43:32–45.

Reitan K. Tissue behaviour during orthodontic tooth movement. Am J Orthod 1960; 46:881–900.

Renfroe EW. Edgewise. Lea & Febiger, Philadelphia, 1975.

Richmond S, Shaw WC, O'Brien KD, Buchanan IB, Jones R, Stephens CD, Roberts CT, Andrews M. The development of the PAR (Peer Assessment rating) index: reliability and validity. Eur J Orthod 1992; 14:125–39.

Richmond S, Roberts CT, Andrews M. Use of the index of orthodontic treatment need (IOTN) in assessing the need for orthodontic treatment pre-

and post- appliance therapy. Br J Orthod 1994; 21:175–84.

Ricketts RM. Planning treatment on the basis of the facial pattern and an estimate of its growth. Am J Orthod 1957; 27:14–37.

Ricketts RM. A foundation for cephalometric communication. Am J Orthod 1960; 46:330–57.

Riolo ML, Moyers RE, McNamara JA Jr, Hunter WS (eds.). An atlas of craniofacial growth: Cephalometric standards from the University School Growth Study. Monograph #2, Craniofacial Growth Series. Center for Human Growth and Development, The University of Michigan, Ann Arbor, 1974.

Romano R (ed.). Lingual Orthodontics. BC Decker Inc., Hamilton, Ont., 1998.

Rondeau BH. The pendulum appliance. J Gen Orthod 1995; 6:22–30.

Ross RB, Johnston MC. Cleft Lip and Palate. Williams and Wilkins, Baltimore, 1972.

Ross RB. Treatment variables affecting facial growth in complete unilateral cleft lip and palate. Part 3: Alveolus repair and bone grafting. Cleft Palate J 1987; 24:33–44.

Roth RH. The straight wire appliance 17 years later. J Clin Orthod 1987; 21:632–42.

Ryan R, Walker G, Freeman K, Cisneros GJ. The effects of ion implantation on rate of tooth movement: an in vitro model. Am J Orthod Dentofac Orthop 1997; 112:64–8.

Rygh P. Orthodontic root resorption studied by electron microscopy. Angle Orthod 1977; 47: 1–6.

Salyer KE, Bardach J. Atlas of Craniofacial and Cleft Surgery. Lippincott-Raven, Philadelphia, 1999.

Sandler PJ, Reed RT. Removable retainers: a modification of the Barrer appliance. Br J Orthod 1988; 15:127–9.

Sandy JR. Tooth eruption and orthodontic movement. Br Dent J 1992; 172:141–9.

Sassouni VA. A classification of skeletal facial types. Am J Orthod 1969; 55:109–123.

Sauget E, Covell DA Jr, Boero RP, Lieber WS. Comparison of occlusal contacts with use of Hawley and clear overlay retainers. Angle Orthod 1997; 67:223–30.

Schmidt Nowara W, Lowe A, Wiegand L, Cartwright R, Perez Guerra F, Menn S. Oral appliances for the treatment of snoring and obstructive sleep apnea: a review. Sleep 1995; 18:501–10.

Schwindling F-P. Jasper Jumper Color Atlas. Schwindling, Merzig, Germany, 1997.

Seligman DA, Pullinger AG. The role of intercuspal occlusal relationships in temporomandibular disorders: a review. J Craniomand Disord Facial Oral Pain 1991; 5:96–105.

Seligman DA, Pullinger AG. A multiple stepwise logistic regression analysis of trauma history and 16 other history and dental co-factors in females with temporomandibular disorders. J Orofac Pain 1996; 10:351–61.

Sergl HG. Festsitzende Apparaturen in der Kieferorthopädie, Carl Hanser Verlag, München, 1990.

Sergl HG, Kerr WJ, McColl JH. A method of measuring the apical base. Eur J Orthod 1996; 18:479–83.

Sergl HG, Zentner A. Theoretical approaches to behavior change in myofunctional therapy. Int J Orofac Myology 1994; 20:32–9.

Severens JL, Prahl C, Kuijpers-Jagtman AM, Prahl-Andersen B. Short-term cost-effectiveness analysis of presurgical orthopedic treatment in children with complete unilateral cleft lip and palate. Cleft Palate Craniofac J 1998; 35:222–6.

Sforza C, Poggio CE, Schmitz JH, Colombo A. Soft tissue facial morphology related to headform: a three-dimensional quantitative analysis in childhood. J Craniofac Genet Dev Biol 1997; 17:86–95.

Shaw WC (ed.). Orthodontics and Occlusal Management. Wright, Oxford, 1993.

Shaw WC, Richmond S, O'Brien KD. The use of occlusal indices: A European perspective. Am J Orthod Dentofac Orthop 1995; 107:1–10.

Schmuth GP. Considerations of functional aspects in dentofacial orthopedics and orthodontics: Sheldon Friel Memorial Lecture. Am J Orthod Dentofac Orthop 1999; 115:373–81.

Schumacher HA, Bourauel C, Drescher D. Frictional forces when rectangular guiding arches with varying edge bevel are employed. J Orofac Orthop 1998; 59:139–49.

Shellhart WC, Lange DW, Kluemper GT, Hicks EP, Kaplan AL. Reliability of the Bolton tooth-size analysis when applied to crowded dentitions. Angle Orthod 1995; 65:327–34.

Sheridan JJ. Air-rotor stripping update. J Clin Orthod 1987; 21:781–8.

Sheridan JJ, Hastings J. Air-rotor stripping and lower incisor extraction treatment. J Clin Orthod 1992; 26:18–22.

Sheridan JJ, LeDoux W, McMinn R. Essix retainers: fabrication and supervision for permanent retention. J Clin Orthod 1993; 27:37–45.

Shetty V, Caridad JM, Caputo AA, Chaconas SJ. Biomechanical rationale for surgical-orthodontic expansion of the adult maxilla. J Oral Maxillofac Surg 1994; 52:742–9.

Shprintzen RJ. The implications of the diagnosis of Robin sequence. Cleft Palate Craniofac J 1992; 29:205–9.

Sillence DO, Rimoin DL, Danks DM. Clinical variability in osteogenesis imperfecta-variable expressivity or genetic heterogeneity. Birth Defects Orig Artic Ser 1979; 15:113–29.

Sinclair PM, Little RM. Dentofacial maturation of untreated normals. Am J Orthod 1985; 88:146–56.

Singer CP, Mamandras AH, Hunter WS. The depth of the mandibular antegonial notch as an indicator of mandibular growth potential. Am J Orthod Dentofac Orthop 1987; 91:117–24.

Slavicek R. Clinical and instrumental functional analysis for diagnosis and treatment planning. Part 9. Removable splint therapy. J Clin Orthod 1989; 23:90–7.

Slomic AM, Bernier JP, Morissette J, Renier D. A craniometric study of sagittal craniosynostosis. J Craniofac Genet Dev Biol 1992; 12:49–54.

Smith RJ, Burstone CJ. Mechanics of tooth movement. Am J Orthod 1984; 85:294–307.

Solow B. The dentoalveolar compensatory mechanism background and clinical implications. Br J Orthod 1980; 7:145–61.

Solow B, Tallgren A. Natural head position in standing subjects. Acta Odontol Scand 1971; 29:591–607.

Sondhi A. Orthodontics and patients with temporomandibular disorders: inform before you perform. Am J Orthod Dentofac Orthop 1999; 115:551–2.

Sonnesen L, Bakke M, Solow B. Malocclusion traits and symptoms and signs of temporomandibular disorders in children with severe malocclusion. Eur J Orthod 1998; 20:543–59.

Sperry TP, Steinburg MJ, Gans BJ. Mandibular movement during autorotation as a result of maxillary impaction surgery. Am J Orthod 1982; 81:116–23.

Staffenberg DA, Wood RJ, Cutting CB, Grayson BH, Thorne CH. Introduction of an intraoral bone-lengthening device. Plast Reconstr Surg 1995; 96:978–81.

Staley RN, Kerber PE. A revision of the Hixon and Oldfather mixed-dentition prediction method. Am J Orthod 1980; 78:296–302.

Stanford CM, Keller JC. The concept of osseointegration and bone matrix expression. Crit Rev Oral Biol Med 1991; 2:83–101.

Stedman's Medical Dictionary (26th edition). Lippincott, Williams and Wilkins, Philadelphia, 1995.

Steedle JR, Proffit WR. The pattern and control of eruptive tooth movements. Am J Orthod 1985; 87:56–66.

Stefani RE. Muscle deprogramming splint. J Gen Orthod 1992; 3:6–11.

Steiner CC. Cephalometrics for you and me. Am J Orthod 1953; 39:729–55.

Steiner CC. Cephalometrics in clinical practice. Angle Orthod 1959; 29:9–29.

Steiner CC. The use of cephalometrics as an aid to planning and assessing orthodontic treatment. Am J Orthod 1960; 46:721–35.

Stockfisch H. Possibilities and limitations of kinetor bimaxillary appliance. Trans Eur Orthod Soc 1971; 317–28.

Stockfisch H. The kinetor. Trans Eur Orthod Soc 1973; 457–61.

Stockfisch H. The Principles and Practice of Dentofacial Orthopaedics. Quintessence Publishing Co., London, 1995.

Stohler CS, Carlson DS (eds.). Biological and psychological aspects of orofacial pain. Volume 29, Craniofacial Growth Series. Center for Human Growth and Development, The University of Michigan, Ann Arbor, 1993.

Stoller AE. The Universal Appliance. The CV Mosby Co., St. Louis, 1971.

Storey E, Smith R. Force in orthodontics and its relation to tooth movement. Austr J Dent 1952; 56:11–18.

Stucki N, Ingervall B. The use of the Jasper Jumper for the correction of Class II malocclusion in the young permanent dentition. Eur J Orthod 1998; 20:271–81.

Tan ST, Mulliken JB. Hypertelorism: nosologic analysis of 90 patients. Plast Reconstr Surg 1997; 99:317–27.

Tanaka MM, Johnston LE. The prediction of the size of unerupted canines and premolars in a contemporary orthodontic population. J Am Dent Assoc 1974; 88:798–801.

Tanne K, Matsubara S, Shibaguchi T, Sakuda M. Wire friction from ceramic brackets during simulated canine retraction. Angle Orthod 1991; 61:285–90.

Ten Cate AR. Oral Histology: Development, Structure and Function (4th edition). Mosby—Year Book, St. Louis, 1994.

Ten Cate AR. Oral Histology: Development, Structure and Function (5th edition). Mosby—Year Book, St. Louis, 1998.

Terry HK. The labiolingual appliance. Am J Orthod 1969; 55:714–33.

Tessier P. Anatomical classification of facial, craniofacial and latero-facial clefts. J Maxillofac Surg 1976; 4:69–92.

Teuscher U. A growth-related concept for skeletal class II treatment. Am J Orthod 1978; 74: 258–275.

Thayer TA, Bagby MD, Moore RN, DeAngelis RJ. X-ray diffraction of nitinol orthodontic arch wires. Am J Orthod Dentofac Orthop 1995; 107:604–12.

Thilander B, Rönning O (eds.). Introduction to Orthodontics (2nd edition). Förlagshuset Gothia AB, Göteborg, 1995.

Thomas PM. Orthodontic camouflage versus orthognathic surgery in the treatment of mandibular deficiency. J Oral Maxillofac Surg 1995; 53:579–87.

Thompson WJ. Occlusal plane and overbite. Angle Orthod 1979; 49:47–55.

Thuer U, Ingervall B. Effect of muscle exercise with an oral screen on lip function. Eur J Orthod 1990; 12:198–208.

Thurow RC. Edgewise Orthodontics (4th edition). The CV Mosby Company, St. Louis, 1982.

Tidy DC. Frictional forces in fixed appliances. Am J Orthod Dentofac Orthop 1989; 96:249–54.

Tolarová MM, Cervenka J. Classification and birth prevalence of orofacial clefts. Am J Med Genet 1998;75:126–37.

Trotman C-A, McNamara JA Jr (eds.). Orthodontic treatment: outcome and effectiveness. Volume 30, Craniofacial Growth Series. Center for Human Growth and Development, The University of Michigan, Ann Arbor, 1994.

Tucker MR. Orthognathic surgery versus orthodontic camouflage in the treatment of mandibular deficiency. J Oral Maxillofac Surg 1995; 53:572–578.

Turp JC, McNamara JA Jr. Orthodontic treatment and temporomandibular disorders: is there a relationship? Part 2: Clinical implications. J Orofac Orthop 1997; 58:136–43.

Turvey T, Hall DJ, Fish LC, Epker BN. Surgical ortho-dontic treatment planning for simultaneous mobilization of the maxilla and mandible in the correction of dentofacial deformities. Oral Surg 1982; 54:491–8.

Turvey TA, Vig KWL, Fonseca RJ (eds.). Facial Clefts and Craniosynostosis: Principles and Manage-ment. WB Saunders Co., Philadelphia, 1996.

Tweed CH. The Frankfort-mandibular incisor angle (FMIA) in orthodontic diagnosis, treatment planning and prognosis. Angle Orthod 1954; 24:121–69.

Tweed CH. Clinical Orthodontics. The CV Mosby Co., St. Louis, 1966.

Uitto V-J, Larjava H. Extracellular matrix molecules and their receptors: An overview with special emphasis on periodontal tissues. Crit Rev Oral Biol Med 1991; 2:323–54.

Vaden JL. The Tweed-Merrifield philosophy. Semin Orthod 1996; 2:237–40.

Valinoti JR. The European activator: Its basis and use. Am J Orthod 1973; 63:561–80.

Van der Linden FPGM. A study of cephalometric bony landmarks. Am J Orthod 1971; 59:111–25.

Van der Linden FPGM. Development of the Dentition. Quintessence Publishing Co., Chicago, 1983.

Van der Linden FPGM. Facial Growth and Facial Orthopedics. Quintessence Publishing Co., London, 1986.

Van der Linden FPDGM. Problems and Procedures in Dentofacial Orthopedics. Quintessence Publishing Co., London,1990.

Van der Linden FPGM. Practical Dentofacial Orthopedics. Quintessence Publishing Co., London, 1996.

Van der Linden FPGM. Orthodontics with Fixed Appliances. Quintessence Publishing Co., Lon-don, 1997.

Van der Linden FPGM, Boersma H. Diagnosis and Treatment Planning in Orthodontics. Quintes-sence Publishing Co., London, 1987.

Vargervik K, Harvold EP. Response to activator treat-ment in Class II malocclusions. Am J Orthod 1985; 88:242–51.

Vargervik K, Ousterhout DK, Farias M. Factors affect-ing long-term results in hemifacial microsomia. Cleft Palate J 1986; 23 Suppl 1: 53–68.

Viazis AD. Comprehensive assessment of anteropos-terior jaw relationships. J Clin Orthod 1992; 26:673–80.

Vig KWL. Orthodontic considerations applied to cran-iofacial dysmorphology. Cleft Palate J 1990; 27:141–5.

Vig KWL. Nasal obstruction and facial growth: The strength of evidence for clinical assump-tions. Am J Orthod Dentofac Orthop 1998; 113:603–11.

Vig KWL, Millicovsky G, Johnston MC. Cranio-facial development: the possible mechanisms for some malformations. Br J Orthod 1984; 11:114–8.

Vig KWL, Burdi AR (eds.). Craniofacial Morpho-genesis and Dysmorphogenesis. Monograph #21, Craniofacial Growth Series. Center for Human Growth and Development, The University of Michigan, Ann Arbor, 1988.

Warren DW. A quantitative technique for assessing nasal airway impairment. Am J Orthod 1984; 86:306–14.

Weiland FJ, Ingervall B, Bantleon HP, Droacht H. Initial effects of treatment of Class II malocclusion with the Herren activator, activator-headgear combi-nation, and Jasper Jumper. Am J Orthod Den-tofac Orthop 1997; 112:19–27.

Wennstrom JL. Mucogingival considerations in ortho-dontic treatment. Sem Orthod 1996; 2:46–54.

Wiltshire WA, Ferreira MR, Ligthelm AJ. Allergies to dental materials. Quintessence Int 1996; 27:513–20.

Winchell B. Orofacial myofunctional therapy for adult patients. Int J Orofac Myology 1989; 15:14–8.

Wolford LM, Hilliard FW, Dugan DJ. Surgical Treatment Objective; A Systematic Approach to Prediction Tracing. The CV Mosby Co., St. Louis, 1985.

Woodside DG, Linder-Aronson S, Lundstrom A, McWilliam J. Mandibular and maxillary growth after changed mode of breathing. Am J Orthod Dentofac Orthop 1991; 100:1–18.

Woodside DG, Metaxas A, Altuna G. The influence of functional appliance therapy on glenoid fossa remodeling. Am J Orthod Dentofac Orthop 1987; 92:181–98.

World Health Organization. Application of the Inter-national Classification of Diseases to Dentistry and Stomatology (3rd edition). WHO, Geneva, 1995.

Worms FW, Isaacson RJ, Speidel TM. Surgical orthodontic treatment planning: Profile analysis and mandibular surgery. Angle Orthod 1976; 46:1–25.

Wylie WL. The assessment of antero-posterior dysplasia. Angle Orthod 1947; 17:97–109.

Wylie WL, Johnson EL. Rapid evaluation of facial dysplasia in the vertical plane. Angle Orthod 1952; 22:165–83.

Xu TM, Lin JX, Kui H, Huang JF. Bite-opening mechanics as applied in the Begg technique. Br J Orthod 1994; 21:189–95.

Yamin-Lacouture C, Woodside DG, Sectakof PA, Sessle BJ. The action of three types of functional appliances on the activity of the masticatory muscles. Am J Orthod Dentofac Orthop, 1997; 112:560–72.

Yen PKJ. Identification of landmarks in cephalometric radiographs. Angle Orthod 1960; 30:35.

Yudelson R. The universal appliance. Am J Orthod 1967; 53:159–81.

Zachrisson BU. Third-generation mandibular bonded lingual 3-3 retainer. J Clin Orthod 1995; 29:39–48.

Zachrisson BU. Clinical implications of recent orthodontic-periodontic research findings. Semin Orthod 1996; 2:4–12.

Zachrisson BU. Important aspects of long-term stability. J Clin Orthod 1997; 31:562-83.

Zarb GA, Carlsson GE, Sessle BJ, Mohl ND (eds.). Temporomandibular Joint and Masticatory Muscle Disorders (2nd edition). Munksgaard, Copenhagen, 1994.

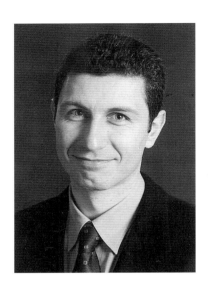

Dr. John Daskalogiannakis received his dental degree from the University of Athens, Greece, and his orthodontic certificate and MSc from the University of Manitoba, Canada. After completing a 2-year fellowship at the Craniofacial Center, The Hospital for Sick Children, Toronto, Canada, he joined the staff of the Department of Orthodontics and Oral Biology at the University of Nymegen, The Netherlands.